THEORY
AND
PRACTICE
IN
HEALTH
EDUCATION

Mayfield Publishing Company

THEORY
AND
PRACTICE
IN
HEALTH
EDUCATION

HELEN S. ROSS

AND

PAUL R. MICO

To Dorothy B. Nyswander, a source of great inspiration to a generation of students and colleagues, among whom we are fortunate in having been two.

RA
440
.R67

Library of Congress Catalog Card Number: 80-82564
International Standard Book Number: 0-87484-406-1

Manufactured in the United States of America
Mayfield Publishing Company
285 Hamilton Avenue, Palo Alto, California 94301

Compositor: Interactive Composition Corporation
Printer and binder: R. R. Donnelley & Sons Company
Sponsoring editor: C. Lansing Hays
Managing editor: Maggie Cutler
Manuscript editor: Barbara Pronin
Designer: Nancy Sears
Production manager: Michelle Hogan

Contents

Tables

Figures

Preface

Written primarily for the undergraduate student, this text presents a survey of theory and practice in the field of professional health education. An introductory chapter explains what health education is and why it is needed. Parts 1–3 focus respectively on individuals, organizations, and social systems, each part containing chapters that explore health-related problems, theories, and activities designed to bring about beneficial change. Part 4 offers one chapter each on planning, methods, and evaluation in health-education practice. The concluding chapter discusses professional aspects of the field and is supplemented by two appendixes containing additional matter of professional interest.

Such is the complexity of human health behavior that neither dogmatic certainty of explanation nor a strictly traditional scheme of presentation has heretofore been possible. It has been necessary, instead, to introduce many behavioral theories, emphasizing those we believe to be most important, and to organize some material, such as several theories relating to community and social behavior, under possibly unfamiliar headings. It cannot even be said that the text's individual, organizational, and social foci are as neatly distinct as our organization suggests, because in reality they untidily overlap, as our own many years of practical experience have amply demonstrated.

Thus, selecting, organizing, and presenting this material has offered a formidable challenge, but we believe that in the attempt to meet that challenge lies the book's greatest strength. By providing a basis for the future codification of the health-education field, it will have continuing value for students and practitioners alike. Our more immediate purpose, however, has been to enhance the knowledge and skills of health educators, thereby to improve the health behavior of the general public. In this pursuit, student-teacher collaboration is essential if the learning process is to be meaningful and dynamic. Those already in practice may wish to test our ideas against their own experience or discuss their pertinence with colleagues.

Two groups of practitioners will find this text to be of use. The first group is composed of health professionals who consider health education to be an important aspect of their work; these include physicians, nurses, social workers, psychologists, nutritionists, schoolteachers, pharmacists, dentists, dental hygienists, sanitary engineers, etc. The second group is composed of health-education specialists, or those who are preparing themselves for this career, whose training is specifically designed to produce expertise in the arts and sciences of health education.

For the authors, writing this book has been an enjoyable and enlightening experience. We would like to express gratitude to the colleagues and students with whom we have shared our ideas and who in turn have guided us in the writing. In particular, we would like to thank the following reviewers: Geraldene Bordman, Norman Craig, Phyllis Ensor, Daniel Girdano, Alan C. Henderson, Marshall Kreuter, Betty Mathews, Meredith Minkler, Richard H. Needle, Ed Roulhac, and Guy W. Stewart. We also owe thanks to C. Lansing Hays, Carole Norton, and Maggie Cutler of Mayfield Publishing Company for their numerous readings of, and suggestions for, the manuscript. We especially wish to express gratitude to Barbara Pronin for her painstaking efforts in editing the manuscript. Finally, we wish also to thank our families for their continuing encouragement and support.

THEORY

AND

PRACTICE

IN

HEALTH

EDUCATION

1

Introduction to health education

The intent of this chapter is to respond to two of the most frequently asked questions about health education: What is it and why is it needed? Addressing the first question, the chapter opens with ten health education vignettes and discusses their common features. A subsection on health education and educators presents definitions of the two and distinguishes between those who engage generally in health education and those who are specially trained in the field. The next subsection suggests a number of problems and promises that characterize the field today. The second part of the chapter establishes the general need for health education by reviewing problems associated with the major determinants of health, by assessing major transitions occurring in the field, and by explaining the implications of these factors for health education.

WHAT IS HEALTH EDUCATION?

Health education in action

• For a couple of hours once a week, with the help of a group facilitator, a group meets in a program designed to assist its members in helping one another live with diabetes. Members learn how to administer their own medications, what kinds of food they can safely eat and how it should be prepared, and how to recognize symptoms that suggest the need for immediate treatment. They also learn how to deal with their anxieties about diabetes, how to adjust to living as diabetics, and how to involve their families and friends in developing a psychosocial system that will provide them with needed support in carrying out their new behaviors.

• Learning how to care for her first-born infant, a young mother watches as a visiting nurse shows her how to bathe the baby, then bathes it herself to demonstrate that she has mastered the technique. Nurse and mother discuss the infant's care and feeding, the immunizations it should receive, how to recognize the symptoms of illnesses that require medical care, and the purpose of attending follow-up infant-care clinics. In this way the mother is made to feel comfortable in discussing her fears about giving adequate care to her baby.

• Having conducted a study of community health problems and needs and identified the inadequacies in the services currently available to them, a group of citizens has met with state and local health officials to explore opportunities for improvement. A primary health-care center has been agreed upon as the best solution for meeting their community's needs. In developing plans for such a center, they have been assisted by health educators, and they are now in the process of implementing these plans.

• The management of an industrial organization in a highly competitive field has endorsed a training program designed to help key managers cope more effectively with problems of stress. Under the guidance of a qualified person who has been employed to conduct the program, managerial personnel are identifying the causes of stress in their organization and exploring how their work environment and working conditions can be altered to minimize the problem. While examining their own personal styles of handling stress, they are learning skills in managing their time more constructively, in organizing and assigning more rational priorities to workloads, in supervising, in delegating responsibilities, even in exercise and weight reduction.

• The board of directors of a health systems agency is engaged in a training program to help its members carry out their responsibilities more effectively. They want to enhance their own interpersonal relationships, communications, and decision making; the quality and productivity of their meetings and the functions of their committees; working relationships with their staff; and their relationships with the constituent groups in their community, as well as with federal, state, and other local agencies. They want to learn more about health care as a system—what health planning is and how to conduct it—and gain a better understanding of the federal and state regulations under which they must operate.

• A team of workers at a primary health-care center is being assisted in improving the overall effectiveness of the center's services. Workers are clarifying their respective roles and functions, sharing leadership responsibility for various services, collecting information from clients and community leaders on ways to improve their services, and involving other staff members in reorganizing the steps and procedures by which clients are served.

• A coalition of national health agencies has formed a national committee for the purpose of promoting legislation that would improve health-education resources and directions emanating from the federal government. To this end they have documented the low level of federal expenditure for health education, catalogued the various programs and agencies within the federal structure that have implications for health education, studied the congressional legislative process, and identified sources of help as well as of possible opposition. Having developed proposed legislation for introduction into Congress, they are gathering support from interested organizations throughout the country.

• In an effort to immunize a specific group of people against a preventable disease, a team of workers carried out a coordinated program of mass communication and community organization by means of the following planned steps. A survey determined existing immunization levels among the groups for whom the program was intended. A plan was developed to identify activities that would ensure the program's success, and a time schedule was established for it. The cooperation of communications leaders was obtained early in the program, and committees were organized throughout the community to help carry it out. Mass communications materials were developed on the basis of known attitudes and motivations and were tested on the target groups. Finally, immunization clinics were given locations and time schedules best suited to fit the needs of those to be reached.

• A student health committee is being assisted in organizing and carrying out a school-wide campaign to improve nutrition (by replacing junk-food machines with dispensers of fruit and milk) and to prevent smoking on school grounds. To obtain the cooperation and support of students and administration alike, committee members are conducting exercises in values clarification with mixed groups of students and faculty and are involving both formal and informal groups in discussing and negotiating a set of related rules.

• The management and union of an industrial firm are being assisted in a program to improve environmental working conditions for all employees. Following a survey of existing conditions, a joint committee has met to confront problematic issues of needs and costs. Committee members have also been meeting with their respective constituent groups in order to keep all company members involved in the process and informed of progress.

These examples of health education in action have three prominent features in common: (1) they are based on a need to understand or improve a situation of concern; (2) activities are undertaken to bring about changes either in people's behavior or in their environment; and (3) those who will be affected by a change effort are involved in the planning and implementation activities.

Collecting information about health problems provides a basis for determining a need for change. This information can be collected informally, by asking people to discuss their problems and needs, or formally, by means of well-designed surveys. In either case, the more accurate the information, the greater the rationale for change. Further, change is far more likely to be constructive and permanent if it is planned rather than undertaken haphazardly. Planning involves setting goals, determining which activities can be carried out to attain those goals, setting priorities for allocating resources, seeking ways of monitoring implementation progress, and evaluating results.

That those who will be affected by a change effort should be involved in its planning and implementation is axiomatic; hence the presence of involvement throughout the examples above. Involvement may take the form of formal boards and committees, informal groups, or merely getting people to participate in providing information, sharing ideas, and utilizing services, all of which may lead to behavioral change. Behavior, in this sense, consists not only of what people do or fail to do but of their attitudes and motivations as these relate to their health. Although not all health behavior needs to be changed, the same processes can be used to reinforce or support constructive behavior.

The examples have another common feature as well: someone is mentioned, or implied, as assisting the learning process, and that person is a health educator. As the examples suggest, health education is a diverse and dynamic field. Although the process is essentially the same in every case, it can be conducted in many different settings and for many different purposes by many different types of health educators. But examples serve only to whet the appetite. They do not satisfy the need to understand the process of health education or the theory and practice behind it. Neither do they explain the making of health educators nor of the profession they have chosen to join.

Health education and educators

There are as many definitions of the term *health educator* as there are health-education specialities, but the definitions vary only slightly. The definition set forth by the World Health Organization's (WHO) Expert Committee on Planning and Evaluation of Health Education Services is accepted throughout the world: "The focus of health education is on people and on action. In general, its aims are to encourage people to adopt and sustain healthful life patterns, to use judiciously and wisely the health services available to them, and to make their own decisions, both individually and collectively, to improve their health status and environment."[1] The WHO Scientific Group on Research in Health Education expanded this by declaring that the objective of health education is

> the development in people of (1) a sense of responsibility for their own health and for that of the community, and (2) the ability to participate in community life in a constructive and purposeful way. The possibility of such responsible participation being carried over into other spheres of life is great. Health education thus helps to promote on the one hand a sense of individual identity, dignity, and responsibility, and on the other hand community solidarity and responsibility.[2]

In any profession, agreement on the meaning of language enables practitioners effectively to comunicate with one another and with their publics. In health education, two major steps have been taken to help develop this agreement. One was the 1972 work of the Joint Committee on Health Education Terminology;[3] the other was the preparation in 1976 of *HEIRS: Thesaurus of Health Education Terminology*.[4]

The Joint Committee on Health Education Terminology, composed of representatives from most of the national professional associations concerned with health education at the time, developed an extensive list of terms whose definitions they had reached agreement on. The list included such terms as: *health education, community health education, community organization (for health), consumer participation (in health planning), group process (in health education), health education of the public, health education program, health-education resources, health environment, health information, health instruction, mass communication (in health), patient education,* and *school health education.**

The types of health educators defined were: *health science educator, public (community) health educator,* and *school health educator.* Among other terms defined were: *private health agency, public health agency, school health education curriculum* and *curriculum guides, school health program, school health services,* and *voluntary health agency.* A review of these definitions provides a descriptive overview of the health-education field.

Health education, then, is an educationally oriented process of planned change which focuses on those behaviors or problems that directly or indirectly affect people's health. The target may vary depending upon the nature

*For definitions, see Glossary.

of the problem being addressed. In some cases it may be focused on individuals themselves in face-to-face or small-group settings. In others, the focus may be on the structures and procedures by which people organize themselves into such social systems as teams, organizations, coalitions, communities, or larger system networks in order to achieve common goals. In still others, the focus may be on such interactive processes as mass communications, needs and motivations, values and ethics, norms and standards, public policy, social planning, problem solving, training, community organization, political action, and the management of conflict.

In any case, health education helps people, or organizes them, to understand their problems better on the assumption that engaging in such processes will lead to behavior more conducive to health. It is a highly sophisticated art and science with a growing body of professional specialists dedicated to its improvement.

As it has here been defined, however, anyone who conducts health education can be regarded as a health educator, and this misapprehension constitutes a serious problem in the field of health education. Although many health-care workers who are not professionally trained in the field are responsible for good health education, many others mistakenly believe themselves to possess such competence and, in failing to seek assistance from specialists, deny their patients or clients needed understanding and help. Even if they have sufficient time to devote to health-education efforts, they may not understand theory well enough to determine which methods or steps are the most appropriate to adopt.

A professionally trained health educator—called a *health education specialist*—has the sole function of planning, conducting, and evaluating health-education programs. The specialist may work in different settings—schools, health departments, hospitals, rural cooperatives, training and continuing education centers, unions, private enterprise corporations, insurance companies, health maintenance organizations, universities, voluntary health agencies, neighborhood health centers, state and federal agencies, or health systems agencies—and may have different titles to correspond to work responsibilities, but the basic function remains the same.

Conceptions of what constitutes basic functions have changed over the years, however, as R. A. Bowman has demonstrated in a compilation of studies concerning the functions of health education specialists in various settings and times.[5] During the second half of the nineteenth century, for example, health educators were principally engaged in preparing lectures, leaflets, pamphlets, exhibits, and news releases. In the first half of the twentieth century, a small group of health educators realized that disseminating health information did not necessarily cause people to change their behavior. At this time—during the 1940s and 1950s—a new philosophy of health education emphasized involving the learner in the learning process. To this end, health educators became more active in community organization processes and began to employ more direct face-to-face methods with individuals.

By the 1960s, with the passage of much national legislation affecting the field of health and the delivery of health services, the functions of health educators had begun to shift toward a greater involvement in policy development, program planning, administration and supervision, consultation, training and continuing education, research and evaluation, and the uses of behavioral science and social science methods. The comprehensiveness of these present-day functions are set forth, in part, in a statement prepared by the California Conference of Local Directors of Health Education.* Although these functions are based on the role of a public-health educator working for local health departments, they show the wide variety of knowledge and skills that specialists must now possess.

Preparation and practice

During the 1970s, changes in life styles, the increased interest in ecology, the escalation of substance-abuse problems, concern for patients' rights, and emphasis on the accountability of health professionals have all had direct implications for the preparation of those who intend to pursue careers in professional health education. For to help individuals adopt better health practices, to help health organizations develop integrated health services and give greater attention to patients' rights, and to assist communities in providing healthier environments, students must now understand the theoretical bases of, and have skills in bringing about, individual, organizational, and community change. Guidelines prepared by the Society of Public Health Education (SOPHE) describe the requirements for entry into professional preparation programs, as well as the basic distinctions among the three primary levels of preparation and practice: the baccalaureate, master's, and doctoral levels.[6]

The baccalaureate is regarded as the basic practicing health-education professional degree. Students entering a baccalaureate program must have a previous foundation of knowledge in human physiology, human ecology and health, human growth and development, social psychology, social or cultural anthropology, and introductory sociology. Baccalaureate degrees include the Bachelor of Arts or of Sciences in Health Education (BAHE, BSHE).

Students entering a master's program must either have a baccalaureate degree in health education or take prerequisite courses that will provide

*See Appendix A.

them with the basic knowledge and skills for pursuing advanced studies in the field. In addition, such students must be capable, at the entry level, of participation in policy formulation, of using research skills to define the educational needs of target populations, and of designing, managing, and evaluating health-education programs. Degrees at the master's level include Master of Public Health (MPH), Master of Science in Health Education (MSHE), and Master of Science in Public Health (MSPH).

Students pursuing a doctoral program must be able to perform the minimum functions associated with both the baccalaureate and the master's and must, in addition, be capable of advanced health-education specialization for research, teaching, and practice. Degrees on completion of this level include Doctor of Education (Ed.D.), Doctor of Philosophy (Ph.D.), and Doctor of Public Health (Dr.P.H.).

The health-education specialist utilizes the knowledge and skills described in the SOPHE guidelines to contribute fundamental resources to the other members of the team or organization. These resources include: (1) facilitating team development processes and organizational change; (2) determining the basic theories involved in developing the solution to a problem and applying these theories to resolve the situation; (3) providing resources for designing, planning, implementing, and evaluating programs of change; and (4) providing resources and methods for reaching and helping consumers/patients, such as mass communications, group dynamics, community organization, leadership training, conference management, and conflict resolution.

Problems and promises

A poorly understood discipline and process, health education rests on the horns of a dilemma. On the one hand, it is regarded by health-care leaders as an essential component of all health-care services, and the promises held up for it have always been great. W. Griffiths has stated that "school health programs can, if well done, prepare individuals to make wiser decisions affecting their own personal health, or possibly even more important, may make them better informed citizens on all facets of health systems in their nation."[7]

R. L. Johnson has observed:

From the scope of health education that I would anticipate, educated people will not be satisfied with learning only the early symptoms of disease or the general maxim of seeking medical care early. . . . People will want to know why the health delivery system is organized the way it is now and what are some alternatives. . . . They will want to know how the health or medical-care dollar in this country is spent, where does most of the money go, and are there cheaper ways of achieving optimum health.[8]

Other authors write: "The ultimate value of health education cannot be measured by ordinary standards or in ordinary periods of time . . . . One bit of health information properly applied may save a life now or forty years from now. . . . That single life may be so valuable to society that this health-education learning may be of greater value than any other bit of learning that the individual may have experienced."[9]

On the other hand, health education has received little financial support to date. As the 1973 *Report of the President's Committee on Health Education* summarized it: "Of more than $75 billion now being spent annually for medical, hospital, and health care, about 92 to 93 percent is spent for treatment after illness occurs. Of the remainder, 4 to 5 percent is spent for biomedical research; 2 to 2½ percent for preventive health measures, and ½ percent for health education."[10]

Included in these figures were the following specifics. Of the $18.2 billion allocated in 1973 for medical and health activities by the U.S. Department of Health, Education and Welfare,* less than one-half of 1 percent was spent for health education; even a smaller fraction was spent of the additional $7.3 billion allocated for health purposes to all other federal agencies; and less than one-half of 1 percent of their budgets was spent by the state- and territorial-level health departments. These figures have not changed significantly since 1973.

Although the needed financial support has not yet materialized, there is at least growing recognition among policy makers that people are not fully using the capacity either to prevent illness or to gain maximum benefit from existing health systems.[11] Effective preventive measures, such as regular blood-pressure checks, sigmoidoscopies, and Pap tests, are ignored by many who could benefit from them, while the cost-effectiveness of other preventive health services, such as tonometry and physical examinations, should be established and put into more extensive use.**

Indeed, a 1972 study by N.B. Belloc and L. Breslow has shown that many diseases and premature deaths—and up to 80 percent of the deaths caused by cardiovascular disease and cancer are premature—can be prevented if people only practice six basic health habits: (1) eating three regular

*The Department of Health, Education and Welfare changed its name to the Department of Health and Human Services in 1979, while this book was in press. The Department of Education is now a separate entity.

**Sigmoidoscopy is inspection of the sigmoid (colon) flexure by the aid of a long tool called a speculum. Tonometry is measurement of tension, particularly intraocular (eye) tension.

meals a day without snacking; (2) practicing moderate exercise at least three times a week; (3) having seven or eight hours' sleep each night; (4) not smoking; (5) maintaining weight at a normal level; and (6) drinking alcohol in moderation if at all.[12]

A 45-year-old man who practices fewer than half these habits has a remaining life expectancy of 21.6 years, while one who practices all or nearly all has a life expectancy of 33.1 years—more than 53 percent longer than the other. According to Belloc and Breslow, the magnitude of this difference is better understood "if we consider that the increase in the life expectancy of white men in the United States between 1900 and 1960 was only 3 years."[13]

It is believed that people who have the knowledge to do so will make far better use of the existing health system and that health education—perhaps even more than medicine with its skyrocketing costs—can help to bridge the gap between what is known to be healthful human behavior and what is actually practiced in our society. In addition, the increased communications accompanying enhancement of knowledge would make both consumers and providers more cost-conscious, thereby helping to control the rising cost of medical care. It is the role of health education to help people develop these knowledges and change their behaviors, and, as will be seen, the need to begin is urgent.

NEED FOR HEALTH EDUCATION

Determinants of health

H. L. Blum has identified four major factors influencing the status of health: heredity, environment, health-care services, and behavior.[14] Heredity is important because genetic traits passed from parents to offspring are partly responsible for determining children's eventual physical and mental capacities. Environment has two related forces, physical and social. Physical environment constitutes a potentially hostile and hazardous force affecting human health, while inequities in social organization create such by-products as poverty, which contributes directly to many health problems. As a field, health-care services is a major force in itself, because how well health problems are addressed depends upon how well services are organized and delivered. These three areas warrant additional discussion here; behavior will be extensively discussed elsewhere in this book.

Heredity Heredity's role in the transmission of certain diseases, such as diabetes, sickle cell anemia, Tay Sach's disease, and some types of mental retardation, holds obvious implications for the field of health education.

More generally, however, to attain optimum health, one must know which hereditary factors exist to affect its status, as well as which actions will make best use of one's physical and mental capacities. In this area, health education is needed to help individuals learn about their own state of health, attain health appraisals, participate in early-detection screening programs, and decide what other actions are required to attain maximum health.

Environment Many problems in the physical environment have direct relationships to health and health behavior.[15] Air pollution, which is caused by the presence of poisonous chemicals discharged from industrial smokestacks, lead and carbon monoxide fumes discharged from petroleum-fueled vehicular exhaust pipes, and gaseous discharges from fires and other sources, can cause asthmatic attacks, allergic reactions, and breathing difficulties that may be hazardous to people with certain types of lung and heart disease. There are, further, more than 300 known toxic substances that can pollute drinking water supplies. Some of these cause gastroenteric diseases; all contribute to the increasing costs and difficulties of providing the public with safe drinking water.

Numerous other environmental problems associated with various forms of land, air, and water transportation hazards cause thousands of disabilities and deaths each year. The high noise levels produced by transportation, heavy industry, construction and electronics cause many people to suffer from nervousness, headaches, and insomnia. Many health hazards are also created by occupational exposure to fumes and dusts, faulty equipment, and such harmful chemical materials as asbestos, beryllium, and vinyl chloride. In addition, more than 500 new chemical compounds are introduced into use each year, many of which are insufficiently tested and safeguarded at the time of their release and are later found to be detrimental to health.

To improve the physical environment, people must become more conscious of safety practices, particularly in the operation of motor vehicles and in the use of machinery or equipment related to everyday occupations. Business and industrial management must become more cooperative in reducing or eliminating the pollutants and other hazards their operations introduce into the environment. Legislators must become more skilled in producing public policy for regulating pollution-producing industries; regulatory agencies must become more effective in applying these policies; citizens must become better informed about the causes and prevention of pollution, as well as better organized to participate in social problem-solving efforts. Through community organization processes, health educators can assist citizen groups in identifying their health problems, as well as in planning and carrying out legislative or voluntary community actions to solve some of them.

It is widely recognized that health is also directly related to socioeconomic conditions in general and to poverty in particular, with its concomitants of low income or unemployment; inadequate or slum housing; poor sanitation, human services, and public facilities; low educational levels; higher costs for food and other necessities; poor self-image and coping skills. According to H. A. Weeks, the 10 to 12 percent of the U.S. population that lives in poverty has twice the normal rate of infant mortality, seven years' less than normal life expectancy, significantly more days of bedridden disability, more hypertension, heart disease, tuberculosis, malnutrition, and stomach cancer.[16] Among Blacks and American Indians, rates of perinatal abnormalities, parasitic diseases, and mental disorders are five times higher than those of whites.

Stress, another major force of the social environment, results from people's inability to cope well with the conditions of their environment or with one another. Blum finds four significant sources of stress.[17]

1. Population density, or overcrowding, contributes to certain chronic diseases, tuberculosis, anxiety, and suicide.

2. Human interaction with the system, or the institutional forms and procedures by which social relationships are organized, is a sociological source of stress that contributes to hypertension and other forms of heart disease.

3. Psychic stress caused by life changes contributes to many emotional disorders and physical illnesses.[18]

4. The stress arising from life-style preference may stem from such behavioral habits as poor nutritional practices, lack of sleep, addiction to tobacco, alcohol, or drugs, overweight, and lack of exercise, or from psychological forces that cause people to become workaholic overachievers, highly competitive, or chronic worriers. Such life styles contribute to a wide range of chronic conditions significantly reducing both the length and quality of life.

Finding solutions to poverty problems requires long-range, large-scale, comprehensive programs that deal with related issues of public policy, economic development, employment, housing, and education while responding at the same time to community health needs. This in turn requires the willingness of agencies to collaborate at national, state, and local levels, the willingness of government and private enterprise to work together for the common good, the development of conditions that will enable the advantaged and disadvantaged to work together toward resolving problems that afflict them both, and some means for the constructive management of social conflict. By utilizing organization development technologies and community organization processes, health educators can assist in assessing the health needs of organizations and communities, in determining goals, establishing objectives, developing and implementing plans for action, and in evaluating the effectiveness of these activities.

Reducing stress-related problems has many implications for health education as well. Most obvious is the need to help people adopt life styles that are conducive to healthy productive lives; but closely allied to this is the equally great need to help people cope more effectively with the stresses created by their personal interactions in organizational, community, and social settings. Health educators can help patients and clients to adopt healthier practices and to cope better with stress by involving them in their own decision-making and learning processes through face-to-face interactions, group discussions, behavioral modification and other methods that will be described later in this book.

Health-care services Clearly, health needs cannot be met if health-care services are unavailable or seriously inadequate, and many current observers believe such services to be in a state of continuing crisis.[19] In 1976, for example, public expenditures for health care exceed $120 billion—more than 8 percent of the gross national product—with hospital costs alone rising at an annual rate of 15 percent. Indeed, the soaring costs of medical care are such as to place its adequate financing in serious jeopardy, although attempts are being made to contain costs by means of legislation.[20]

Unfortunately, high costs have not resulted in the bringing of adequate services to all people, such as those who live in rural communities or inner cities. Physicians and dentists prefer to practice where resources are available to provide quality service, and these resources are organized around medical centers located in metropolitan areas. Rural practitioners who have moved to cities or retired from practice have not been replaced by young graduates because the latter also want to practice where resources are to be found. In consequence, rural populations face the prospect of emergency illnesses or accidents without readily available help.

For people in inner cities, the resources exist but may not be used for one reason or another. Either the poor cannot get to them because of lack of transportation or health-care offices are not open during evenings or weekends when people are not working. Often, too, so complex and bewildering is the array of available services that even the most knowledgeable people have difficulty knowing where to seek what they want.

Where health services are accessible, they may be unacceptable to patients or clients because of racial, cultural, or ethnic barriers, their depersonalized character, or the inability of staffs to communicate effectively with those who are not fluent in English. Compounding these difficulties is the lack of accountability that may characterize the administration of health services. Here, decisions concerning which services are to be offered or which facilities are to be built may be made with little regard to basic needs; increased costs may be passed on to consumers instead of being directed toward increasing the efficiency of operations; and the quality of care may be insufficiently exposed to evaluative measures that would improve future performance.

Although the United States is generally accorded the distinction of having the highest level of medical technology in the world, that technology is not being applied well enough to its citizens. In point of fact, the U.S. now ranks seventeenth among nations on the basis of a variety of comparative measures. In the People's Republic of China, for example, the infant mortality rate is less than half that for nonwhites in New York and Detroit and almost a third less than that for whites throughout the United States, the reason for this being the intensive prenatal care that is practiced in China.[21]

This is not to suggest that there is a paucity of proposed solutions, however. L. Corey, M. F. Epstein, and S. E. Saltman have categorized six areas which they believe require attention.[22]

1. Though all people have difficulty obtaining needed services, special efforts should be made to see that the elderly and poor are provided with medical care.
2. Financial barriers to health care must be removed. Levels of service should not be based on the ability of clients to pay or not to pay.
3. Health services should not be delivered sporadically, at scattered locations, and under different organizational arrangements but on a comprehensive, coordinated basis.
4. Health service should no longer be disease oriented but should place greater emphasis on health maintenance and prevention.
5. Because health problems and the programs needed to resolve them are alike complex, interdisciplinary efforts and provider-consumer cooperation are essential.
6. While many methods for improving health-delivery services to selected segments of the public have been successfully demonstrated in the past, these must be greatly expanded in order to improve services for all people.

In this area, particularly, there is an acute need for the public to join with the community of health providers at national, state, and local levels, and in all disciplines, to help solve problems of health-care costs and of inadequate service to poor, aged, and rural populations. Health educators can assist by helping to mobilize the consumer through their community organization, by introducing group-work skills, and by imparting planning, implementation, and evaluation skills as well.

Transitions in health care

The field of health care is highly dynamic and is currently undergoing transitions affecting such fundamental matters as philosophy, policy, administration, organization, personnel, patients, and consumers (see table 1).

TABLE 1
Transitions in Health Care

| Transition Area | Transitions | | Impacts |
	From	To	
Philosophy	Health is a privilege	Health is a right	Values
Policy	Fragmented and locally determined	Comprehensive and federally established	Private interests
Administration	Professional service	Business management	Measurement of effectiveness
Organization	Solo practice and acute care	Group practice and primary care	Systems development
Costs	Professionally determined	Third-party insurance-determined	Power and control
Personnel	Specialists	Generalists and extenders	Roles
Patients	Dependency	Partner	Relationships
Consumers	Passive recipient	Active participation	Planning

Philosophy During the early years of health care in this country, those who could afford private medical care had the best that was available. The poor were provided with some free public-health, inpatient, or ambulatory services, particularly at teaching hospitals where medical school students learned the practice of medicine by studying and treating such patients. For the middle class, health care was a privilege which they could neither afford to buy nor were eligible to receive free.

Since World War II, however, the philosophical focus has centered increasingly on the belief that health care is not a privilege but a right, a belief that has been expressed in the preamble of most health measures presented to the public ever since. With the advent of health insurance and the general broadening of health-care services, health has been brought within the reach of most middle-class workers and has also improved delivery of services to the poor. But a right that cannot be exercised is not a right, and many people who wish to exercise the right to health are unable to do so for financial reasons. This problem has created sharp differences in values regarding health.

Organized medicine's general position is to resist the expansion of publicly supported health services, perceiving this as a further movement toward socialized medicine. Conservative groups, observing that an ever-growing proportion of private income goes for taxes that pay for free health services to others, likewise resist such expansion. Health-care leaders, concerned that a wide gap continues to separate levels of health between the advantaged and disadvantaged, promote government-supported strategies that they believe will close the gap. Finally, consumers who cannot afford to pay for health care accept the belief that health is a right and insistently demand that services be made available to them. This conflict in values makes problem-solving efforts exceedingly difficult at all levels.

Policy A relationship exists between policy and philosophy insofar as dominant values are often reflected in policy development. When private medical care was the norm and organized medicine had the greatest influence on the delivery of health services, health policies were made locally, and federal policies consisted basically of laws governing the containment of communicable diseases. As the belief has grown that health is a right, the federal government has assumed increasing responsibility for devising standards and policies that ensure equal quantity and quality of services for all people.

The growing role of the federal government has led to widespread recognition that more comprehensive approaches are needed for the resolution of health problems, a realization that is reflected in the creation of broader, more integrated policies. At the same time, however, the effect of policy transition has been to sharpen differences between federal and private interests. Organized medicine has been joined by some members of the health insurance industry in taking political and legislative action to protect their common or respective interests.

Administration The administration of health-care services has been changing gradually from a professional-service approach to an approach based on business management. The professional-service approach, often administered by physicians, generally regards the proper measurement of health care as the extent to which treatments are successful and patients are cured. Such administrators attempt to provide more and better facilities and resources. They respond to increased costs by requesting larger budgets or by justifying increased costs to consumers.

The business-management approach, administered by nonphysicians trained in the management sciences as well as in health care, regards the proper measurement of health care in terms of productivity and cost-effectiveness of the services provided. Managers attempt to control the use of resources and to deliver services more economically.

This administrative transition has increased tension between those committed to providing quality service and those committed to providing quantity service. For as health-care systems become more organized along the lines of business models, as in the case of health maintenance organizations (HMOs), physicians become employees rather than independent private practitioners, patients and clients are regarded as consumers, and care is prepaid by insurance or fees. HMOs are prepaid health-care plans, providing services as needed only to their members, who pay fixed monthly or annual fees.

Organization Closely related to administrative transition is a transition in the way health services are organized. For many years, basic community health services consisted only of the offices of private physicians and of a community-supported hospital for treating the acutely ill. Because these fragmented services left many needs unmet, a shift has been occurring toward group practice and primary health-care centers.

Group practices are formed by private physicians who come together to share common office-support costs and to develop teams of specialized medical resources for the purpose of providing their patients with more comprehensive services. These are often called clinics. Primary health care centers, such as HMOs and neighborhood health centers, offer ambulatory consumers a comprehensive range of preventive, diagnostic, treatment, and rehabilitation services (hospitalization is generally regarded as secondary care). Introduced during implementation of the antipoverty programs of the

1960s, neighborhood health centers provide primary-care services to the populations of inner-city poverty areas and are usually governed by boards of directors composed of residents of those neighborhoods.

This organizational transition has increased the need to develop systems that integrate primary, secondary, tertiary, and other specialized or supportive health services into planned, cooperative, coordinated, comprehensive relationships. To help bring about such coordination, health-systems agencies (HSAs) have been organized at regional (usually multicounty or metropolitan) levels throughout the country.

Although the long-range planned development of integrated resources may eventually enable all people to exercise their right to health, resistance to planning can be great, especially among groups whose self-interests run counter to a plan for rational regional growth. When comprehensive planning blocks self-interest forces, systems development can become a highly politicized issue.

Personnel One of the primary transitions currently affecting health-care personnel is in the area of role modification and change. Owing to a higher level of training and to medical licensure, the physician was once automatically regarded as the leader of a health team. Because training to produce highly specialized professionals is long and costly, however, they are often in short supply, particularly in rural areas and inner-city neighborhoods. For this reason, an approach gaining increased support involves educating intermediary aides and assistants to carry out the professional's less technical, more routine functions by means of preparation in specific short-term training programs. The professionals in turn take on the function of managing and supervising their aides.

Another aspect of role transition in health care centers on the pressures associated with specialized or generalist practice. As health personnel become more highly trained and experienced, they tend to specialize in specific skills and functions. But as public pressures increase for more comprehensive or better integrated human services, professionals and aides alike find greater acceptance in pursuing general or family practice than in specialization.

Thus, the physician (or dentist, pharmacist, nurse, etc.) is now increasingly a member of a team in which both leadership and more routine functions are shared, depending upon the needs of the patient or client. Because people generally resist changing their work patterns, however, such role changes have not been easily made but have been accompanied by role-oriented confusion and conflict. Accommodating them has meant increased reliance on team-building and role-negotiation processes

Patients Busy health professionals often lose sight of their patients' individual needs and believe that by merely telling them what to do, and expecting their compliance in carrying out prescribed treatments, their health problems will be satisfactorily resolved. There is abundant evidence, however, that patients do not follow doctors' orders simply because they have been told what to do, that fostering a dependency relationship means doing for patients increasingly more that they could be doing for themselves, and that the promotion of health requires people to understand what they can do for themselves.

Educated patients are better patients, and today's patient or client has shifted from being a passive recipient of services to one more responsible for personal health care, becoming in effect a partner in the health-care transaction. If it is to be successful, such a partnership requires extensive investment toward a common goal. Providers must relinquish the role of telling and take on the more difficult task of helping. Patients must relinquish their dependency and take increased responsibility for their own care and treatment. Again, however, such changes in mutual perception and expectation are not easily made.

Consumers Until recent years, the prerogative for health-care decision making rested chiefly with professionals, the assumption being that they better understood health problems and how to solve them. The problems have not been resolved, however, and now consumers themselves must assist in the problem solving. Voluntary health agencies, which have their own boards of directors, have long demonstrated the rationale for community leadership participation.

- In order for basic health needs to be met, consumers should participate in identifying those needs.
- In order for health programs to be useful to the public, consumers should be involved in planning their design, organization, and delivery.
- In order for health-care services to be adequately financed, consumers, who pay health-care bills and taxes, should participate in determining the costs.
- In order for right-to-health to become a reality, consumers must be involved in shaping that right.
- In order for the democratic principle of local self-determination to be realized in health care, consumers must participate in the democratic processes by which health-care decisions and policies are made.

The consumer, then, is changing from a passive recipient to an active participant, and this has greatly affected the ways and means of contemporary health care. Guidelines for defining providers and consumers have become highly specific. Planning processes have become more consumer oriented than ever before, with citizen participation in all planning steps, from needs assessment and goal setting to programming, implementation, and evaluation. Federal and state governments are increasingly requiring that program implementation be under the control of local boards, the majority of whose membership is made up of consumers. In addition, consumer-advocacy and self-interest groups have become vigorously active in promoting their own needs and in attempting to influence health-care decision making wherever and however they can.

As a result of this transition, tensions between providers and consumers have increased, particularly as conflicts over what is needed and what should be done are heightened by mutual distrust. The success of the consumer transition could transform the face of health care; its failure could force federal and state governments to rescind some of their decentralized authorities. In the meantime, health education has important contributions to make during this period of change.

Health educators must help consumers to become more active and to accept responsibility for influencing right-to-health policy. Educators themselves must take on greater responsibility for facilitating processes of transition and change within the health-care field, employing their team-building and problem-solving skills to help health-care teams work together more effectively against resistance to change and urging toward constructive resolutions the processes by which health care is organized and delivered.

COMMENTARY

In our society, health care has historically been undertaken with a single purpose: to cure disease, thereby to delay death as long as possible, an approach that accounts for the character of the breakthroughs that have characterized the field's evolution over many years. Since the turn of the century, life expectancy has increased from age fifty to more than age seventy. There has been a steady decline in morbidity and mortality rates among the communicable diseases, particularly with respect to typhoid fever, smallpox, diphtheria, bubonic plague, tuberculosis, whooping cough, measles, scarlet fever, the dysenteries, and tick-borne diseases. Maternal mortality has been reduced and infant deaths cut as well.

Medical-technical advances have been both rapid and remarkable. The discovery of new antibiotics and drugs has helped to prevent disease and prolong life. Chemotherapy has given hope to the mentally ill and diabetic, as well as to those with certain types of heart disease and cancer. Transplants of organs and tissues have also prolonged lives. Throughout the first half of the twentieth century, official and voluntary health agencies have contributed to advances in public-health laboratory services, statistical services, environmental sanitation services, immunizations, antibiotics, public-health nursing services, and health education.

On the other hand, there is widespread evidence of drug abuse; increasing incidence of venereal disease; premature deaths resulting from treatable chronic diseases; accidents as a leading cause of injury and death among children, youth, and young adults; high obesity and low physical fitness at all ages; increasing pollution of natural resources; needless suffering and wasted money owing to the blundering of quacks and faddists; and a general lack of knowledge about health in everyday life.

The historical approach has been one of medical-technical development: discovery of more effective drugs and treatments, development of better equipment and facilities, preparation of more highly skilled and knowledgeable health-care personnel, and improvement in the organization and delivery of health-care services. But these alone are no longer able to impel major improvements in the level of health, which must come about as a result of dramatic changes in the health behavior of people themselves. Health education is an important element in helping to bring about these changes, and the next three parts of this book will be devoted to illuminating the health-education process.

REFERENCES

1. World Health Organization, *Health Education*, p. 6.
2. Ibid., pp. 6–7.
3. The Joint Committee on Health Education Terminology met in Chicago for two three-day sessions each, on 1–4 March and 13–16 September 1972. It was composed of representatives of the American Academy of Pediatrics, American Association of Health, Physical Education, and Recreation, American College Health Association, American School Health Association, Public Health Education and School Health sections of the American Public Health Association, and the Society for Public Health Education.
4. U.S., Department of Health, Education and Welfare, Public Health Service, Center for Disease Control, *HEIRS: Thesaurus of Health Education Terminology*, prepared for the Bureau of Health Education by the editorial staff of *Health Education Monographs*, Johns Hopkins University School of Hygiene and Public Health, Baltimore, Md., 1965.
5. R. A. Bowman, "Changes in the Activities, Functions, and Roles of Public Health Educators," *Health Education Monographs* 4, no. 3 (Fall 1976): 226–45.
6. Society for Public Health Education, "Guidelines for the Preparation and Prac-

tice of Professional Health Educators," *Health Education Monographs* 5, no. 1 (Spring 1977): 75–89.

7. W. Griffiths, "Health-Education Definitions, Problems, and Philosophies," *Health Education Monographs*, no. 31 (1972), pp. 7–12.

8. R. L. Johnson, "Health Education: Ramifications and Consequences," *Health Education Monographs*, no. 31 (1972), pp. 19–21.

9. American Association of Health, Physical Education, and Recreation, "A Point of View for School Health Education," *Journal of Health, Physical Education, and Recreation*, no. 33 (1962), p. 26.

10. President's Committee on Health Education, *The Report of the President's Committee on Health Education*, p. 25.

11. U. S., Congress, House, Committee on Interstate and Foreign Commerce, *Report No. 94–1007: National Health Promotion and Disease Prevention Act of 1976*, 94th Cong., 2d sess., 1976, p. 5.

12. N. B. Belloc and L. Breslow, "Relationship of Physical Health Status and Health Practices," *Preventive Medicine* 1, no. 3 (August 1972): 415–21.

13. Ibid., pp. 419–20.

14. H. L. Blum, *Expanding Health-Care Horizons*, p. 63.

15. Ibid., pp. 49–51.

16. H. A. Weeks, "Income and Disease: The Pathology of Poverty," in *Medicine in a Changing Society*, ed. L. Corey, M. F. Epstein, and S. E. Saltman, p. 53.

17. Blum, *Expanding Health-Care Horizons*, pp. 51–54.

18. For an insightful analysis of life changes, see G. Sheehy, *Passages: Predictable Crises of Adult Life* (New York: E. P. Dutton & Co., 1976).

19. Corey, Epstein, and Saltman, *Medicine in a Changing Society*, pp. 37–39.

20. The Hospital Cost Containment Act of 1977 was introduced to Congress as H.R. 6575. The message proposing the act was delivered on 25 April 1977.

21. L. Woodstock, "Health-Care Goals for Americans: 1975," in Corey, Epstein, and Saltman, *Medicine in a Changing Society*, p. 45.

22. Ibid., p. 8.

PART ONE
HEALTH
EDUCATION
AND
INDIVIDUALS

2

*Problems in
individual
health behavior*

3

*Theories of
individual
behavior*

4

*Programs for
individual
change*

Particularly if health problems have an attitudinal or behavioral basis, health-care workers tend to place all the responsibility for them on the shoulders of the individual, implying that such problems can be resolved by means of individual education. Although they are often correct, this book maintains that some problems require other approaches, and much of the following text is devoted to exploring these.

Nevertheless, individuals do exercise considerable responsibility for their own health behavior, however constructive or destructive it may be. Documenting the results of that behavior is not difficult, and chapter 2 reviews data that suggest both the nature and extent of individual health problems. Accounting for behavior—or explaining why individuals behave as they do—is a complex matter, however, and chapter 3 attempts to select from an extensive field those behavioral theories thought to be most relevant to health education.

Finally, while it is logical to assume that health education for individuals is conducted on an individual basis, more often the focus is on bringing individuals together into group settings or on employing other strategies for reaching several persons at the same time. In these cases the purpose is still to enable individuals to change their behaviors in ways conducive to better health, and chapter 4 describes several health-education programs that have individual behavioral change as their primary goal.

2

Problems in individual health behavior

SOME INDIVIDUAL PROBLEMS

• *Although it is known that cervical cancer can be detected and successfully treated in its early stages, and although the Pap test takes only a few moments to administer, only 5 percent of women over the age of twenty have a Pap test every year.* [1]

Throughout the nation the American Cancer Society's staff and volunteers direct considerable energy toward combating this problem, producing films, brochures, and publicity releases for radio and television and making extensive use of mass communications media in general. Health department programs continually address this concern, as do physicians, health maintenance organizations, hospital personnel, neighborhood health centers, healthmobiles, multiphasic screening programs, and the like. Women's health groups likewise include this vitally urgent preventive health measure in their programs. Why, then, do so few women respond to these efforts?

• *Although 95 percent of the recurrences of rheumatic fever can be prevented through appropriate use of antibiotics, 18,000 people die annually from rheumatic fever because they have not had the appropriate treatment.* [2]

Among numerous other groups and agencies, the American Heart Association devotes considerable educational effort toward addressing this problem, but the number of disabilities and deaths remain staggeringly high. Why do those who are potential risks for rheumatic fever not seek diagnosis? Even more important, why do those who know they have the disease fail to get treatment that would prevent recurrence and serious related consequences?

• *Although hypertension can be controlled on a large scale and blood pressure reduced in selected population groups, only half the people who suffer from hypertension are aware of the problem, while few of those who are aware of it follow the prescribed corrective practices.*[3]

Hypertension is one of the major causes of heart disease, which is the leading killer of people today, and the efforts exerted to educate people about this problem far outweigh those devoted to other health problems. People are repeatedly enjoined to have the type of physical examination that leads to discovery of hypertension and to follow prescribed corrective practices once hypertension has been diagnosed. If people are aware of these messages, why do most of them not respond?

• *Although smoking, drinking, obesity, irregular meals, physical inactivity, and lack of sleep are known to cause earlier death among those who practice even two or three of these habits, many people refuse to change behaviors that are obviously hazardous to their health.*[4]

Since 1964, smoking has declined among people twenty-five years of age and older, particularly among men, though teenage smoking has increased, particularly among women. In 1974 the per capita consumption of cigarettes for the U.S. population eighteen years of age and older was 4,270, the highest since 1963.[5] Further, an estimated 9 million Americans are alcoholics or problem drinkers.[6] Alcohol plays a role in half the nation's highway fatalities, half of all its homicides, and one-third of its suicides. In lost work, property damage, and use of health and welfare services, the cost to society of alcohol abuse exceeds $15 billion.[7]

Nutritional problems range from malnutrition and obesity to quality and safety of food supply. Malnutrition can be a cause of fetal prematurity and immaturity and is often associated with learning disabilities among young children. Obesity, which may affect 30 percent of Americans, increases susceptibility to diabetes, hypertension, arthritis, pulmonary dysfunction, angina, and gall bladder disease. Coronary heart disease appears to be associated with increased intake of saturated fats and cholesterol. Potential hazards exist, too, in foods with certain additives, fortifiers, artificial colors and flavoring.[8]

Finally, this nation's sedentary way of life also constitutes a serious health problem for the 45 percent of adults who do not exercise. Habitual physical inactivity is thought to contribute to hypertension, premature aging, poor musculature, mental tension, coronary heart disease, and obesity.[9] Yet so insistent are the informational and educational campaigns addressing such problems that no one can claim ignorance of their relation to health. Why then, do the problems persist in such great numbers? Why do people continue to pursue destructive practices, and what must the health educator know who would work in this area?

• *A 1966 review of thirty-one studies on patient compliance with medical advice revealed more than 30 percent noncompliance in 86 percent of the studies and more than 50 percent noncompliance in 33 percent of the studies, resulting in untold wastes of medical-care resources, as well as in unnecessary disease and death.*[10]

Noncompliance means that patients do not follow the advice of their physicians or other health-care personnel in taking medications over a period of time, in returning to the doctor's office or clinic for scheduled checkups or further treatment, in electing present surgery that might obviate more serious future surgery, or in changing harmful to helpful behavior. In this situation especially, where it can be assumed that patients have been told plainly what they should or should not do, why do they not comply?

• *During the past ten years the percentage of children protected against polio has declined steadily. In 1973, two out of five children aged one to four were not adequately protected, with the result that there is now a potential for outbreaks of a serious communicable disease that had previously been under control.*[11]

Here is an excellent example of medical technology's having advanced far beyond people's ability to understand and take advantage of it, for no child should ever have to suffer from a disease that is preventable by immunization. Although school health, public health, and private medical practitioners have worked hard to educate people on the necessity for immunizing their children, the data reveal great numbers of children still unprotected. Why?

In general, all leading causes of death have behavioral implications. Heart disease reflects, among other things, poor food choices, use of cigarettes, and lack of exercise. Lung cancer and emphysema are associated with smoking; diabetes, with excessive eating; cirrhosis of the liver, with excessive drinking.[12] Drug addiction and venereal diseases take a heavy toll among teenagers and young adults, while an inability to cope with life's stresses affects people of all ages. Individual behavior lies at the core of many of these situations, and the weight of the evidence points overwhelmingly toward poor health behavior.

Health education, a process for shaping healthful behavior, involves applying the behavioral and social sciences to health-care problems. While there are no easy solutions to these problems, research is constantly under way to discover more about human behavior and how it can be changed. The challenge for health educators is to understand this research and to learn how to apply it effectively.

PROBLEMS FOR HEALTH EDUCATION

Such is the complexity of human nature, with its interrelated problems and interdependent behavioral processes, that no one discipline has ever been sufficient to deal comprehensively with its totality. The practical alternative has been to study segments of the totality, to trace the relationships among the segments, and in this tentative way to approach an understanding of the whole. To this end, health education has utilized theory derived from a variety of behavioral and social sciences, including psychology, social psychology, psychiatry, sociology, anthropology, and political science.

At its annual meeting in 1974 the American Public Health Association conducted a symposium examining the relationship to a broad range of disease processes of such social conditions as urban living, socioeconomic status, social disorganization, conflict, and stability, showing that many diseases and deaths are both directly and indirectly attributable to psychosocial factors.[13] In 1975 the World Health Organization called for a strengthening of its programs on the basis of its recognition that psychosocial factors can modify the outcome of health education.[14] These activities reflect a growing awareness that the social and behavioral sciences, however compartmentalized their initial studies of human behavior may have been, are now gradually broadening their perspectives to include more of the behavioral whole.

The U.S. Public Health Service believes that changes in the nation's health status will come about more from changes in personal life style and from control of environmental problems than from additional personal health-care services. Because health-care needs can be reduced through efforts that educate people about their ability and responsibility for protecting their own health,[15] health education demands particular attention and support. The current theme of the Public Health Service is prevention, and four areas of importance are being stressed: health education, nutrition, child health, and environmental health.[16]

Here it must be observed, however, that the necessity of choosing between broad and narrow perspectives for review purposes confronts the authors with a dilemma in expository approach. On the one hand, some dimensions of behavior are so inextricably interrelated with others that it is difficult to separate them and make an arbitrary assignment of one set of theories to one particular chapter. On the other hand, despite some overlapping among them, individual, organizational, and social behaviors are each distinct enough to be discussed separately, and it is useful to do so even though theories proliferate and scholars may disagree on the fundamental meanings of certain elements in the existing body of behavioral knowledge.

For review purposes, for example, the numerous theories relating specifically to individual behavior can be categorized into eight bodies: personality, developmental, perception, motivation, learning, attitude change, problem solving and creativity, and group dynamics. Personality theory is important in exploring the effects of heredity, environment, and self-aspects of personality on people's basic capacities. The patterning of development throughout the life cycle tells how growth occurs under combined internal and external forces. Perception theory is important in clarifying why individuals accept or reject health-education messages, depending upon their selective perception processes.

Emotion and motivation theory help to characterize an individual's humanness, the feelings that must be expressed and needs that must be met. Learning theory enables health educators to know how people learn so that they can design better individual programs. Because attitudes help to shape individual behavior, health educators must also know how attitudes are formed and can be changed. Problem-solving and creativity theory illuminates how people approach a problem, develop an idea, work on it, and decide which solution to choose. Finally, group dynamics theory illustrates how people behave in groups and how groups themselves influence individual behavior.

By G. Lindzey, C. S. Hall, and R. F. Thompson, however, personality theory alone has been subclassified into nine additional areas: psychodynamic, social psychological, trait, type, cognitive, behavior, self, and existential.[17] Advanced by Sigmund Freud (1856–1939) and Carl Jung (1875–1961) among other early psychologists, psychodynamic theory emphasizes inborn predispositions, unconscious motivation, and infantile complexes. Social psychological theory, developed by Alfred Adler (1870–1937), Erich Fromm (1900–1980), Harry Stack Sullivan (b. 1892), and Karen Horney (1885–1952), emphasizes the role of sociocultural factors and interpersonal relations in personality development.

Trait theory, described by Gordon Allport (1897–1967) and R. B. Cattell, relates personality development to innate traits and learned dispositions. W. H. Sheldon (b. 1898) correlated three dimensions of personality with three dimensions of physique to produce what he called type theory. Cognitive theory, devised by G. A. Kelley (1905–1966), asserts that personality is defined by personal constructs, or the way in which an individual interprets his world.

A. Bandura (b. 1925), R. H. Walters, B. F. Skinner (b. 1904), N. E. Miller, and J. Dollard regard habit as the key concept in behavioral theory. Self-theory and the actualization of self were described by Abraham Maslow and K. Goldstein (1878–1965). M. Boss (b. 1903) advanced the existential theory, which asserts that individuals can be whatever they want to be and are themselves responsible for realizing their own potential.

In addition to these theories, Freud, Jung, Sullivan, and Erik Erikson have all described various stages of personality development, while R. J. Corsini has developed a partial listing of no fewer than seventy-eight personality theories.[18] Despite this substantial body of theory, however, some issues are still being debated, such as the ways in which personality develops, the role of conscious and unconscious processes, the influence of heredity and environment, and the importance of situational factors in human behavior.[19] For if much is known about observable human behavior, much still remains to be learned about that which is not observable.

Observable behavior consists of actions or reactions that occur visibly in given situations, such as whether an individual does or does not smoke, is friendly or hostile, laughs or cries, is helpful or uncaring. Likewise observable, much interactive behavior involving two or more persons may occur within a family or social group setting, at work on the job, at play in the neighborhood, while voting in elections or discussing current issues and events. Beneath the observable surface, however, lay heredity and genetics, feelings and perceptions, likes and dislikes, wants, needs, and motivations, beliefs and values, knowledge and skills, education and experience, culture and climate—factors which can neither be seen nor ignored and which health educators must take into account when constructing educational programs for patients.

Further, none of the behavioral theories is alone sufficient to serve the general needs of health educators, who must attempt to organize parts or groups of theories in ways that are relevant for developing programs and strategies that relate to individual behavior. Such programs and strategies should be founded on three precepts:

1. Programs should be individualized for the learner, a principle based on theories of personality development, attitude formation, and perception.

2. Strategies should take into consideration individual intellectual and emotional growth and self-determination, a principle based on theories of self-actualization and creativity.

3. Strategies should facilitate individual change toward more affirmative health behavior, a principle based on theories of motivation, experienced-based learning, attitude and behavioral change, group dynamics and problem-solving processes, and models of change processes.

Psychologist and philosopher Kurt Lewin is generally credited with originating the thought that there is nothing so practical as a good theory. The theories that have been selected for discussion in chapter 3 are those that have the greatest meaning for health education, and meaningfulness will here be measured by practicality: what makes sense for the health educator who works with patients, community leaders, or in-service trainees in pursuit of individual behavioral change.

REFERENCES

1. S. K. Simonds, "Health Education as Social Policy," *Health Education Monographs* 2, no. 1 (1974): 1–10.
2. Ibid.
3. Ibid.
4. N. B. Belloc and L. Breslow, "Relationship of Physical Health Status and Health Practices," *Preventive Medicine* 1, no. 3 (August 1972): 415–21.
5. U.S., Department of Health, Education and Welfare, *Forward Plan for Health FY 1977–81,* HEW Publication no. (OS) 76–50024, June 1975, p. 7.
6. Ibid., p. 101.
7. Ibid., p. 100.
8. Ibid., p. 103.
9. Ibid., p. 112.
10. M. S. Davis, "Variations in Patients' Compliance with Doctors' Orders: Analysis of Congruence between Survey Responses and Results of Empirical Investigations," *Journal of Medical Education* 41, no. 11 (1966): 1038–39.
11. U.S. Department of Health Education and Welfare, *Forward Plan for Health FY 1978–82,* HEW Publication no. (OS) 76–50046, August 1976, p. 74.
12. Ibid., pp. 14–18.
13. C. B. Bahnson, "Behavioral Factors Associated with the Etiology of Physical Disease," *American Journal of Public Health* 64, no. 11 (November 1974): 1033–55.
14. V. Djukanovic and E. P. Mach, *Alternative Approaches to Meeting Basic Health Needs in Developing Countries,* pp. 7–25.
15. U.S., Department of Health, Education and Welfare, *Forward Plan for Health FY 1978–82,* p. 36.
16. Ibid., p. 69.
17. G. Lindzey, C. S. Hall, and R. F. Thompson, *Psychology.*
18. R. J. Corsini, *Current Personality Theories.*
19. Lindzey, Hall, and Thompson, *Psychology,* pp. 29–47; see also B. F. Skinner, *Science and Human Behavior.*

3
Theories of individual behavior

Such is the diversity and complexity of knowledge about individual human behavior that space permits only a few of the many existing concepts and theories to be presented here. Even this broad range of information cannot embrace the totality of human behavior, however, but can only reflect our fragmented approaches to the study of it, the different questions asked by different researchers, and the different perceptions gained by different thinkers. Health educators must attempt to integrate this knowledge as they formulate strategies that will assist them in changing people's health behaviors. Programs that incorporate many of the theories and principles presented here will be discussed in chapter 4.

EIGHT THEORIES

Personality theory

Gordon Allport's definition of personality, offered more than forty years ago, is still standard: "Personality is the dynamic organization within the individual of those psychophysical systems that determine his characteristic behavior and thought."[1] Three of the basic forces that help to share this dynamic organization are heredity, environment, and self, each of which will be discussed in turn.

Heredity Heredity is responsible for two aspects of individual development: (1) the physiological process of reproduction and growth, which influences the development of the fetus from conception to birth, and (2) the genetic structuring of chromosomes, which is unique to each individual. Chromosomes are made up of DNA (deoxyribonucleic acid) molecules which carry the genes that determine an individual's physical attributes.[2] While it is now known that certain diseases, such as sickle cell anemia, Tay Sach's disease, diabetes, and some forms of mental retardation are the result of heredity, genetic effects on personality development are still being studied.

Although all species of life must adapt to changing environmental forces if they are not to become extinct, the adaptation process normally requires a gradual shift over countless generations. Today, however, the hazards to which the human organism is exposed can so affect the genetic structures of one generation as to produce changes among the offspring of the next. The inability of many expectant mothers to tolerate thalidomide, for example, produced a generation of deformed infants before the cause of this tragedy could be discovered, while radiation-induced genetic disorders arising from the atomic bombings of Hiroshima and Nagasaki are still being documented among the survivors and their descendants.

Contemporary research is amassing much knowledge about such basic structures as DNA, genes, and chromosomes and how these can be modified or changed both to preserve and to enhance life. In regard to heredity, health education also has important roles to play. First, it can help potential parents become aware that genetic defects may exist in their familial histories and motivate them to seek genetic counseling before becoming parents. Second, it can help to organize and conduct screening programs of possible genetic problems so that early diagnosis can lead to early treatment.

Environment Theorists generally agree that environmental forces—forces originating outside the individual—are very important in shaping personality development. These forces exhibit three dimensions.

1. Physical environment includes the geographical factors that affect people's lives, such as terrain and climate, land and water resources, and population density.
2. Sociocultural environment includes the basic culture or subculture in which the individual grows and develops, the organized beliefs and values that dominate this group, the individual's position or role in the sociocultural setting, and the conditions that govern interpersonal interactions among family members, peer groups, and work groups.
3. Socialization environment includes communication processes, role

expectations, and values formulation and clarification, as well as the influence of such organized structures as schools, churches, and places of work, all of which affect the way individuals perceive and respond to their world.[3]

When sociocultural and socialization forces are at the center of organization and community social-change theories, the health educator is primarily concerned with the nature and shaping of these forces. With regard to personality development, however, concern centers on internal and external forces alike, exploring how the individual adjusts and develops as a result of their impingement on the self.

Self   The structure of self has special importance for health education because it offers a theory base for influencing change at the individual level. In this context, the term *self* denotes how individuals perceive themselves in terms of identity, worth, esteem, and effectiveness, or in terms of realistic knowing, doing, achieving, and being; how they experience events and interpret them either to reinforce or alter earlier perceptions; how they develop consistency and continuity of purpose; and whether they see their own selfhood as unique. In clarifying the structure of self, two theories are useful: self-concept and self-determinism.

W. Beatty has developed a self-concept theory of learning which integrates personality development, motivation, and learning in a single construct.[4] According to Beatty, the self-concept is an organization of self-images perceived through the appraisals or feedback of others. On the basis of this perceived self, the individual develops a concept of adequacy—i.e., how to behave in order to be effective. The perceived self and adequate self together make up the self-concept.

Where aspects of the two selves overlap, there is confirmation of these aspects of the self-concept. For the most part, however, the two selves do not overlap, and resolving the discrepancies between them by striving to become more like the adequate self is the source of motivation. The process of reducing these discrepancies—of using feedback and taking action to determine which behaviors will lead to the adequate self—is called learning.

Beatty identifies four areas of organized experience and learning—worth, coping, expressing, and autonomy—as contributing to the resolution of these discrepancies and the attainment of individual maturity. (1) By experiencing love or other forms of inclusion, the individual gains a sense of self-worth without an accompanying sense of defensiveness. (2) By learning how to do something that previously could not be done, the individual feels better able to cope effectively. (3) By means of the affective (i.e., pleasant or unpleasant) experiencing of sensations, the individual becomes more self-expressive and relatively freer of tension and anxiety. (4) By making autonomous choices, the individual develops a greater range of choices for controlling his own future. Although not all discrepancies may be resolved in the mature individual, enough progress will have been made for him to redirect his attention toward resolving some of the discrepancies that exist between society in general and people in particular.

Self-determinism is a theory developed by the field of humanistic psychology, whose adherents believe that human beings, unique in their individual responses, behaviors, attitudes, beliefs, and values, are also potentially self-actualizing. Taking issue with Freudian psychoanalytic theories which emphasized the bad/irrational aspects of man, humanistic psychologists urged recognition and development of the inherently good/rational aspects of human behavior. Rejecting Skinnerian theories of behavioral conditioning, which in their view either oversimplified or ignored the individual's internal psychological make-up, they believed that man has a significant measure of freedom for self-determination.[5]

Gordon Allport, in particular, has criticized the behavioral sciences for postulating an empty organism who is impelled by drives and molded by environmental circumstances but is incapable of creating or living in a democracy. In his view, democratic theory assumes that man possesses a measure of rationality, a portion of freedom, a generic conscience, personal ideals, and a sense of unique self-worth.[6]

The work of Carl Rogers, too, has greatly influenced the thinking and methodological development of applied behavioral scientists, especially those who work in client-centered counseling and small groups.[7] For Rogers believes that personality develops from experience, which he defines as everything that is accessible to the organism's awareness. He believes further that individuals tend naturally toward growth and wholeness, so that, when ambiguous experiences are clarified for them, they will choose a path toward self-maintenance, self-enhancement, and self-actualization.

Both the self-concept theory of learning and the theory of self-determinism have important implications for health education. The first theory should guide health educators who are designing patient-education programs to select methods that will enable patients to experience their own self-worth, cope with their illnesses, express themselves in fuller and more unique ways, and exercise independence from, rather than dependence upon, health providers. The second theory, which asserts that people can make deliberate choices about their personal lives and health behavior,[8] legitimates the role of health education in helping people to make more informed choices. Many self-help groups in this country have been organized around the concept of self-determinism.

All the concepts of personality development advance the view that individuals who are raised in a positive environment, who possess a strong sense of self and an awareness of personal competencies, have a greater chance than others of becoming self-actualized. They assume further that the more individuals practice habits that attune the body to the actualized self, the likelier they are to want to pursue the goal of staying healthy.

Developmental theory

Two principal bodies of theory attempt to explain individual development of identity.[9] Structuralists, concerned with *why* behaviors occur, believe that internal rules guide all behavior, that rules change as the person develops, and that identity development is the joint product of maturation and experience.

Behaviorists, concerned with how behaviors can be *changed,* offer two strategies. (1) B. F. Skinner and his followers believe that observable behaviors can be changed by a manipulation of rewards;[10] that is, people will behave in ways that enable them to feel meaningfully rewarded and will discontinue behaviors that are ignored. (2) A. Bandura and his followers believe that children, in particular, change their behaviors because of a desire to emulate role models who are being rewarded for their behaviors, in this way learning that they will be rewarded for similar behaviors.[11] Some diet-education programs are based on behavioral concepts, the dieter being rewarded for weight loss by peer support and improved physical appearance.

Among the eminent writers who have contributed to the study of the developmental process is Erik Erikson, who asserts that the ego is shaped by society and that the individual, undergoing a process of constant challenge and growth, is preprogrammed to go through eight developmental stages.[12] Normally the individual moves inevitably from one stage to the next, struggling through the transitions, and becomes fully mature and realized only after passing through the eight stages successfully.

J. C. Coleman has developed a six-stage process of developmental tasks based in part on the concepts of Erikson and R. Havighurst[13] but translated into specific behaviors that characterize each of the stages (see table 2).

Knowledge of the various stages of development and of the meaning of roles can guide health educators in developing their programs and in behavioral counseling as well. Programs can be organized for parents whose children are at stages where they are developing attitudes about health and health practices. Here, health educators can not only help parents become role models for their children but can themselves serve as role models by practicing what they preach. Finally, rewarding good behavior or attempts at change should be a routine part of educational procedure as health personnel work with patients, students, and neighborhood residents alike.

TABLE 2
Coleman's Developmental Tasks

1. Early Childhood
   0–6 Years

   Acquiring a sense of trust in self and others. Developing healthy concept of self. Learning to give and receive affection. Identifying with own sex. Achieving skills in motor coordination. Learning to be member of family group. Beginning to learn physical and social realities. Beginning to distinguish right and wrong and to respect rules and authority. Learning to understand and use language. Learning personal care.

2. Middle Childhood
   6–12 Years

   Gaining wider knowledge and understanding of physical and social world. Building wholesome attitudes toward self. Learning appropriate masculine or feminine social role. Developing conscience, morality, a scale of values. Learning to read, write, calculate, other intellectual skills. Learning physical skills. Learning to win and maintain place among age-mates. Learning to give and take and to share responsibility.

3. Adolescence
   12–18 Years

   Developing clear sense of identity and self-confidence. Adjusting to body changes. Developing new, more mature relations with age-mates. Achieving emotional independence from parents. Selecting and preparing for an occupation. Achieving mature values and social responsibility. Preparing for marriage and family life. Developing concern beyond self.

4. Early Adulthood
   18–35 Years

   Seeing meaning in one's life. Getting started in an occupation. Selecting and learning to live with a mate. Starting a family and supplying children's material and psychological needs. Managing a home. Finding a congenial social group. Taking on civic responsibility.

5. Middle Age
   36–60 Years

   Achieving full civic and social responsibility. Relating oneself to one's spouse as a person. Establishing adequate financial security for remaining years. Developing adult leisure-time activities, extending interests. Helping teenage children become responsible and happy adults. Adjusting to aging parents. Adjusting to physiological changes of middle age.

TABLE 2 (continued)

---

6. Later Life | Adjusting to decreasing physical strength. Adjusting to retirement and reduced income. Adjusting to death of spouse and friends. Meeting social and civic obligations within one's ability. Establishing an explicit affiliation with age group. Maintaining interests, concern beyond self.

Tasks at All Periods | Developing and using one's capacities. Accepting oneself and developing basic self-confidence. Accepting reality and building valid attitudes and values. Participating creatively and responsibly in family and other groups. Building rich linkages with one's world.

SOURCE: From *Psychology and Effective Behavior* by James C. Coleman. Copyright © 1969 by Scott, Foresman and Company. Reprinted by permission.

Perception theory

Perception is regarded as a basic psychological process because without it there would be no memory, thinking, or learning. Technically, perception involves the following sequence of events. An object emits energy that stimulates a sensory organ; the sensory organ codes the energy into the language of nerve activity; and the nerve activity is conveyed to the brain, where its processing results in perception of the object. In this context, *attention* denotes conscious focus on the object that stimulates the sensory organ; *perception* denotes how things look, sound, feel, taste, or smell.[14]

From the viewpoint of health education, perceiving is the process by which people select, organize, and give meaning to the internal and external stimuli affecting them. Selective perception, which determines which messages people will accept or reject,[15] is especially important here insofar as the educational process cannot even be initiated unless the message has been perceived in the first place.

Not only do people tend to screen out or reject information that makes them uncomfortable or that lacks personal meaning for them, but messages that are received may become distorted because people see what they want to see, perceiving only those elements that coincide with their needs, interests, or expectations. Health educators can therefore benefit from pretesting their messages and modifying them if need be, so that what is transmitted in an educational program has the best chance of being selectively perceived.

Motivation theory

Motivation becomes important after the perceptual process has had a chance to function, for motivation is a further process of utilizing any means that will have the effect of stimulating action. Motives take the form of drives and incentives which initiate behavior aimed at fulfilling basic human needs.

Drives   Drives are divided into two classes: primary and learned.[16] The source of a primary drive is an inborn organic disturbance, such as hunger, thirst, drowsiness, cold, or lack of oxygen; its motive is to reduce or eliminate the disturbance by eating, drinking, obtaining warmth, or breathing. While there is general agreement among scholars about the nature and source of primary drives, the nature and sources of learned drives, such as achievement and approval, form a complex and controversial area of study. Differences of opinion are reflected in the following hypotheses.

• All drives—a hunger for power as well as a hunger for food—are innate and originate in bodily tensions, the individual merely learning the best ways of satisfying them. Having learned ways of satisfying them, the individual becomes conditioned to continuing the reinforced behaviors because of their external rewards. When these rewards cease, basic needs are met in other, more rewarding ways.

• Learned drives are not drives at all but are behaviors that displace the customary means of satisfying a primary drive—as sexual tension, for example, is often displaced into such nonsexual activities as sports, work, or the exercise of political power. Although originating as displaced behaviors, learned drives become functionally autonomous through repetition and reinforcement. Thus, an individual may begin to smoke because of a desire to conform to social norms but continues the habit because it becomes satisfying in its own right.

• All behaviors—whether smoking, drinking, or power seeking—are motivated by anxiety, and the behaviors are merely instrumental ways of reducing it.

Incentives   Incentives, or external motivators, also take two forms. Those that help a person to satisfy needs and realize potentials are termed *facilitative;* those that attempt to impose behaviors alien to a person's needs or potentials are termed *coercive.* Beyond this distinction, however, there is little clarity or agreement about the nature or use of incentives. What may be facilitative for one person may be coercive for another; while, even for the same person, what might be facilitative at one point might be coercive at another point.

In studying family-planning programs, in which individuals are encouraged to plan for spacing and limiting the size of their families, M. Minkler has made some interesting observations about the use of incentives, such as monetary or other rewards, in inducing a favorable attitude change toward birth control. (1) Where a client perceives himself to have a free hand in decision making about a given family-planning behavior, lower incentives tend to be more effective in producing attitude change. (2) Where a client perceives himself to have no choice in deciding matters of family planning, higher incentives produce a greater amount of attitude change.[17] For health educators, the important aspect of these observations is that programs should utilize a variety of methods to meet individual needs.

Psychological needs The term *drives* refers to the source of motivation; the term *needs* refers to the goal of behavior (e.g., hunger is a drive, food is a need). Although psychological needs are vitally important in relation to health, it is difficult to state with certainty just what these needs are. Empirical studies undertaken to determine psychological health would have first to deprive people of their needs and then assess the results, experiments which for ethical reasons are clearly not easy to carry out.

Still, some psychologists have attempted to identify and describe psychological needs. Erich Fromm has identified five basic needs that he regards as inborn, objective, and uniquely human:

1. the need for *relatedness:* to create satisfying relationships based on mutual caring, respect, sympathetic understanding, and responsibility in place of the animal's instinctive ties with nature;
2. the need for *transcendance:* to become a creative person rather than a creature of instinct;
3. the need for *rootedness:* to belong, to be in close relationships with others;
4. the need for *identity:* to be unique through personal creative efforts or to be identified with others who are unique and creative;
5. the need for a *frame of orientation,* or a stable and dependable way of perceiving and apprehending the world.[18]

Humanistic psychology isolated self-actualization as a basic human need, a concept that was first championed by K. Goldstein[19] although Abraham Maslow is perhaps its best-known proponent. Maslow begins by identifying two kinds of needs: (1) basic needs, such as those arising from hunger, thirst, or sexual tension, and (2) metaneeds for such abstract qualities as goodness, beauty, justice, order, and unity. Although basic needs take precedence, metaneeds must also be met before a person can feel fulfilled.[20]

FIGURE 1
Maslow's Hierarchy of Needs

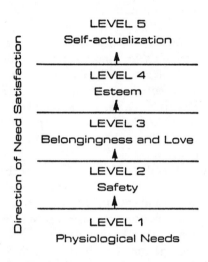

SOURCE: Adapted from Robert E. Schell and Elizabeth Hall, *Developmental Psychology Today*, 3d ed. (New York: Random House, 1979), p. 41.

Maslow's theory of self-actualization is based on the hierarchical relationship of five basic needs: physiological, safety, identity, esteem, and self-actualization (see figure 1).

Usually the starting point for motivational theory, physiological needs include such life sustainers as food, water, oxygen, activity, and sleep; physiologically motivated behavior is most highly observable in infants. Safety needs, which emerge after basic physiological needs have been met, include protection from physical harm and the alleviation of threat; safety-motivated behavior is commonly observed in children. Identity needs, which surface when physiological and safety needs have been fairly well gratified, include giving and receiving affection, a sense of belonging, a desire for identity, and the recognition accorded by membership in social groups—love-motivated needs generally associated with adolescents and teenagers.

When a desire for self-confidence, self-respect, and a sense of self-worth becomes dominant, esteem needs emerge, and these are usually associated with young adults, who strive for higher status and more material gains.

Finally, self-actualization needs reflect a desire for full development of one's capacities and potentialities—a desire to become all that one is capable of becoming—and this desire is associated with the individual's maturation (a major point in Beatty's self-concept theory).

Three additional theories of motivation should be noted here. The maintenance theory holds that living systems endeavor to maintain their physiological and psychological variables within a range essential for survival;[21] that is, a certain level of sensory input is essential for human survival, and an individual strives to increase it when it falls below the needed level.

The dissonance theory, whose major proponent is L. Festinger,[22] holds that the process of choosing between conflicting information produces psychological dissonance, which the chooser is impelled to reduce because of the discomfort it creates. (This will be discussed in greater detail in connection with attitude-change theory).

The emotion theory asserts that all emotions except the depressive ones are states of psychophysiological arousal, agitation, and excitement produced by a variety of internal and external stimuli. Insofar as they stimulate as well as direct behavior, emotions are also motives, unless they are so intense that they disrupt meaningful behavior.[23]

Clearly, health education has much to learn from these various theories of motivation. Knowledge of basic drives and motives, for example, is essential in working with those who have special needs, such as alcoholics, drug users, and overeaters, the poor and unemployed, the adolescent and aged. Here, maintenance theory can be used to support and reinforce desirable behaviors. At the same time, dissonance theory can alert the educator to the dangers of overloading the system by presenting information (smoking is harmful) that so contradicts the client's present apprehension (smoking is enjoyable) as to invite the possibility of message rejection.

If wisely used, emotion theory is also important in health education; for if fear, anxiety, and stress can be easily used to gain patient compliance with a prescribed treatment, the same emotions can contribute significantly toward preventable diseases and death. H. Selye has shown that asthma, various heart conditions, ulcers, and migraine headaches are among a number of stress-related disorders suffered by people, called the "worried well," in whom no organic disease can be found and who therefore use costly health services needlessly.[24] Further, fear-arousal techniques to gain patient compliance have been shown to have only limited success. Some individuals respond to them only if they can take action immediately, otherwise repressing their fears and either delaying action or taking no action toward preventive health behavior.[25]

Behavioral science trainers and health educators still use Maslow's five-level hierarchy as a theoretical base for discussing motivation and self-actualization, for Maslow's theory of self-actualization and Beatty's self-concept theory are both fundamental to the applied health-education concept of wellness. Although a variety of methods are required if health-education programs are to meet the needs of individuals at all stages of their development, educators can assume that the more the patient or consumer experiences self-actualization, the likelier he is to pursue positive health behaviors. Unlike the disease-orientation process which encourages the practicing of healthful behaviors in order to prevent disease, self-actualization encourages healthful behaviors by enabling people to utilize their own capacities more fully.

Learning theory

Simply defined, learning is a process of gaining knowledge, comprehension, or skill through experience or study. It can be a rudimentary process of conditioning in which a stimulus evokes a response until the response becomes automatic, or it can be a complex process involving reasoning, imagining, abstracting, and problem solving. Because health education must concern itself with the latter process in developing individualized learning experiences for patients or consumers, this section will present some of the principles of, and conditions for, learning while reviewing several learning theories and applications.

Learning process According to J. C. Coleman, the complex learning process must take four factors into account: the learner, the task, the procedure, and the learning situation.[26]

Beyond question, the subject's willingness to learn, the efficiency of the learning process, and the extent of the learning that takes place will all be greatly influenced by what the learner brings to the learning situation. For learning will be limited or expanded by: (1) the subject's previous learning or resources; (2) the subject's basic motivations for learning, which include the tendency to apprehend what relates directly to purpose and to feel rewarded by a sense of satisfaction in learning; (3) the subject's frame of reference, which will determine what is perceived and learned; and (4) the subject's personal maturity and adjustment, which will affect such factors as patience, concentration, and objectivity.

The type of task to be learned, its size, complexity, and clarity, and the conditions and procedures under which learning is to take place—in short, the learning situation itself—must also be factored into the equation. Both method of approach and ease of learning will be influenced by the type of task to be undertaken; whereas a verbal skill may be mastered in one session, for example, acquiring a motor skill may require practice over a longer period of time. Obviously, too, learning will be easier when the body of material to be learned is small and simple, when the learner is at least somewhat familiar with its content, and when the learning task is clearly defined. Finally, learning will be facilitated by establishing a fixed time and place for it and by using the best resources and facilities available.

To effect desirable individual changes among participants, health educators must carefully plan, organize, and administer the learning experience, building a background and motivational climate to guide and extend it and helping to transfer learnings to enrich life experiences. Throughout the process, feedback is important in providing swift access to a knowledge of ongoing results. By monitoring progress, feedback can serve as an index to reward or punishment, thereby aiding the reinforcement and transfer of positive learnings.

Experiential learning theory   D. S. Kolb views learning as a four-stage cycle that includes concrete experience, observation and reflection, formation of abstract concepts and generalizations, and testing the implication of concepts in new situations.

In the first stage, learners are actively involved in exploring, testing, and accommodating themselves to the learning problem. In the second stage, they endeavor to maintain this involvement but become reflective observers as well, examining the problem from every perspective and in every detail in order to apprehend its wholeness, in this way attaining an image that can be reduced to its component parts. In the third stage they employ inductive reasoning to analyze the problem and reformulate it as a personally meaningful theory or concept. In the fourth stage they employ deductive reasoning to test the theory or concept, thereby developing a notion of what actions should be taken to resolve the problem. They then return to the first stage, this time with a specific hypothesis to be tested in a new experience.

Close observation reveals that the learning process is here depicted as a resolution of dynamic tensions between concrete experience (involvement) and abstract conceptualization (detachment) along one pole and between active experimentation (actor) and reflective observation (observer) along the other. Because these bipolar tensions are not stable, people do not develop ideally at all four stages but develop individualized learning styles that are strong in some areas and weak in others.

These individualized styles can be characterized as *divergers, convergers, assimilators,* and *accommodators.* Divergers are concrete and reflective and learn through inductive reasoning. Convergers are active and abstract and learn through deductive reasoning. Assimilators are reflective and abstract and learn inductively. Accommodators are concrete and active and learn enactively.

In Kolb's view, then, learning is a continuous process; learning situations will be determined by the individual's particular learning style; and an environment is responsive to learners if it (1) permits them to explore freely and provides an opportunity to discover a problem; (2) gives them immediate information about the consequences of their actions; (3) is self-pacing, i.e., if it allows events to occur at a rate largely determined by the learners; (4) permits them to make full use of their capacity for discovering various kinds of relations; and (5) is structured so that they are likely to make interconnected discoveries about the physical, cultural, and social worlds. For health educators, the experiential learning model is exceptionally useful in developing individualized learning experiences.[26a]

Cognitive, affective, and action domains The authors of *Taxonomy of Educational Objectives* have formulated a hierarchical classification system showing that an individual's level of learning rises as learning activities successively occur in the cognitive, affective, and action domains of the learning process.[27] The cognitive domain relates to the learner's ability to deal with knowledge or information on an intellectual basis; the affective domain involves ways of handling emotions; the action domain embraces actions that relate specifically to health behavior.

The cognitive domain is arranged into six processes, which, ranging from the simplest to the most complex, include knowledge, comprehension, application, analysis, synthesis, and evaluation. Knowledge denotes the recollection of factual information. Comprehension emphasizes understanding the message being communicated. Application means putting the message to use. Analysis involves reducing the message to its component parts and examining their meaning in relation to the whole. Synthesis involves integrating the parts into a pattern, while evaluation requires making judgments on the basis of standards or other criteria to measure the message's overall effectiveness.

Centering on values, attitudes, interests, feelings, and emotions, the affective domain also ranges from simple to complicated processes: receiving, responding, valuing, organization, and value complex. Receiving denotes the ability to recognize the presence of stimuli in the environment. Responding means reacting to the stimuli, whether in affirmative, negative, or neutral ways. Valuing involves degree of acceptance of the stimuli. Organization pertains to the individual's process of judging the situation and establishing a system of dominant values. Value complex denotes the establishment of consistent behavior within this system of dominant values. Finally, the action domain embraces all health behavior, including neuromuscular motor skill, or acts that require neuromuscular coordination.

An example of dieting will help to illustrate the three domains of the learning process. In the cognitive domain, individuals who want to lose weight must first know which foods will contribute to that goal, understand why these foods are helpful, have access to such foods, and be able to determine by analysis which portions of the diet are best suited to their particular needs. They must then establish a pattern of diet maintenance and periodic weighing to check whether weight is in fact being lost. In the affective and action domains, individuals may recognize that there are societal rewards for slenderness and respond affirmatively to these rewards. Accepting the values that attach to giving rewards for weight loss, they will eventually develop a value system of their own which involves engaging in actions that will lead them to an overall healthier condition.

Attitude-change theory

Studies of communications aimed at producing attitude change have given thought to three variables: the validity of the source of the communication, the nature of the communication itself, and the characteristics of the audience to whom the communication is directed. With regard to the first variable, it has been found that the greater the prestige and credibility of the source of a communication, the greater will be the change in attitude.[28] (Consideration must also be given, however, to the so-called sleeper effect, or delayed attitude change, a phenomenon that may occur because the message receiver detaches the communication from its source over the course of time, recalling the former but not the latter.)

The nature of the communication itself is another significant variable insofar as its effectiveness will depend upon the kind and intensity of emotion it arouses. As suggested earlier, high fear-content messages that instruct the receiver to take some specific action tend to be more effective than those that merely provoke anxiety. To demonstrate, a 1953 study described by I. L. Janis and I. Feshback required high school students to attend dental hygiene lectures under conditions of either great fear, moderate fear, or no fear. Study results indicated that the greater the fear aroused by the message, the less likely were the students to accept it.[29]

Of equally great importance to communication effectiveness are the psychological characteristics of the audience to whom the communication is directed, for attitude-change attempts must address themselves to the individual's psychological functioning. Among other cognitive consistency theories, F. Heider's balance theory asserts that because individuals like consistency in their relationships and environment, confrontation with dissimilar messages can produce a state of conflict and psychological imbalance. To restore harmony, the individual must either alter his own attitudes or the attitudes of others or must change his environment.[30]

L. Festinger's studies on cognitive dissonance likewise demonstrate that an individual who is confronted with psychologically inconsistent ideas, attitudes, beliefs, and opinions is motivated to reduce the tension by taking action.[31] Thus, a person who enjoys smoking, but who is disturbed by the evidence linking smoking to lung cancer, will attempt to reduce the unpleasant tension produced by this opposition either by ceasing to smoke or by ignoring the research and evidence, claiming that the pleasure of smoking outweighs its risks.

Attribution theories deal with attitudes and traits that are attributed to oneself or others when judgments are based on limited information. By way of demonstration, M. D. Storms and R. E. Nisbett administered a placebo pill to two groups of people suffering from insomnia. One group was told that the pill's calming effect would enable them to fall asleep readily; to the other group the pill was described as an excitant that would delay but not prevent sleep. Unable to sleep, members of the first group attributed their wakefulness to internal factors and concluded that they had serious cases of insomnia. Members of the second group, though likewise wakeful, attributed their temporary sleeplessness to an external factor—the pill—and were able to fall asleep sooner.[32]

Thus, if they are to effect desirable attitude changes toward health behavior, health educators must recognize that the prestige and credibility of a communication source can affect a message's acceptance, that a message's persuasiveness will depend upon its content and emotional appeal, that high fear-content messages may only provoke anxiety and rejection of the message, and that the completeness or incompleteness of information can affect attitudes as well. In this connection, it has also been shown that those who hold moderate attitudes are more susceptible to change than are those who hold extremist attitudes.[33] Further, because attitudes are influenced by the groups to which people belong, individual attitudes can sometimes be changed either by changing group norms or by influencing the individual to join a different group.[34]

Problem-solving and creativity theory

D. Krech and his associates group problem situations into three structural categories: explanation, prediction, and intervention.[35] Explanation involves a fairly well structured stimulus situation in which most of the necessary information is present for understanding why a specific event has occurred. Prediction involves a less-structured situation in which certain conditions are set forth for the purpose of anticipating an event that has not yet occurred. Still less structured, invention involves creating a novel set of conditions that will bring about a specified event. To some degree, all these situations involve perceptual processes, here viewing perception as a form of guided or controlled thinking to achieve realistic adaptation to an external challenge.

In explanation situations, in which the stimulus patterns are usually well structured, the problem-solving approach tends to be highly perceptual. In prediction situations, the fact that stimulus structures exist but are fewer, weaker, and less defined can work either for or against perceptual problem solving; i.e., whereas the less clearly defined structures make it easier for the individual to break away from unworkable approaches, the presence of relatively strong structures still provides some accurate information on which to base workable solutions. Invention situations, in which perceptual processes have less play, make greater demands on the individual's past learning and experience.

Problem-solving approaches can be generally characterized in terms of trial-and-error, gradual analysis, and insight processes. Trial and error is a haphazard process in which approaches are so tentative, unrelated, and confused that the individual may neither recognize that a solution has been found nor know how to duplicate it in the future. Gradual analysis is a process of making rational, systematic, step-by-step progress, carefully checking each step before moving to the next. Insight is the sudden perceptual awareness of having discovered a solution. Though insight may occur after a period of trial and error or of gradual analysis, in this case the solution is recognized and understood and offers direct transfer to other, similar problems.

How a problem is approached may determine whether a solution will be found at all, as well as what sort of solution it is likely to be. Often, however, people are greatly impeded in their approaches by the following common difficulties:

1. Inability to define a problem clearly enough to work on it effectively
2. Adopting mistaken attitudes and assumptions that limit information and tend to be self-perpetuating
3. Oversimplifying by either overlooking or ignoring key elements
4. Accommodating a rigid mental set by failing to look at a problem in other than one highly particularized way
5. Adopting a defensive orientation in which the desire to prove one's point, rationalize errors, or protect one's feelings obstructs a clear view of the problem
6. Allowing emotion or stress to distort rational thought processes.

Although problem solving is an ordinary part of everyday life, while creativity focuses on producing new concepts, understandings, and methods, both require a search for uncommon responses. According to D. W. MacKinnon, creativity must fulfill three conditions. First, it must involve an idea that is novel or at least infrequent. Second, it must fit a situation, solve a problem, or accomplish some recognizable goal. Third, it must sustain the original insight, or an elaboration or evaluation of it, to the fullest extent.[36]

Further, J. P. Guilford has identified three kinds of thinking—deductive, inductive, and evaluative—as being creative.[37] By means of deductive thinking, which is based on information already at hand, the individual is able to discern previously unnoticed relationships among units of information. Inductive thinking requires adding new elements or hypotheses to existing information and imagining the possible consequences of alternative solutions. Evaluative thinking requires judging an idea's appropriateness and making any necessary revisions before it is shaped into final usable form.

In health education, perceptual awareness and insight are very important factors in problem solving, and there can be no question that people are likelier to change their behaviors when they are personally involved in the problem-solving process. Because individuals learn in different ways, however, health educators must design programs and methods that accommodate these differences. A method such as group discussion, for example, may help to reduce individuals' defensiveness about smoking or overweight so that they can deal more effectively with their emotions and move toward more positive health practices.

Although problem-solving competence depends above all on the individual's personal maturity, there are several means by which health education can assist the process. These include devising a basic problem-solving strategy or theory that the individual will find useful in approaching problems; employing logic based on sound assumptions and on words that accurately convey what is meant; obtaining help from others, such as health educators or counselors, who can facilitate the problem-solving process; and encouraging group problem solving on the assumption that several people working on a problem together will be more successful than one individual working alone.

Group dynamics theory

Because so much of health-education practice takes place in group settings, group dynamics probably holds more meaning for the field than any other body of theory presented in this chapter. Group dynamics is the study of the nature and development of groups, of the interrelationships of group members, and of the relationships of groups with other groups and within larger institutions as well. Although group dynamics theory relates to individual, organizational, and community change alike, it is introduced here to facilitate an understanding of discussions based upon its principles in later chapters.

One cannot but notice the current proliferation in public life of encounter groups, sensitivity groups, psychotherapy groups, drug and alcohol therapy groups, general discussion groups, task forces, and the like. Indications are that this emphasis on group work will heighten and increase in the future. Certainly, most students being prepared for health-education roles today study group dynamics. Many are trained in its general methodology as part of their formal academic preparation, or they acquire group knowledge and skills in short-term training workshops as part of their professional development. Others become familiar with basic processes simply by taking educational or leadership roles in groups.

That focus on small groups as a field of study and practice is an ever-growing preoccupation of Western behavioral science is also revealed by the increasing number of writings that deal with group phenomena. In a 1953 study, R. T. Golembiewski described as "explosive" the number of such writings published shortly after World War II.[38] In her 1971 doctoral dissertation reviewing the literature dealing with research on T-groups, H. S. Ross confirmed a continuing trend in work and publication on the topic of groups.[39]

But this bountiful growth in the field of small-group theory makes it difficult for health educators to select those orientations having the greatest meaning for practice. D. Cartwright and A. Zander, for example, have identified eight different theoretical orientations to group theory,[40] while M. E. Shaw has suggested the addition of at least one more.[41] The following pages will focus on five theories which the authors believe have particular relevance for health education: interaction theory, systems theory, psychoanalytic orientation theory, empirical/statistical orientation theory, and field theory, the last focusing particular attention on the concept of force-field analysis.

First, however, several important observations should here be recorded. (1) Because groups provide behavioral norms (expected standards) to which members commit themselves, members who deviate from these norms risk losing their membership, while behavioral-change interventions that require such deviation will encounter strong resistance. (2) Because groups can influence members' perceptions of reality (especially in ambiguous situations), as well as their attitudes and behaviors, members use their groups as a touchstone against which to evaluate external communications or attempts at influence. (3) Groups provide members with a sense of identity definition, a sense of belonging, and, for those who may be suffering fear, anxiety, or stress, a sense of safety and security as well.[42]

Interaction theory Interaction (or exchange) theory, whose major proponents are J. W. Thibaut and H. H. Kelley, is based on a consideration of three elements: activity, interaction, and sentiment.[43] Activity refers to the work or behaviors that the group undertakes, such as planning a health program or learning to cope with heart disease problems. Interaction pertains to the exchanges that occur among group members; sentiment, to the feelings members have about their working together.

Interaction theory is based on the assumption that the group exists solely for the participation and satisfaction of its members; hence group processes are analyzed in terms of the modifications or changes that individuals make in solving their interdependency problems. Clearly, members who feel that a group is satisfying their own needs while also accomplishing the group task at hand are the likelier to commit themselves enthusiastically to change, a principle that is useful to the effective functioning of health education committees and task forces.

Systems theory Systems theory differs from interaction theory insofar as analysis focuses on the linkages between inputs to the group's function, output from its efforts, and the roles that members play in their work together. In this regard, I. D. Steiner, the foremost proponent of systems theory, has identified three variables: (1) task demands, or the requirements imposed upon the group by the nature of the task to be accomplished; (2) resources, meaning the knowledge, skills, experiences, or tools that individual members make available to the group; and (3) process, or the steps and procedures by which the group carries out its task.[44]

Steiner's theory is based on a productivity model which holds that actual productivity equals potential productivity minus losses due to faulty process. This equation provides a basis for showing how individual contributions do or do not contribute to the group's productive performance; it identifies the major variables that can affect group productivity; and it suggests that group process cannot enhance group productivity unless each member's resources are fully utilized.

Health educators find systems theory useful when working with groups on issues of health concern; on issues of productivity, such as the development of plans, reports, research, and evaluation; and on other problem-solving situations that require the group's creative resources and energies to be organized and focused.

Psychoanalytic orientation theory Psychoanalytic orientation, which originated in Freudian psychology, is concerned with the individual's motivational and defensive processes within interpersonal group relationships. Proposed by W. C. Schutz in his formulation of a Fundamental Interpersonal Relations Orientation (FIRO) model, the theory identifies three characteristics that group members exhibit in their interpersonal relations: inclusion, control, and affection.[45]

Inclusion denotes the need for an individual to be accepted as a group member and to experience a sense of togetherness with the others. Control refers to people's ways of influencing or managing the behaviors of others or the decisions and actions of the group as a whole. Affection refers to the emotions, ranging from close to distant relationships, that develop and are expressed among group members. The FIRO model is especially useful when health educators are conducting experiential learning experiences with groups or are helping a board or team to function more effectively.

Empirical/statistical orientation theory Originally called group syntality theory by R. B. Cattell, who was one of its prime developers,[46] empirical/statistical orientation theory was given its present name by D. Cartwright and A. Zander as they explored the concept further in their own work.[47] In either case, the theory relies on analysis of individual behavior and on statistical procedures for achieving a better understanding of group behavior.

Cattell's theory concerns itself with the characteristic traits of individual members, with the collective personality of the group, and with how the group organizes itself to carry out its purpose, employing the term *synergy* to denote the sum of the individual energies brought to the group. Some of this energy (called *maintenance synergy*) must be used to establish and maintain cohesive harmony in group interrelationships, while the remainder (called *effective synergy*) is devoted to carrying out the group's purpose. Groups that experience a great deal of conflict and that use their synergy for maintenance purposes are likely to be ineffective in attaining their goals, a principle that is helpful to health educators who work in areas of conflict resolution.

Field theory Facilitating group change means being able to diagnose the forces at work in a given situation, and one of the most useful tools for such diagnosis is Kurt Lewin's force-field analysis, an idea originally conceptualized by Lewin in 1948 and described further in 1961.[48] Field theory—the application of force-field analysis to an understanding of group behavior—suggests that the ongoing forces within a group situation are mutually influential and accessible to systematic analysis.

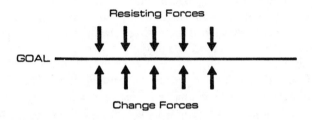

FIGURE 2
Lewin's Force-Field Concept

Resisting Forces

GOAL

Change Forces

SOURCE: This figure, like the many variations developed by other practitioners, is derived from the work of Kurt Lewin, *Field Theory in Social
Science*, eds. Darwin Cartwright (New York: Harper & Bros., 1951), pp.
188–237.

For Lewin, behavior is the result of two sets of forces working constantly
against each other either in the individual or in the interdependent situation
(see figure 2). *Change forces* produce pressure to move toward a desired goal;
resisting forces produce pressure to resist the driving forces.

When driving forces are strong and restraining forces weak, behavior
will be toward attaining the goal. When driving forces are weak and restraining forces strong, behavior toward goal attainment will be blocked.
When driving and restraining forces have equal weight, the individual or
situation becomes immobilized and no action is possible. In all three cases,
however, the *total* weight of the combined forces remains constant; it is the
shifting of weights that causes one set of forces to diminish in proportion to
the other set's gain.

When properly applied, force-field analysis can help the health educator
understand why behavior is being motivated or blocked and can also
suggest three strategies for effecting change: (1) increasing the weight of the
driving forces, (2) decreasing the weight of the restraining forces, or (3)
simultaneously increasing the former and decreasing the latter. The first
strategy would help smokers, for example, to place greater emphasis on
good reasons for not smoking; the second would help them understand why
they are resisting change and attempt to problem-solve their reasons for
resistance; the third would attempt to do both at once.

Force-field theory suggests, however, that change resulting solely from
increased driving-force pressures is likely to be only temporary because
when pressures are relaxed or dropped the individual will tend to revert to

the previous behavior. In this situation the restraining forces usually remain present in some form and, if not resolved, will tend to regain their former strength when driving pressures are lifted. On the other hand, change resulting solely from decreased restraining-force pressures has a far greater likelihood of attaining permanency because it reduces or removes resistance to change. Helping people to air their feelings and concerns and involving them in problem solving *without* increasing pressure to change enables them to understand their resistance, leading to a better chance for desirable change to occur.

More of an action-planning procedural process, Lewin's unfreezing-to-refreezing theory covers five phases of learning and change: unfreezing, problem diagnosis, goal setting, new behavior, and refreezing.[49] Individuals who are ready to consider change, such as a smoker who has decided to try quitting, are said to be undergoing an "unfreezing" of previously well established behaviors or situations. Problem diagnosis means trying to achieve a better understanding of the problem by, for example, questioning why one smokes, determining what type of smoker one is, and conducting a force-field analysis around the goal of ceasing to smoke.

Once the problem is better understood, goal setting is a critical step in planning behavioral change. When goals have been established, the individual can experiment with new behaviors, trying various alternatives and practicing those found to be most desirable. For the smoker this may mean gradually tapering off, entirely ceasing to smoke immediately, or seeking other forms of oral gratification, such as chewing gum. "Refreezing" has occurred when the new learning has become a routine part of the individual's ongoing behavior—when nonsmoking, for example, has become so habitual as to be taken for granted.

COMMENTARY

To this point, behavioral theories having particular relevance for health education have ranged from the physiological origins of personality development through the complex workings of group dynamics. As noted in the opening paragraphs of the preceding section, research has developed a vast and growing body of theory on the nature, formation, composition, size, structure, development, and effectiveness of groups, and health educators cannot but profit by familiarizing themselves with this material.

Research has shown, for example, that people join groups as one way of satisfying individual needs. If a need exists for group affiliation, if group activities are attractive and rewarding, and if the individual values the group's goals, the likelihood is great that the group will influence the individual's behavior, for group interaction has a powerful potential for inducing individual change.[50]

At the same time, however, group interaction tends to produce group norms, deviations from which can cause members either to persuade the recalcitrant person to conform or to reject him altogether.[51] There is evidence that an individual is likelier to conform to group opinion when other members are in unanimous agreement; if even one member declines to make a judgment, conformity behavior within the group diminishes.[52] In general, then, group interactions must meet both individual and group needs if full participation by members is to continue.

Like group norms, group structure and composition also reflect the needs of individuals within the group. Studies on group structure reveal that persons who have strong needs for a safe environment tend to develop hierarchical structures, while those who have strong needs for esteem tend to develop egalitarian structures.[53] Group-composition studies indicate that individuals who are affirmatively oriented toward other people enhance group morale, interaction, and cohesion, whereas unconventional, unpredictable, or anxious persons tend to inhibit effective group functioning.[54] High-cohesion groups interact better than low-cohesion groups,[55] although groups composed of persons with diverse abilities perform more effectively than those whose members have similar abilities.[56]

Factors ranging from the physical size and setting of groups to the nature of communication networks have also been shown to affect group performance. Not only does participation diminish as a group increases in size,[57] but even seating arrangements can affect communication patterns. Individuals seated across from one another interact more often than they do with people seated elsewhere. Moreover, a certain territoriality can develop in group settings, with individuals tending to choose the same seating area or chair from one meeting to the next.[58] It has been found, too, that group morale is higher in decentralized than in centralized communication networks because the former are more efficient when a group's problems are complex.[59]

Finally, studies have shown that groups proceed through distinct developmental stages, that in complex situations group problem solving tends to be more effective than individual problem solving, but that groups generally take more time to complete tasks than do individuals working alone. It has been found, in addition, that decisions made by individuals after group discussion has occurred are usually riskier than those made before the exercise of group discussion.[60]

So complex a process is behavioral change, however, that only by integrating several theories and concepts can its permutations begin to be understood. The integration of such diverse elements into a collective strategy to help produce a desired result is called a *model,* and three of these will be described briefly in the next section: the Health Belief Model, originally proposed to help explain individual health behavior; the Personal Choice Model, which arose from studies on smoking; and the Typology of Behavioral Leverage Points, developed to aid in the reduction of cardiovascular risk.

INTEGRATIVE MODELS

Health belief model

The Health Belief Model, developed in the 1950s to explain preventive health behavior, focused on the relation of health behavior to utilization of health services.[61] Greatly indebted to Kurt Lewin, who believed that the world of perceivers determined the actions of perceivers,[62] health-belief researchers included in their model a heavy component of the behaving individual's perceptual world and motivation. But they concentrated on the individual's current dynamics, believing that prior experience exercises influence only insofar as it is still represented in the individual's present state of affairs.[63]

The Health Belief Model, which has recently been revised to include general health motivation, distinguishes illness behavior and sick-role behavior from health behavior. Illness behavior is defined as any activity undertaken by persons who *feel* ill to discover what is wrong and what can be done about it. Sick-role behavior is any activity undertaken by persons who consider themselves to *be* ill for the purpose of getting well. Health behavior is any activity undertaken by persons who believe themselves to be healthy for the purpose of detecting and preventing disease in any asymptomatic stage.[64]

The model itself is interactive (i.e., each step affects the others) and is based on three primary dimensions: the individual's readiness to comply with treatment, the motivating and enabling forces that determine what the individual will do, and the compliance behaviors actually exhibited.

Readiness depends upon three sets of related variables: belief in a vulnerability to illness and estimations of the degree of threat; motives to reduce the threat with related goals for good health; and belief that compliance with recommended behaviors will reduce the threat and lead toward good health.

Modifying and enabling factors include such forces as the individual's personal characteristics, the nature and extent of the changes and costs that are likely to be involved, the nature and extent of interactions with health personnel, the feelings or attitudes attached to those interactions, and the effect on the individual of previous experience and social pressure.

These combinations of factors are believed to determine the likelihood of compliance with recommended behaviors, and the Health Belief Model has, in fact, been shown to be reliable in predicting compliance. Further research is needed, however, on which to base health-education interventions and strategies.[65]

Personal-choice behavior model

Research on smoking habits has revealed that people smoke for a variety of reasons: for pleasurable stimulation and oral gratification, to diminish feelings of anxiety and stress, because of an unawareness of physical addiction, or because psychological addiction has caused the withdrawal of cigarettes to produce a sense of deprivation or loss. Although educational programs to help people stop smoking have been developed and tested throughout the United States for at least a decade, millions of people continue to smoke, either because they have deliberately chosen not to quit or because they have been unable to break the habit.

D. Horn has termed this *personal-choice behavior,* a phenomenon that includes many more or less socially acceptable ways of either coping with or enhancing life. When personal-choice behavior is inappropriate or abusive, however, it may create problems for the individual and society alike. Horn's framework for examining these problems, called the Personal-Choice Behavior Model, identifies four stages in the movement toward individual change: initiation, establishment, maintenance, and cessation.[66]

Smoking usually begins when people are young. Its initiation may derive from curiosity, the availability of cigarettes, the likelihood of peer approval, or a desire to rebel against adult authority, although research reveals that smoking is more common among the children of smokers than of nonsmokers.

Establishment of smoking on a continuing basis may be influenced by cost-benefit balance, common perceptual stereotypes, or personal psychological factors. Cost-benefits range from expanded opportunities for social interaction to the pleasurable feelings associated with relaxation of tension. Perceptual stereotypes are influenced by the attractive models and popular personalities whom advertisers employ to boost cigarette sales. Psychological factors include the individual's internal conflict over whether to conform to the demands of authority figures or to maintain personal control over one's own destiny.

Smoking maintenance is usually the result of a habit or dependency. A habit is a tendency to repeat a behavior without thinking about it; dependence denotes an increasing desire or need for the effects produced by the behavior. Whether cessation occurs will depend upon such factors as a perception of the psychological uselessness of smoking, of the dangers of continued smoking, or of the environmental forces that support efforts toward change.

From the Personal-Choice Behavior Model health educators can infer the following steps for inducing individual change toward nonsmoking: (1) promoting positive attitudes toward nonsmoking among youth, giving special attention to peer-group norms and to parents who are modeling role behavior for their children; (2) forming discussion groups that can help the individual cope with decisional conflicts about smoking; (3) employing behavioral modification techniques to break dependency patterns; and (4) helping the smoker to perceive the threat to his health, to feel capable of behavioral change, and to regard such change as contributing to personal mastery of his own behavior and destiny.

Typology of behavioral leverage points

To help reduce the high incidence of preventable or modifiable cardiovascular disease and death, medical practitioners have been encouraged to make more extensive use of behavioral science knowledge. To this end, D. Stokols has developed for application purposes a model characterizing the types of interventions that are most relevant for reducing cardiovascular risk (see table 3).

Interventions are categorized on the basis of two dimensions. (1) Intervals of social influence (shown horizontally) consist of three major periods: the early socialization period (presumably childhood or young adulthood), the adult precoronary period (before the onset of illness), and the adult postcoronary period (after the onset of illness). (2) Levels of intervention (shown vertically) are twofold: micro (at the level of interpersonal or family relationships) and macro (at the social/community level).

At the early socialization microlevel, the health-education intervention is aimed primarily at parents who are models of aggression, impatience, and overarduous habits, who practice poor health behaviors, and who impart patterns of delayed gratification and self-reward. At the corresponding macrolevel, the intervention is aimed at television and other media that promote violence, intense competitiveness, overambition, and other habits destructive to health. The intervention is likewise aimed at schools, which influence behavioral patterns by means of peer-supported influences and structural constraints. A strategy aimed at producing a structural constraint might influence the school board to forbid the installation of cigarette or junk-food machines in schools.

Adult precoronary socialization is essentially diagnostic in character and occurs at the microlevel primarily through the doctor-patient relationship;

TABLE 3
Typology of Behavioral Leverage Points for the
Reduction of Cardiovascular Risk

Intervals of Social Influence

	Early Socialization	*Adult Precoronary Disease*	*Adult Postcoronary Disease*
Micro	*Family, Peer Interactions*	*Doctor-Patient Relationship (diagnostic)*	*Doctor-Patient Relationship (therapeutic)*
	modeling of coronary-prone behavior delay of gratification vicarious learning of self-reward patterns verbal-behavioral discrepancies of the model	activation of attentional mechanisms use of I-E Scale in prediction of noncompliance personal characteristics of the physician covert sensitization psychological reactance	overattentiveness to risk with onset of symptomatology covert desensitization participant modeling multiple modeling
Macro	*Media, Educational Systems*	*Community Health-Screening Programs*	*Rehabilitative Programs*
	media modeling of coronary-prone behavior health-supportive potential of T.V.; dissemination of risk-factor information personal causation training in school settings	informational appeals perceived vulnerability specificity of recommendations media modeling	establishment of reference group; social comparison processes vicarious reinforcement situational modification of expectancies for success

Levels of Behavior Intervention

SOURCE: D. Stokols, "The Reduction of Cardiovascular Risk: An Application of Social Learning Perspectives," in *Applying Behavioral Science to Cardiovascular Risk*, ed. A. J. Enelow and J. B. Henderson (New York: American Heart Association, 1975), p. 137.

61

at the macrolevel, primarily through community health-screening programs. Adult postcoronary socialization, which is characteristically therapeutic, occurs at the microlevel through the physician-family interaction. At the macrolevel, primary influences are organizations offering postcoronary counseling and rehabilitation services.

The use of this model for developing health-education programs in schools, churches, and youth organizations, as well as with physicians and community leaders, is self-evident. Stokols believes, however, that before the future of some social-learning hypotheses can be firmly established, long-term field-experimental investigations must be conducted in health settings.[67]

COMMENTARY

Out of all these various concepts and theories emerge the following principles and conditions[68] which must be taken into consideration by every health educator who is working to produce individual learning and change.

• *Individuals are themselves their own richest resource for learning.* All human beings are repositories of personal ideas, feelings, attitudes, and experiences which together comprise a rich vein of resources for problem solving and learning. Learning is maximized when their thoughts and feelings are in harmony, when the concepts they are taught are relevant to their personal needs and problems, and when they are themselves directly involved in the learning process. People become more responsible as they actually assume responsibilities and become more independent as they actually experience success.

• *Learning is also a collaborative, cooperative, evolutionary process.* As individuals are exposed to the alternative behavioral models employed by others, they are better able to modify and refine their personal styles toward greater effectiveness. To achieve this, learning situations must promote free and open intercommunication and shared evaluation.

• *Because behavioral change often causes people to relinquish old and comfortable ways of thinking, believing, and valuing, health educators must create conditions that foster new learning and effective change.* Again, this means encouraging individuals to become voluntarily involved in planning their own programs for change—determining program content, deciding which issues are to be explored, and formulating criteria to measure their own progress. It means making individuals aware of their own unique contributions to the learning process while at the same time making programs flexible enough to allow time for an exploration of alternative solutions.

Finally, because group interactions inevitably produce some degree of confrontation and challenge, the search for alternative solutions will be greatly facilitated if it is conducted in a nonthreatening ambiance and accompanied by self-openness rather than self-concealment, by mutual respect and trust, by acceptance of different ideas, and by recognition that error is a natural and even helpful part of the learning process. In the field of health education, many such programs are being conducted today, and some of the more characteristic of these will form the subject of chapter 4.

REFERENCES

1. G. W. Allport, *Personality*, p. 28.
2. J. C. Coleman, *Psychology and Effective Behavior*, pp. 41–43.
3. Ibid., pp. 52–60.
4. W. Beatty, "Emotions: The Missing Link in Education" (Paper presented at Conference on Issues in Human Development: Present and Future, at Institute for Child Study, University of Maryland, 20 April 1968).
5. Coleman, *Psychology and Effective Behavior*, pp. 22–23.
6. G. W. Allport, *Becoming*, pp. 99–101.
7. C. R. Rogers, *On Becoming a Person*.
8. Beatty, "Emotions," pp. 4–5.
9. Coleman, *Psychology and Effective Behavior*, pp. 22–24.
10. B. F. Skinner, *Science and Human Behavior*, pp. 45–283.
11. A. Bandura, "Influence of Models' Reinforcement Contingencies on the Acquisition of Initiative Responses," *Journal of Personality and Social Psychology* 1 (1965): 589–95.
12. E. Erikson, *Childhood and Society*, pp. 247–74.
13. R. Havighurst, *Developmental Tasks and Education*, pp. 1–98.
14. G. Lindzey, C. S. Hall, and R. F. Thompson, *Psychology*, pp. 90–135.
15. A. L. Knutson, *The Individual, Society, and Health Behavior*, pp. 159–79.
16. Lindzey, Hall, and Thompson, *Psychology*, pp. 342–64.
17. M. Minkler, "The Uses of Incentives in Family Planning Programmes; A Study of Competing Theories Regarding Their Influence on Attitude Change," *International Journal of Health Education* 19 (supp.), no. 3 (July-September 1976): 1–11.
18. E. Fromm, *The Sane Society*, pp. 30–63.
19. K. Goldstein, *The Organism*.
20. A. H. Maslow, *Toward a Psychology of Being*, pp. 177–200.
21. R. Dubois, *Man Adapting*.
22. L. Festinger, *A Theory of Cognitive Dissonance*.
23. Lindzey, Hall, and Thompson, *Psychology*, pp. 367–89.
24. S. R. Garfield, "The New Medical Care Delivery System," *Scientific American*, April 1970, pp. 15–23.
25. S. Radelfinger, "Some Effects of Fear-arousing Communications on Preventive

Health Behavior," *Health Education Monographs*, no. 19 (1965), pp. 2–15; B. J. Roberts, "A Framework for Consideration of Forces in Achieving Earliness of Treatment," *Health Education Monographs*, no. 19 (1965), pp. 16–32; and I. L. Janis and I. Feshback, "Effects of Fear-arousing Communications," *Journal of Abnormal and Social Psychology* 48 (1953): 78–92.

26. Coleman, *Psychology and Effective Behavior*, pp. 378–96.

26a. Kolb, D. A., and Fry, R., "Toward an Applied Theory of Experiential Learning," in *Theories of Group Process*, ed. by C. L. Cooper (New York: John Wiley and Sons, 1975).

27. B. S. Bloom, ed., *Taxonomy of Educational Objectives. Handbook 1: Cognitive Domain*; and D. K. Krathwahl, B. S. Bloom, and B. B. Masia, *Taxonomy of Educational Objectives. Handbook 2: Affective Domain*.

28. C. I. Hovland and W. Weiss, "The Influence of Source Credibility on Communication Effectiveness," *Public Opinion Quarterly* 15 (1951): 635–50.

29. Janis and Feshback, "Fear-arousing Communications," pp. 78–92.

30. F. Heider, "Social Perception and Phenomenal Causality," *Psychological Review* 51 (1944): 358–74.

31. Festinger, *Theory of Cognitive Dissonance*, pp. 1–31.

32. M. D. Storms and R. E. Nisbett, "Insomnia and the Attribution Process," *Journal of Personality and Social Psychology* 16 (1970): 319–28.

33. T. H. Tannenbaum, "Initial Attitude toward Source and Concepts as Factors in Attitude-Change through Communication," *Public Opinion Quarterly* 20 (1965): 413–25.

34. K. Lewin, "Group Decision and Social Change," in *Readings in Social Psychology*, ed. G. Swansom, T. M. Newcomb, and Z. L. Harlety, pp. 197–211.

35. D. Krech, R. S. Crutchfield, and N. Levson, *Elements of Psychology*, pp. 252–60.

36. D. W. MacKinnon, "Assessing Creative Persons," *Journal of Creative Behavior* 1, no. 3 (1967): 291–304.

37. J. P. Guilford, *The Analysis of Intelligence*, pp. 61–122.

38. R. T. Golembiewski, *The Small Group*, pp. 17–33.

39. H. S. Ross, "Changes Effected in Cross-Cultural T-Groups," (Doctoral diss., University of California at Berkeley, 1971).

40. D. Cartwright and A. Zander, eds., *Group Dynamics*, pp. 26–27.

41. M. E. Shaw, *Group Dynamics*, pp. 16–17.

42. S. K. Simonds, "Emerging Challenges in Health Education," *International Journal of Health Education* 19 (supp.), no. 4 (October-December 1976): 9.

43. J. W. Thibaut and H. H. Kelley, *The Social Psychology of Groups*, pp. 9–168.

44. I. D. Steiner, *Group Process and Productivity*, p. 166–86.

45. W. C. Schutz, *FIRO*; and idem, *Joy*, pp. 13–33.

46. R. B. Cattell, "Concepts and Methods in the Measurement of Group Syntality," *Psychological Review* 55 (1948): 48–63.

47. Cartwright and Zander, *Group Dynamics*.

48. K. Lewin, *Resolving Social Conflicts*; and idem, "Quasi-Stationary Social Equilibria and the Problem of Permanent Change," in *The Planning of Change*, ed. W. G. Bennis, K. D. Benne, and R. Chin, pp. 235–38.

49. Lewin, "Quasi-Stationary Social Equilibria," pp. 235–38.

50. Cartwright and Zander, *Group Dynamics*, pp. 49–60; and Shaw, *Group Dynamics*, pp. 82–108.

51. S. E. Asch, *Social Psychology*, pp. 450–501.

52. Ibid.

53. Shaw, *Group Dynamics*, p. 285.

54. W. W. Haythorn, "The Composition of Groups: A Review of the Literature," *Acta Psychologica* 28 (1968): 97–128.

55. D. M. Goodacre, "The Use of a Sociometric Test as a Predictor of Combat Unit Effectiveness," *Sociometry* 14 (1951): 148–52.

56. P. R. Laughlin, L. G. Branch, and H. H. Johnson, "Individual versus Triadic Performance on a Unidimensional Complementary Task as a Function of Initial Ability Level," *Journal of Personality and Social Psychology* 12 (1969): 144–50.

57. F. Frank and L. R. Anderson, "Effects of Task and Group Size upon Group Productivity and Member Satisfaction," *Sociometry* 34 (1971): 135–94.

58. R. Sommer, *Personal Space*, pp. 3–58; and F. L. Strodtbeck and L. H. Hook, "The Social Dimensions of a Twelve-Man Jury Table," *Sociometry* 24 (1961): 397–415.

59. Strodtbeck and Hook, "Twelve-Man Jury Table," pp. 412–14.

60. Shaw, *Group Dynamics*, pp. 97–109.

61. I. M. Rosenstock, "Historical Origins of the Health Relief Model," *Health Education Monographs* 2, no. 4 (Winter 1974): 328–35.

62. Lewin, "Group Decision and Social Change," pp. 197–211.

63. Rosenstock, "Health Belief Model," pp. 354–84.

64. M. H. Becker, ed., "The Health Belief Model and Personal Health Behavior," *Health Education Monographs* 2, no. 4 (Winter 1974): 409–19.

65. U.S., Department of Health, Education and Welfare, *Proceedings of the National Heart and Lung Institute Working Conference on Health Behavior*, HEW Publication no. (NIH) 76–868, 12–15 May 1975, pp. 41–46.

66. D. Horn, "A Model for the Study of Personal-Choice Health Behavior," *International Journal of Health Education* 19, no. 2 (1976): 89–98.

67. D. Stokols, "The Reduction of Cardiovascular Risk: An Application of Social Learning Perspective," in *Applying Behavioral Science to Cardiovascular Risk*, ed. A. J. Enelow and J. B. Henderson, pp. 133–46.

68. Adapted from G. Pine and P. Horne, "Principles and Conditions for Learning in Adult Education," *Adult Leadership* 18, no. 4 (October 1969): 108–34.

4

Programs for individual change

Health education attempts to integrate diverse theories into rational activities or programs for the purpose of encouraging healthful public behavior. The programs described in this chapter are all examples of theory in action, though not every theory introduced in chapter 3 will be directly reflected here: some will be specifically identified, while others will be implicit in the programs presented.

Before describing these programs, however, the term *program* itself should be defined. One useful definition has been developed by the United Way of America in surveying the criteria used by local United Way organizations in defining their programs. According to this definition, a service is a program when:

1. it is a structured part of the organization's operation, such as a special department with a regularly assigned staff or an organized set of policies and procedures related to an identifiable program
2. it serves one of the organization's primary rather than subsidiary or ancillary objectives
3. it is consistent with the organization's purposes as stated in its articles of incorporation or bylaws or based on formal board action

4. it is a standard recognized structure having a comparable form in other, similar organizations
5. it involves more than a nominal amount of support, revenue, and expenditure
6. it lends itself to program-service accounting and budgeting, to service measurement, and to priority ranking and review.[1]

These criteria characterize health-education programs for inpatient, outpatient, and self-help groups alike. As illustrated by table 4, patient education fostering individual behavioral change is a program priority for both the Federal Bureau of Health Education[2] and the National Center for Health Education.[3] Self-help programs emphasizing preventive health behavior must utilize the resources of health education in addressing their needs as well.

TABLE 4
Overview of Program Priorities for the Federal Bureau
of Health Education and the National Center
for Health Education

	Bureau of Health Education	National Center for Health Education
Individual Behavior	(1) Patient education in health and mental-care institutions	(3) Patient education
Organizational Behavior	(2) School health education (3) Occupational health education	(1) Health education in the work place
Social Behavior	(4) Community health education (5) National health and health-related agency programs (6) Mass media and health education	(2) P.L. 93–641: Health Planning and Health Resources Development
General	(7) Standards for health education and promotion	

INPATIENT PROGRAMS

Inpatient (i.e., in-hospital) education programs are based on the premise that patients have a right to know the current status of their health, what they can do to achieve optimum health and prevent recurrence of illness, and what community resources are available to help them achieve these ends. In 1976 the Society for Public Health Education presented an elaboration of this premise in a position statement on patient/family education programs, in which the following points were prominent.

1. Recognizing that an informed patient is an essential member of a health-care team, comprehensive health-care delivery systems should regularly include educational programs as an integral part of high-quality care.

2. To ensure that an organized, practical, helpful approach is taken, the responsibility for patient education should be assigned, in larger settings, to a committee composed of qualified health professionals representing the several multidisciplinary departments or services required for developing sound content.

3. Whatever the setting—whether an inpatient or outpatient department, community clinic, doctor's office, or skilled nursing facility—the patient should participate in establishing relevant educational objectives.

4. Insofar as the availability of resources sets boundaries on the development of patient-education programs, patients and their families should be informed of both the system and accessibility of care, as well as of the role of both factors in aspects of treatment or prevention of illness.

5. Because determining the effectiveness of the program is of paramount importance, goals must have specific objectives expressed in terms that are measurable for purposes of evaluation. Recording the educational prescription, approved by the physician or clinic manager, as part of the patient's record is important in assessment and evaluation processes.[4]

Before going to an example of a specific in-hospital health education program, the reader should examine figure 3, which shows a patient-education planning model prepared for the Department of Health, Education and Welfare by the American Public Health Association's Committee on Educational Tasks in Chronic Illness. For this model affirms that health-education programs should take closely into account five of the principles emphasized in chapter 3 of this book: (1) that individuals will act when their needs are being met and when they are involved in decision making; (2) that people are better able to change their behaviors when they understand and accept a program's goals; (3) that people act when they can relate an educational situation to their own lives; (4) that patients should be involved in carrying out their own programs; and (5) that patients learn and can be motivated by feedback.

Program for diabetic patients

From 1973 to 1976, under three and one-half years of grants from the California Regional Medical Program, St. Mary's Hospital and Medical Center in San Francisco conducted an in-hospital health education program for diabetic patients. The only criterion for referral was that the patient be hospitalized with a primary or secondary diagnosis of diabetes. Figure 4 shows how the program was conducted.

1. An in-hospital physician referred one of his patients to the program, believing that the latter could benefit from participation in it.
2. Since the teaching was done by a staff team composed of a nurse, dietitian, pharmacist, social worker, and chaplain, each of these visited the patient to assess his educational needs in their individual areas of specialty.
3. The full team then met to pool their assessments and identify the changes that would be needed for the patient to comply with the prescribed therapeutic regimens.
4. Team members next worked individually with the patient, teaching from flexible lesson plans, reinforcing one another's emphases, and, in general, tailoring the total service to the patient's needs.
5. At the conclusion of the teaching, the team met again to evaluate the effectiveness of their activity and to decide which plans or instructions should be incorporated into follow-up care. Because the patient's physician was unable to attend this meeting, he was given a full report so that he could reinforce the team recommendations on discharging the patient.
6. Two months after discharge, a team member made a follow-up contact with the patient to determine whether the new knowledge and behavior had become integrated into his life style.

In general, the staff handled difficulties that arose very well. Communication with non-English-speaking patients was difficult, for example, and translation costs were high for informational brochures written in languages other than English. In addition, some patients could neither read nor write in any language. Understanding how important it is that patients meet their health needs in relation to their own social and environmental settings, team members demonstrated great creativity in using various audiovisual and

FIGURE 3
Patient-Education Planning Model

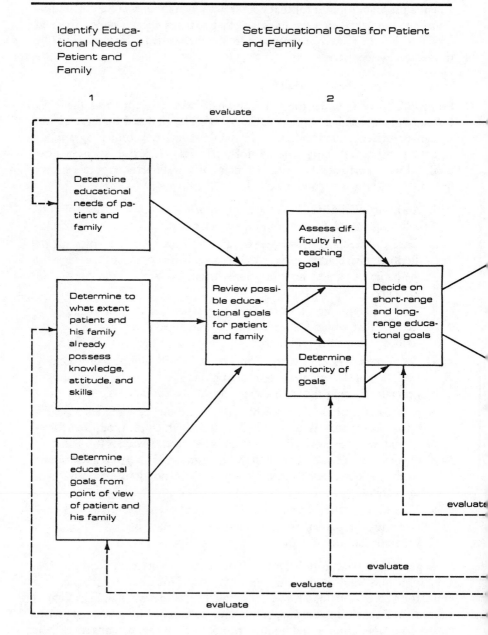

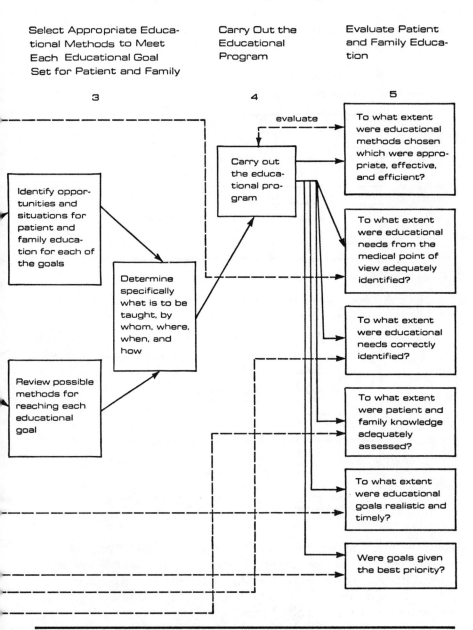

Select Appropriate Educational Methods to Meet Each Educational Goal Set for Patient and Family

3

Carry Out the Educational Program

4

Evaluate Patient and Family Education

5

Identify opportunities and situations for patient and family education for each of the goals

Determine specifically what is to be taught, by whom, where, when, and how

Review possible methods for reaching each educational goal

Carry out the educational program

evaluate

To what extent were educational methods chosen which were appropriate, effective, and efficient?

To what extent were educational needs from the medical point of view adequately identified?

To what extent were educational needs correctly identified?

To what extent were patient and family knowledge adequately assessed?

To what extent were educational goals realistic and timely?

Were goals given the best priority?

SOURCE: Adapted from U.S. Department of Health, Education and Welfare, *A Model for Planning Patient Education: An Essential Component of Health Care*, HEW Publication, no. (HRA) 76–4028, 1972.

FIGURE 4
Education Flow Chart for In-hospital Diabetic Patients

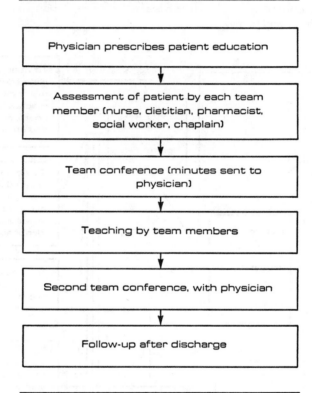

SOURCE: Adapted from E. Bernheimer and L. H. Clever, "Experiences Implementing Patient Education in an Outpatient Clinic" (Report submitted to California Regional Medical Program, St. Mary's Hospital and Medical Center, San Francisco, 1974–75).

NOTE: Bernheimer suggests dropping the second conference, which did not prove to be very effective.

nonverbal means of communicating with those who had language or literacy problems. If program results showed that such patients ultimately learned little about the nature of their disease or its treatment processes, they nevertheless did change their behaviors in ways that resulted in significant weight loss and improved blood-pressure readings.

Initially, too, the staff had expected immediate and dramatic changes in patients' health behavior. As they began better to understand the processes of motivation and behavioral change, however, and to appreciate how difficult it is for people to alter deeply rooted life styles, they became more accommodating of patients' efforts. The patients in turn liked the program, not only because it taught them how to take better care of themselves but also because of the attention it gave them. As Erich Fromm has observed, to relate to and be respected by others is a basic human need;[5] hence the importance of a support system in bringing about individual behavioral change.

Although the St. Mary's program had received its initial impetus from an influential staff physician, it was not accepted until concerns about protecting the doctor-patient relationship had been resolved. In addition, effecting role changes bothered some staff members at first, while finding enough time to devote to educational efforts remained a continuing problem for all. The program, then, was begun on a low-priority, low-acceptance basis, so that the first proceeding was to create an environment for change.

To this end, four committees were organized which included more than sixty members of the hospital staff. A Medical Advisory Committee was responsible for setting educational policy and establishing educational objectives. An Allied Health Advisory Committee developed and tested the curriculum, lesson plans, and interview forms. An Evaluation Committee considered the best ways of measuring the program's effectiveness. A Steering Committee composed of the heads of the nursing, dietary, pharmacy, and social service departments suggested issues to be considered and arranged the order of business.

Although hospital staff members carried out the educational activities, a qualified health educator acted as educational coordinator. Assisting the staff in organizing the program and developing workable procedures included sharing knowledge and experience from related programs elsewhere in the country, helping to orient the participating staff to the program, helping to solve problems as they arose, and interviewing the participating staff to help evaluate program results. On the gradual success of the St. Mary's program, E. Bernheimer notes:

In the process of developing the curriculum and system, communication improved between members of different allied health professions, and mutual respect grew. Of equal importance was the opportunity for learning that occurred. All shared in the writing of the curriculum. An important principle of involvement by those conducting the program was observed. More about diabetes was learned, and an appreciation was gained for each other's expertise, in the discussions of the revised drafts. Slowly, an atmosphere of trust developed, and this was reflected in more open discussions at committee meetings. This did not occur immediately; it took months.[6]

OUTPATIENT PROGRAMS

On a nationwide basis, outpatient (i.e., ambulatory patient) visits are currently seven times greater than inpatient visits. For the poor and aged, especially, emergency rooms and outpatient departments have become the first line of treatment. At the same time, however, many people use these services who do not really need them, posing a serious problem for the equitable delivery of such services to those who do need them. For both these reasons, the outpatient service is increasingly being viewed as a potentially useful setting for patient education.

The outpatient department

In planning an educational program for an outpatient department, five pragmatic factors must be taken into consideration: (1) the characteristics of the outpatient staff (number, type, qualifications, responsibilities); (2) the characteristics of the outpatient population (number, types, type of care needed, patients' readiness for learning); (3) the contact time of staff and patient; (4) the availability of space; and (5) the availability of audiovisual equipment. Above all, however, inpatient and outpatient programs must complement each other and exhibit continuity. The following instance will illustrate how inpatient and outpatient teachings can be mutually complementary.

A new diabetic inpatient may be so anxious about his diagnosis or so ill from hyperglycemia as to be relatively insusceptible to learning in this setting, though he must nevertheless be given sufficient inpatient education to enable him to begin managing the disease. Once he has had time to adjust psychologically and to work with diabetes management for a couple of weeks, he should be given the opportunity to pursue additional classes as an outpatient; for now that teaching can be built on concepts already practiced, he will be better prepared for, more receptive to, and readier to act upon the prescriptions of the educational process. Having completed an in-depth course on diabetes, he can receive continual updating during office visits with his physician or return visits to the outpatient clinic.

Continuity, too, can be promoted when a hospital develops a comprehensive system in which both inpatient and outpatient services are employed in fostering health education. Activities may include:

1. Using closed-circuit television to disseminate general health information to inpatients
2. Introducing individualized, disease-related inpatient education programs which provide the basic information needed for hospital discharge

3. Augmenting this basic teaching with an in-depth, disease-related out-patient education series

4. Holding monthly sessions on an outpatient basis to provide members of the community with information on health promotion, health maintenance, and general disease awareness.

Such a system assures that patients' needs are being met at all stages of the illness/health continuum. An established curriculum assures, moreover, that all health professionals and departments will know what is being taught.

Among other continuity links, patient-education flow sheets can be used in both inpatient and outpatient settings to document the patient's needs, what he was taught, and what his responses were to the teaching. Making this form available to all teaching professionals facilitates communication continuity when the patient has already received some inpatient teaching and is to have outpatient follow-up sessions. If he is rehospitalized, the in-house staff will be able to measure his educational progress on the basis of his outpatient record. In some hospitals, clinical specialists are teaching individuals on an inpatient basis and then following up on them as they attend clinic sessions or outpatient classes.

On the principle that patients are more likely to pay attention to messages that bear directly and immediately upon their personal lives—to absorb messages about diabetes when they are being tested for diabetes, for example—many outpatient departments are making extensive use of on-the-spot educational materials. This includes providing informational pamphlets in waiting-room racks, enabling waiting patients to view educational films, and developing health-education libraries or ambulatory media centers where patients can pace their own learning while making use of a wide variety of media.

Because these media alone are not often effective in changing individuals' behavior, health professionals are available to answer questions, reinforce learning, and discuss the application of new learning to everyday life. In this connection, J. M. Scanlan has described a program in which teenage volunteers were used to help educate patients in a nutrition clinic's waiting room by showing films on nutrition (as well as on nonnutrition and nonhealth), discussing nutrition and infant health with patients, inviting guest speakers to the clinic, and distributing hand-out educational materials.[7]

On the principle that people also learn by interacting, health-education departments offer a wide variety of interactive programs in the outpatient setting, including group classes, support sessions, community seminars, and health-education fairs. At a small rural hospital that does not have a well-defined outpatient department, evening group classes can be held in the hospital cafeteria. Whatever the setting, however, it is the health professional who is ultimately responsible for making health education an integral part of the patient's care, and, for this reason, planning, coordinating, and teaching roles must be clearly distinguished in advance.

The worried well

Approximately 60 percent of those currently under the care of physicians believe themselves to have physical ailments that are not borne out by medical examination.[8] These patients, known as the "worried well," are usually diagnosed as functionally ill, or psychosomatic, and they consume far too much of the time of health personnel who include treatment of their complaints as a traditional part of medical practice.[9]

While many aspects of this problem remain puzzling, two facts are clear. First, the worried well have great difficulty in dealing with their anxieties directly and therefore express them indirectly in the form of physical ills, though for the most part not consciously aware that they are doing so. In serious cases it is possible for such people to become sufficiently ill as genuinely to require medical treatment.

Second, health-care organizations and personnel are basically oriented toward finding disease and treating it. When unaware that they have a worried-well patient on their hands, they make extensive and costly efforts to determine what the physical problem might be. When aware that the patients are among the worried well, they all too frequently humor them with placebo treatments. Even when they wish to treat such patients differently, they may not know what other approaches are useful.

At work in this problem are various driving and resisting forces as these have been defined by Kurt Lewin in his work on force-field analysis.[10]

1. Many patients who want to be physically well need help in learning to deal directly with the emotional source of their difficulties. But most are unaware that their problems are emotionally based and therefore resist efforts to move them from medical to educational or therapeutic approaches to wellness.

2. Since many health-care personnel work more with the organically ill than with the psychosomatically ill, some prefer merely to give the latter a pill and send them home than to devote time to attempting to change their behaviors, especially since there is a serious deficiency of educators or therapists for conducting educational programs. But since the worried well tend to place excessive reliance on authority figures for problem-solving directions, even this perfunctory treatment reinforces an overdependency of the patient on the physician.

3. Most health-care administrators strive to make the most efficient use of their available resources, especially insofar as this reduces health-

care costs. But to sustain institutional operations on a financially sound basis, some administrators find it necessary to maintain high patient-loads, and the worried well constitute an inexhaustible source of potential patients.

A pilot program Recognizing that people who suffer from emotional stress make significantly greater use of inpatient and outpatient services than do those who suffer from physically based health problems, health-care administrators at the Kaiser-Permanente Medical Care Center in Oakland, California, sought in 1972–74 to determine whether alternative modes of care could be found and used effectively by paraprofessional personnel.[11]

To this end, a patient program was planned by a team composed of a physician, a psychiatrist, a nurse educator, and a health-education specialist. In most patient programs the health-education specialist serves as program coordinator and as consultant to the nurse educators. In this case, however, for demonstration purposes, the specialist worked directly with groups of worried-well patients in an ambulatory setting. The approach involved holding six ninety-minute group discussion meetings scheduled one week apart, each dealing with a specific phase of learning and change. This approach was based on the surmise that a minimal intervention, if specially designed, could not only bring about behavioral change but be cost-effective as well.

The program was based on the assumptions that supportive short-term discussion groups conducted by trained paraprofessionals could assist patients in verbalizing and sharing their feelings, in discerning the relationship between emotions and physical complaints, and in finding alternative ways of resolving their problems in order to reduce their reliance on physician services. The series of six discussion sessions, based on Lewin's unfreezing-to-refreezing theory,[12] provided an opportunity for these assumptions to be explored and tested.

At the discussion sessions, with the assistance of the other team members, the health-education specialist aimed at:

1. Creating a relaxed, comfortable atmosphere that would facilitate the learning process
2. Encouraging patients to express their individual feelings and opinions in order to foster a climate of independent learning
3. Encouraging patient interaction for the purpose of promoting mutual learning, helpfulness, and support
4. Encouraging emphasis on current rather than past distresses to avoid creating a psychotherapeutic environment and patient dependence on the health provider

5. Avoiding the assumption of a didactic/authoritarian role in order to discourage any development or continuation of patient-doctor dependency relationships

6. Avoiding personally interpretative or judgmental remarks or offering problem diagnosis or treatment advice that would inhibit the development of patients' independence

7. Sharing her own feelings as a peer-member of the group in order to facilitate the group's active dynamics.

The health educator or nurse educator who guides such groups should be trained in group dynamics methodology, for, as the following review implicitly suggests, the six discussion sessions made use of a variety of the behavioral theories introduced in chapter 3 of this book.

Session 1: All patients filled out a card explaining what they hoped to get from the program, what their major health concerns were, and what people should know about them in order to work with them. Patients were then paired off to share their responses, and, when the pairs felt comfortable with each other, they shared their responses with the group as a whole. General discussion occupied the remainder of the session.

Session 2: This session was designed to meet patients' immediate needs by enabling them to have their most pressing health questions answered by a physician selected by the team. During the first half-hour, patients worked in subgroups to formulate their questions. The remaining hour was spent interacting with the physician, the health-education specialist ensuring that all patients' concerns were addressed.

Session 3: The purpose of the third session was to help patients better understand their feelings and interpersonal interactions in relation to forces of authority, affection, and social relationships. At the beginning of the session a FIRO-B test was administered, which is designed to assess the individual's behavior toward, as well as the behavior desired from, others in three areas of interpersonal interaction: inclusion, affection, and control.[13] When test results had been interpreted, patients posed questions about their scores and devoted the remainder of the session to sharing the questionnaire results with one another.

Session 4: At the fourth session patients reflected on their relationships with others in terms of inclusion, affection, and control, discussing the sources of pent-up anger, resentment, and frustration as these feelings surfaced, and beginning to decide whether, as well as how, to change this aspect of their behavior in ways more conducive to personal satisfaction. At times, role playing helped them to explore alternative ways of handling anger-arousing situations. At this session patients became more in touch with their feelings and began to wonder whether their problems were not more emotional than physical.

Session 5: Although part of this session was sometimes used to continue work on issues or discussions carried over from the FIRO-B sessions, most of the time the group was ready to proceed to new work—in this case, strengthening self-identity. Given sheets of paper, patients were told to write in silence as many responses as they could formulate to the question, Who am I? and were given examples bearing on the roles one plays in family, work, or social settings or the knowledge and skills one possesses. After the responses had been written, paired sharing was followed by group sharing, the members having had enough experience at this point to explore, confront, and discuss one another's perceptions. Patients generally left this session in a reflective state of mind.

Session 6: During the final session, group members explored various alternatives for obtaining whatever additional help they might need after the program series had ended. Members were encouraged to formulate their own specific plans of action and to share them with the group in open discussion.

Several series were conducted as part of the Kaiser-Permanente pilot program, and follow-up studies on the participating patients indicated that the program had met its educational, research, and cost objectives. Although the limited number of participating patients must qualify a broad affirmation of achievement, related literature has tended to support the Kaiser-Permanente findings.[14-24]

On the supposition that many individual ills can be abated by behavioral changes, pilot studies have also been undertaken to determine whether use of a client-held health record, called a Personal-Life Health Plan (PLHP), will encourage individuals to take more and better responsibility for their own health.[25] In addition to containing most of what is customarily to be found in a medical record, the PLHP has material dealing with the individual's own past health history and family health history and includes tables of physiological measurements, tables of individualized morbidity and mortality risks, and a personalized health-maintenance plan.

Based on concepts of self-determinism, the PLHP helps to clarify the steps of identifying existing or potential health problems, seeking out their causes, and taking action to overcome them. Because the pilot studies have indicated that a significant percentage of individuals will use PLHPs and that physicians and nurse practitioners will incorporate them into their routines of care, plans are now under way to conduct a more comprehensive controlled experiment to obtain a more detailed picture of implementation results.

SELF-HELP GROUPS

Although the terms *self-care* and *self-help* are often used synonymously, health educators, especially, should be aware that there are differences between them. While the precise meaning of *self-care* is still an issue of considerable debate, in the health-care field its application generally encompasses self-education about health maintenance and disease prevention, self-diagnosis and treatment of disease, and self-rehabilitation activities.[26-39] In its most frequent usage, the term is applied to the self-observation, diagnosis, and treatment activities of groups that are attempting to develop healthful new life styles.

Self-help differs from self-care in aiming to help individuals improve their psychosocial capacities to function effectively. In this sense, self-help means enhancing one's personal insights, interpersonal skills, coping and problem-solving methods, and learning and change processes. It means, in short, attaining wellness by learning to live effectively with one's own best means for living.[40]

Typology

In general, self-help groups are neither organized by an agency, such as a hospital or health department, nor sponsored or endorsed by any outside organization. Organized around the support-system concept, they are self-sponsored and self-directed units composed of people who share a well-defined common purpose and core of mutual experience. Although professionals may be used to help them work together better, for the most part they draw upon their own collective knowledge, experience, and skills to achieve specific ends.

Based on his view of their purposes and membership composition, L. H. Levy has categorized self-help groups into four types.[41] Type 1 groups exist to control or change personal conduct toward such problems as drug addiction, alcoholism, or chronic obesity; examples include Synanon, Alcoholics Anonymous, and Overeaters Anonymous. Type 2 groups seek mutual help in coping with a common stress problem such as divorce or terminal disease; examples are Parents without Partners, Mended Hearts, Mastectomy Inc., The Stroke Club, Laryngectomy Inc., Make Today Count, and Recovery Inc.

Type 3 groups, exemplified by various homosexual, racial-ethnic, and women's groups, are oriented toward enhancing members' self-esteem and toward raising public consciousness or gaining social legitimacy for their particular causes. According to H. I. Marieskind and B. Ehrenreich, approximately 1,200 groups in the United States, with tens of thousands of participants, identify themselves with the women's health movement alone.[42] Type 4 groups share self-actualization goals and employ experientially based variations of Gestalt and sensitivity training;[43] examples include parent-effectiveness training groups, holistic health discussion groups, physical fitness groups, and encounter groups.

A. Gartner and F. Reissman have developed a different typology.[44] Here, Type 1 groups are engaged in rehabilitative work, helping members adjust to posttreatment situations, and include, in addition to those already mentioned, the United Ostomy Association and the Fraternity of the Wooden Leg. Type 2 groups are organized around the concept of behavioral modification and include Weight Watchers, TOPS, and Smokenders. Type 3 groups, such as Emphysema Anonymous, the Arthritis Foundation, and the American Diabetes Association, are occupied with the care of incurable diseases. Type 4 groups focus on prevention and case finding and are being demonstrated on an informal level by groups of hypertension-prone people and groups for self-examination of breasts. Type 4 groups might also be said to include exercise classes, jogging groups, swim clubs, and groups devoted to Yoga and other meditative practices.

Gartner and Riessman mention, in addition, subgroups for the parents, spouses, and children of those who are in one or another of the four categories. Alcoholics Anonymous, for example, offers Alanon for the spouses and Alateen for the children of alcoholics. All these support groups, which are very important in helping individuals to change their behavior, are consumer-intensive; that is, the self-help member functions as both a deliverer and receiver of services.

Issues for health education

While it is difficult to separate self-care from self-help, it is important for health educators to discern the fine line between them, especially now that various questions are being raised about their relationship.[45] L. S. Levin, for example, has called attention to the following questions.

1. What will be the impact of increased self-care on the doctor-patient relationship and particularly on the doctor's sickness-legitimizing role?

2. What are the criteria defining the effective limits of self-care and of medical care?

3. At what point and with what safeguards can physician responsibility appropriately be transferred to lay persons?

4. What is the likelihood that some health professions will see self-care as an opportunity for transferring routine tasks that carry only modest economic and social rewards?

5. What incentives can be introduced into current social and health systems to encourage greater development of self-care education?

6. What will be the effect of increased self-care on consumer costs, and how will economic benefits be redistributed?

7. In short, will self-care create more problems than it will solve?[46]

In response, Levin believes that "a negative potential exists for exploitation by interests which would limit movements for more equitable and higher quality health services, but should not obscure the positive potential for a strengthened partnership in health between the lay and professional worlds."[47]

Lois Pratt has observed that though professional and business ideology has been unfavorably disposed toward the development of self-care, many families may nevertheless assume health-care functions when they believe themselves to be equal to its demands.[48] Indeed, families will obtain growing support for self-care activities from self-help groups themselves, as well as from organized political-action efforts undertaken by the consumer movement, minority rights, organizations, and groups striving to demedicalize health care, and possibly by a movement focusing directly on family protection.

Richard Grant has described how family and self-help educational courses were developed to promote better utilization of health services in underserved rural areas.[49] The courses helped local citizens acquire experience and skills in identifying community health-education deficits, in developing programs to reduce these deficits, and in engaging local health-care providers more actively in community health-care problems.

Organizing the overall program required assessing the needs and interests of community members with the help of a community advisory committee, planning and scheduling the courses, selecting instructors, initiating publicity, and conducting and evaluating the course sessions. Evaluation indicated that those who had completed the courses knew more, were better able to apply their knowledge, and demonstrated more appropriate utilization behavior than did those who had not participated in the courses.

Although it has been questioned whether it is ethical for health-education specialists to help self-care groups accomplish their purposes, the self-care field must become better organized and studied before this question can be answered. It seems clear, however, that if such groups are to provide an alternative for those who prefer not to utilize traditional health-care resources, their educational needs and functions should be assessed and responsive programs designed to assist them.

Since the goal of self-help groups is to promote optimal health, assistance by a health educator having knowledge of group behavior and skills for facilitating group operations would seem to be both appropriate and helpful. The health educator can usefully intervene in any of several ways:

1. as a full-fledged member who participates in group activities to fulfill personal needs
2. as a temporary facilitator who helps the group to get started and who leaves when members can proceed on their own
3. as a consultant who meets with the group or its appointed leaders for specific problem-solving or technical-assistance intervention
4. as an organizer seeking to help the group address a larger community problem
5. as a trainer helping group members improve their membership functions and problem-solving skills.

More particularly, the health educator can help groups address and answer numerous questions pertaining to organizational, task, and operational considerations and can also assist in clarifying ground rules that will contribute to overall group effectiveness (see table 5).

Because self-help groups do succeed in helping some individuals to learn and change, they are almost certain to multiply in the future, and health

---

TABLE 5
Questions for Self-Help Groups

Organizational Considerations:

How large should the group be?

How often and where should it meet?

Should it have a definite leadership structure, with elected officers serving specific terms, or should leadership be informal, perhaps on a rotating basis?

Should group purposes, membership lists, and records of meetings be committed to writing?

Should dues be charged?

Should an official procedure exist for accepting new and releasing old members?

Task Considerations:

Is the group to carry out a specific program or task affecting nonmembers or to limit its effects to members only?

What is the program or task, how should it be done, and what will be the roles of various members in carrying it out?

How will results be measured, and how will the group use this information?

TABLE 5 (continued)

Operational Considerations:

Should the group have an established agenda?

How long will meetings last, and how are they to begin and end?

How should an idea be introduced into and treated by the group?

How should problem solving be accomplished and decisions made?

How can the group recognize and deal with the fact that a meeting is not going well?

Ground Rules:

What happens if a member is unable to attend a meeting?

During meetings, will members be allowed to come and go as they please, or should they agree to remain throughout the meeting?

Should members sit in a circle so that they can see one another's faces as they speak?

How can openness, honesty, and trust be established?

How should such detrimental behaviors as interrupting, blaming, arguing, imposing, and judging be handled, and is angry or violent physical contact to be condoned?

Will it be permissible to give and receive feedback on behaviors and their effects?

---

educators are likely to number among their more valuable resources. Not all health behavior can be approached on the basis of individual change, however. Some problems require the change process to focus on a broader plane, and for this reason Part 2 will explore health education within the context of organizations.

REFERENCES

1. United Way of America, *UWASIS II*, p. 9.
2. U.S., Department of Health, Education and Welfare, Public Health Service, Center for Disease Control, *The Priorities of Section 1502: Papers on the National Health Guidelines. Health Education and Public Law 93–641*, prepared for the Bureau of Health Education by H. G. Ogden, HEW Publication no. 77–641, 1977.
3. D. J. Merwin, "The National Center for Health Education" (Speech presented at National Conference on Hospital-based Patient Education, Chicago, 9–10 August 1976).

4. Society for Public Health Education, "SOPHE Position Statement on Patient and Family Education," *SOPHE News & Views* 5, no. 2 (April 1976): 2–3.

5. E. Fromm, *The Sane Society*.

6. E. Bernheimer and L. H. Clever, "Experiences Implementing Patient Education in an Outpatient Clinic" (Report submitted to California Regional Medical Program, St. Mary's Hospital and Medical Center, San Francisco, 1974–75), pp. 4–5.

7. U.S., Department of Health, Education and Welfare, Public Health Service, Center for Disease Control, *Using a Nutrition Clinic's Waiting Room for Patient Education*, prepared for the Health Resources Administration by J. M. Scanlan, 1976.

8. D. Mechanic, "Social-Psychological Factors Affecting the Presentation of Bodily Complaints," *New England Journal of Medicine* 21 (1972): 1132–39.

9. H. S. Ross, F. B. Collen, and K. Soghikian, "Health-Education Discussion Groups for 'Worried Well' Patients in an Ambulatory Setting," *Health Education Monographs* 5, no. 1 (Spring 1977): 51–61.

10. K. Lewin, "Quasi-Stationary Social Equilibria and the Problem of Permanent Change," in *The Planning of Change*, ed. W. G. Bennis, K. D. Benne, and R. Chin, pp. 235–38.

11. Ross, Collen, and Soghikian, " 'Worried Well' Patients," pp. 51–61; and P. R. Mico and H. S. Ross, *Health Education and Behavioral Sciences*, pp. 10–12.

12. Lewin, "Quasi-Stationary Social Equilibria," pp. 235–38.

13. W. C. Schutz, *FIRO*, p. 58; and idem, *FIRO-B Questionnaire*.

14. P. D. Buchanan, *The Leader Looks at Individual Motivation*.

15. J. P. Campbell and M. D. Dunnett, "Effectiveness of T-Group Experience in Managerial Training and Development," *Psychological Bulletin* 70 (1968): 73–104.

16. N. A. Cummings and W. T. Follette, "Brief Psychotherapy and Medical Utilization: An Eight-Year Follow-Up" (Department of Psychiatry, Kaiser Foundation Hospital and Permanente Medical Group, San Francisco, n.d.).

17. J. Danforth et al., "Group Services for Unmarried Mothers: An Interdisciplinary Approach," *Children* 18, no. 2 (1971): 59–64.

18. P. W. Doziey, J. O. Loken, and J. A. Field, "T-Group Influence on Feelings of Alienation," *Journal of Applied Behavioral Science* 7, no. 6 (1971): 724–31.

19. G. Egan, *Encounter*.

20. S. R. Garfield, "The New Medical Care Delivery System," *Scientific American*, April 1970, pp. 15–23.

21. R. J. House, "T-Group Education and Leadership Effectiveness: A Review of the Empirical Literature and a Critical Evaluation," *Personnel Psychology* 20 (1967): 1–32.

22. U. Rueveni, "Using Sensitivity Training with Junior High School Students," *Children* 18, no. 2 (1971): 69–72.

23. E. H. Schein and W. G. Bennis, *Personal and Organizational Change through Group Methods*.

24. D. Stock, "A Survey of Research on T-Groups," in *T-Group Theory and Laboratory Method*, ed. L. P. Bradford, J. R. Gibb, and K. K. Benne, pp. 395–441.

25. R. Giglio et al., "Encouraging Behavior Changes by Client-Held Health Records" (Paper presented at Annual Meeting of American Public Health Association, Miami, 17–21 October, 1976).

26. L. S. Levin, A. H. Katz, and E. Holst, *Self-Care*.

27. L. Pratt, *Family Structure and Effective Health Behavior: The Energized Family* (Boston: Houghton Mifflin Co., 1976).

28. J. Gaver, *How to Help Your Doctor Help You* (New York: Pinnacle Books, 1975).

29. D. Sobel, *Everyday Guide to Your Health* (New York: Grossman Publishers, 1973).

30. L. Weed, *Your Health Care and How To Manage It* (Essex Junction, Vt.: Essex Publishing Co., 1975).

31. Boston Women's Health Book Collective, *Our Bodies, Ourselves: A Book by and for Women*, 2d ed. (New York: Simon & Schuster, 1975).

32. H. Z. Bennett, ed., *The Well Body Student Health Manual* (Berkeley and Los Angeles: University of California Press, 1974).

33. K. W. Sehnert and H. Eisenberg, *How to Be Your Own Doctor (Sometimes)* (New York: Grosset & Dunlap, 1975).

34. R. Lang, *The Birth Book* (Palo Alto, Calif.: Genesis Press, 1972).

35. L. H. Levy, "Self-Help Groups: Types and Psychological Processes," *Journal of Applied Behavioral Science* 12, no. 3 (1976): 310–22.

36. L. H. Levy, "Forces and Issues in the Revival of Interest in Self-Care: Impetus for Redirection in Self-Care," *Health Education Monographs* 5, no. 2 (1977): 115–20.

37. R. Grant, S. Fonaroff, and L. H. Levy, eds., "Issues in Self-Care," *Health Education Monographs* 5, no. 2 (1977): 108–89.

38. H. I. Marieskind and B. Ehrenreich, "Toward Socialist Medicine: The Women's Health Movement," *Social Policy* 6, no. 2 (September-October 1975): 34–42.

39. A. Gartner and F. Riessman, "Self-Help Models and Consumer-Intensive Health Practice," *American Journal of Public Health* 66, no. 8 (August 1976): 783–86.

40. Levy, "Self-Help Groups," pp. 310–22.

41. Ibid., p. 312.

42. Marieskind and Ehrenreich, "Toward Socialist Medicine," p. 34–42.

43. Levy, "Self-Help Groups," p. 313.

44. Gartner and Riessman, "Self-Help Models," p. 783–786.

45. Grant, Fonaroff, and Levy, "Issues in Self-Care," pp. 108–14.

46. Ibid., p. 119.

47. Ibid., p. 115.

48. L. Pratt, "Changes in Health-Care Ideology in Relation to Self-Care by Families," *Health Education Monographs* 5, no. 2 (Summer 1977): 121–35.

49. Grant, Fonaroff, and Levy, "Issues in Self-Care," pp. 145–60.

PART TWO
HEALTH
EDUCATION
AND
ORGANIZATIONS

5

Problems in organizational behavior

6

Theories of organizational behavior and change

7

Programs in organizational health education

There are several good reasons why health educators should become knowledgeable about organizational theory and practice. First, because health-care services are themselves provided through organizations such as hospitals and neighborhood health centers, the quantity and quality of such services will inevitably be affected by the purposes and practices of the service organization. Second, as employees of these organizations, health educators can enhance their own effectiveness by gaining an understanding of organizational behavior. Third, because the health of employees in general is often affected—indeed, sometimes subjected to hazard—by the nature and stresses of their work, the office or factory has been shown to be an excellent setting in which to conduct health education.

As the following pages will show, organizations are far more than just places of work. As forces for behavioral change, they are as important to study and understand as are individuals in particular and the community at large. The three chapters composing Part 2 are designed to contribute to such study and understanding. Chapter 5 will focus primarily on health problems within the organizational setting. Chapter 6 will discuss theories of organizational behavior and change. Chapter 7 will give examples of health-education programs that are aimed at producing behavioral change in organizations.

5

Problems in organizational behavior

INTRODUCTION

To the individual and the community, which most health educators have traditionally regarded as the two primary targets for health-education services, this book adds a third target—the organization. Organizations exhibit a variety of external forms, as indicated by the many terms that are used to distinguish them: *corporation, company, agency, institution, association* or *society, center* or *clinic, foundation, body,* and so forth.* They can be very small or very large; currently operational or currently dormant (though still considered operational as long as certain legal forms are filed annually on their behalf); made highly visible to the public by means of educational, public relations, or marketing programs, or deliberately concealed from the public eye. Although usually established by means of articles of incorporation, charters, bylaws, or various quasi-legal documents, they can be easily dissolved by means of either voluntary or enforced closure.

In broader, more conceptual terms, however, an organization can be described as a social-legal structure for enabling input resources to be converted into output products for the purpose of gaining income or other compensation, either directly or indirectly, in return. When the organization's purpose is to manufacture a material product, this may be ac-

*For definitions, see Glossary.

complished by means of an assembly-line process in which specially trained personnel convert raw materials or parts produced by others (input) into packaged products (output) for distribution to places where they can be sold to customers. When the purpose is to provide needed human services,* units of specially trained personnel may either provide the services themselves or support those who will provide direct services. In either case, personnel, equipment, and money are brought into play, though types and amounts may vary considerably.

The organization is a *social* structure in that personnel must interact continually during the input-to-output process. These interactions may be positive forces that enable the organization to function smoothly, or they may be negative forces that inhibit organizational effectiveness. The organization is a *legal* entity in that it must file articles of incorporation with the Office of the State Secretary establishing its name and specific type (e.g., corporation, limited partnership, etc.), identifying its purposes, products, or services, and stating whether it will or will not be profit making. In addition, almost all organizations are subject to a variety of federal, state, and local laws and regulations governing their operation.

There are many reasons why health educators should have a sound working knowledge of organizational functioning, not the least of which is that they are themselves employees of organizations. While it can be assumed that all health organizations exist to serve public needs, how well the needs are met depends upon how well they function. Health educators usually become involved in determining how education is to be conducted, which includes such matters as budgetary and personnel allocation, but other factors influence the quantity and quality of services as well.

These factors include the health organization's basic policies and goals and how programs and services are organized and delivered; whether a specific health-education office will be established and where it will be placed within the overall organizational structure; and to what extent employee training and development programs will be carried out. Clearly, then, the better that health educators comprehend the organization as a basic behavioral entity, the better they will be able to fulfill their own membership roles.

Health educators generally begin their careers as junior employees carrying out well-defined tasks as part of a health-education service unit. They usually work under the direct supervision of a more experienced or advance-educated employee and are expected to cooperate with other members of the unit, with other members of the organization, and with the

---

*The term *human services* refers to the broad category of these organizations. Although this book is concerned with health-care organizations, a specific area of human services, the two terms are often used interchangeably.

clients to whom services are being extended. At this stage they must familiarize themselves with, and adapt themselves to, the organization's basic structure, functions, policies, and procedures, both formal and informal, and learn which other organizational entities it relates to at federal, state, and local levels of government.

As they learn and mature, they move to the positions of greater responsibility and leadership. They become supervisors of personnel, participate more actively in internal management, and devote more of their time to such administrative functions as planning and developing programs, budgeting, reporting, problem-solving and evaluating efforts. Of necessity, in short, they become more aware of the organization as a whole and more involved in helping it to run effectively. This in turn helps assure that the health-education services they manage will address the problems or needs of people in other organizations as well.

It is well known, for example, that certain types of employment, such as coal mining or work requiring exposure to asbestos or radioactive materials, are highly hazardous to employees' health. In recent years it has been recognized also that on-the-job stress can damage employees' health and lead to such further problems as alcoholism and drug abuse. For these reasons, health educators for many years have used the organization as a valuable setting in which to educate employees and to help them cope with the conditions under which they must work.

However, if a hazard-related organizational problem has a technological cause—if there are flaws in equipment or hazards attending the preparation of raw materials, for example—the most direct solution may require expensive technological change. In this case the health educator may be limited to making others aware of the causal relationship, suggesting alternative solutions, encouraging the strict enforcement of existing safety rules and regulations, and helping employees to develop better safety and prevention practices of their own.

Organizational stress, on the other hand, can be caused by many factors:

1. poor work-allocation systems which burden employees with too much work too rapidly
2. poor decision making which results in decisions that are either untimely or unhelpful in problem solving
3. poor internal planning which neither prevents crises from occurring nor allows sufficient time for coping with them
4. poor work norms which lead to lack of cooperation and other counterproductive behaviors among employees
5. poor reward systems which cause people to feel punished for mistakes made but unrewarded for work well done.

In such cases, health educators can help employees change the conditions that evoke such stress.

In the past, initiating employee health-screening programs or safety campaigns in other organizations required little more than knowing the name of their appropriate officials to be contacted for program approval and support. Today, however, with the growing emphasis upon helping people to understand and cope with organization-related health problems, health educators must become increasingly well informed about how people learn and change in organizational settings. They must also understand the organization's production processes in order to reach employees when they are readiest to learn and when productivity will be least disrupted.

Finally, health educators should realize that the organization's environment is a dynamic field of competing social, economic, and political pressures which separately or together influence its readiness to participate in educational activities. It helps to know, for example, that organizations are likelier to lend themselves to such activities during periods of prosperity than during periods of financial difficulty, and are likelier still when such activities are proposed at a time of public concern about health issues. Furthermore, it helps to know that planning for educational programs will involve not only employees and management but labor unions and employee associations as well. Finally, health educators may be competing with other health agencies for an organization's time and attention, and this may involve negotiating collaborative programs with those other agencies.

To the question of whether the organization is an appropriate setting for intervention by health educators, the authors respond with an emphatic *yes*. To repeat: Organizations are social structures exhibiting behavioral modes that can positively or negatively affect both the quality of their products or services and the health of their employees. Because health education can have a positive influence on behavior, it should address itself to organizational problems along with its other functions. The remainder of this chapter will therefore focus on problems affecting administration, control, and delivery of services within the setting of the health-service organization, and on problems affecting the health of those who work in organizational settings in general.

ORGANIZATIONAL PROBLEMS

Administration and control

Health-care administration is ideally directed toward making the best use of organizational planning, management, and evaluation techniques to enhance the quantity and quality of services that organizations make available. Unfortunately, however, many of the administrative and management problems that plague organizations in general are common to the health-care field as well.

At the top, for example, it may be questioned whether the board of directors adequately represents the clientele being served. Between the board and top administrators there may be concern about who makes policy and is responsible for implementation. Between top administrators and middle managers there often exist questions about the exercise of responsibility and delegation of authority. Between middle managers and line personnel there may be concern about supervisory functions, performance ratings, and the distribution of rewards and punishments. Finally, line personnel are frequently concerned about problems of autonomy and their own sense of distance from the organization's upper levels.

As in other organizations, too, health-care personnel are susceptible to the frailties of interpersonal and intergroup processes. Personnel want to be involved in policy formulation and decision making that will affect both their working environments and their lives. All too often, however, communication breakdowns create confusion and actions based on misinformation. Interdepartmental conflicts and competition for scarce resources become counterproductive to the organization's goals. Ineffective meetings create disenchantment among participants. Cliques and self-interest groupings produce disharmony. Insensitivity to the feelings, values, and needs of minority personnel heightens tensions and intergroup animosities. Crisis-oriented ways of working produce emotional outbursts and angry confrontations, and so on.

At the same time, health-care personnel have behavioral problems that are unique to their profession—among them, tensions that arise from a personally vague sense of mission. Although emergency-care units often have life-or-death missions, seldom does the organization as a whole confront missions of such dire urgency. Hospitals and neighborhood health centers alike provide many human services, and support many overhead costs, that are not directly related to matters of life and death.

Inevitably, too, tensions arise as personnel tend to develop a tunnel view of organizational goals that lends heightened justification to their own roles and functions—as surgeons, for example, will perceive their own roles as having greater justification than the roles played by social workers. Finally, all health-care workers have the uneasy feeling that they may not be doing as much or as well as they should. Under all these conditions it is extremely difficult for an organization to develop the climate of experimentation that can facilitate initiation of a change effort.[1]

To the extent that health care *is* oriented toward life-or-death issues, however, the system has tended to be hightly structured and autocratic. Treatment decisions are based on clear-cut diagnostic data, and, because the skills to collect, analyze, and base decisions on those data are largely invested in medical specialists, the health professions have long dominated the health-care field. Although the authoritarian approach enables decisions to be implemented as quickly as possible, it allows little or no tolerance for nonscientific or extrarational responses. According to Robert Reiff, it also leads to a monopolization of power whose effect is to keep knowledge and skills out of the reach of the public.

The resources which the helping professions can mobilize, i.e., the bases of their power, are primarily their knowledge and skills. But they have also constructed a system of organizations and institutions, private offices, hospitals, clinics, professional schools, and more, which constitute their material resources. In addition, they dominate those who run and maintain those institutions. The medical profession, for instance, controls not only its clients but also its nurses, technicians, secretaries, clerks, security police, etc. Ultimately, however, their power resides in their knowledge and skill. And obviously, if one is granted power on the basis of a monopoly of knowledge and skills, then one has a vested interest in keeping them from the public; for the more knowledge the public acquires, the less firm the basis of the authority granted. Thus, the helping professionals guard the core of their knowledge, making no real effort to share it with the public.[2]

The behavioral approach to organizational problem solving, on the other hand, requires collaboration between client and consultant through a joint exploration of problems, of alternative courses of action, and of decision making. Because this approach is time-consuming, sometimes experimental, and always somewhat ambiguous, however, strong resistance to it can be expected from those oriented to the highly structured approach.

Thus, the authoritarian approach of the physician-expert is in conflict with the client-participation approach employed by social workers, physical and occupational therapists, mental health workers, and patient educators. The treatment mode of operation is at times in conflict with the preventive mode. Internal power struggles between boards of directors, nonphysician administrators, and physician medical directors are in conflict with shared leadership and intergroup collaboration approaches. Only in recent years, however, have policy makers been confronted with the issue of consumer control.

The development of neighborhood health centers administered by consumer-controlled health associations was made possible in the early 1960s by the U.S. Office of Economic Opportunity's War on Poverty program, with its legal requirement for the maximum feasible participation of residents to be affected by the program. The subsequent Model Cities programs created by the Model Cities Demonstration Act of 1966 increased the emphasis on consumer participation.

For health administration, the implications of this trend became clear when the Comprehensive Health Planning Act of 1965 (P.L. 89–749) required the majority of members of comprehensive health-planning boards to be composed of consumer representatives. Later federal legislation, such as the National Health Planning and Resources Development Act of 1974 (P.L. 93–641), amended and strengthened in 1979, carried the concept even further by dissolving P.L. 89–749 agencies and creating the present health-systems agencies.

Although laws may change behavior by forcing choices among options, seldom do they change the basic attitudes, beliefs, values, or motivations underlying behavior. Questions of who should control the organizational administration of health services—the professionals who have the knowledge and skills for delivering services or the consumers for whom the services are intended—remain controversial in most areas of the present health system. The most effective answers will arise from a problem-solving process that enables similarities to be emphasized, differences to be accepted, and attitudes to be changed.

Delivery of services

Much concern has centered also on the question of how personnel resources should be organized for the better delivery of health services. In this case a potential solution may have been found in the increasingly widespread reliance on health-care teams. Health teams have experienced a phenomenal growth during the past few years as a result of a great many problematic changes in health care and related fields.

• Changes in patient care have required that previously fragmented delivery of separate categorical services by separate workers be brought together into comprehensive arrangements for primary health care.

• National programs for the delivery of health services have changed from conventional categorical medical models to models requiring interdisciplinary team arrangements and other innovative strategies, as evidenced by the growth of neighborhood health centers, health maintenance organizations, national health-service corps, area health-education centers, and health-systems agencies.

• Community health services have shifted from centralized clinics and ambulatory departments to decentralized neighborhood health centers.

• Health-care management theory and practice have moved administrators from autocratic to more participatory-democratic styles of leadership.

• Academic preparation of health and medical workers has replaced an emphasis on autonomous roles with an emphasis on team settings.

• Medical personnel practice has been moving from solo arrangements to group practice and ambulatory clinic arrangements. In a corollary development, doctors are perceiving themselves less as high-status elitists and are growing more attuned to peer-level relationships with nondoctors.

• The shift in need toward less highly specialized and more readily accessible health-care personnel has led to the creation of new personnel roles and functions in aiding or extending the work of specialists or in performing new technological skills.

• Increased sensitivity on the part of health-care organizations toward issues of racism, minority and women's rights, and consumer participation has had the effect of introducing more minority members into the health professions and of altering work relationships within the field.

• A change in human attitude toward work situations—from an acceptance of subjugation to a need for self-esteem—has motivated health-care workers to seek more meaningful roles and functions in the delivery of services.

• Health problem-solving has shifted from a specific-disease orientation to a consideration of the complex relationship between disease and such factors as race, poverty, poor housing, and poor education, thereby making extremely difficult any simplistically clear-cut measurement of success.

• Consumers and patients have changed from passive recipients to active participants in planning and treatment processes, in this way affecting the development of primary roles in the health team.

• The financing of medical services has changed from fees for physician services to fees for health-care services, particularly by means of third-party insurance payers, which, by reimbursing either the consumers or the providers for service costs, has legitimated new team roles for increasingly more allied health professionals.

Five types of teams are to be found in operation today.

1. *Crisis-oriented teams* are organized around saving or prolonging lives, as in the cases of the severely burned, the severely injured, or for those needing organ transplants. These teams are found in technologically sophisticated health-care facilities where the management decision-making structures are sharply delineated and personnel roles are clearly defined.

2. *Client-oriented teams,* more life enhancing than life saving, are organized around individual problem solving for comprehensive patient care, primary care, family care, or home-care practices. These teams are found in hospital-based clinics, neighborhood health-care centers,

mental health centers, rehabilitation centers, and nursing homes, and they usually reflect less clarity of role, function, purpose, and management structure than do crisis-oriented teams.

3. *Service-oriented teams* are organized around the delivery of groups of services, such as maternal and child-health, family-planning, and general-practice services. They are found in outpatient clinics, health departments, and group medical practices, and they often exhibit still less clarity in regard to purposes and procedures.

4. *Intervention-oriented teams* are organized to reach specific populations-at-risk in public housing developments or among migrant workers, the aging, and those suffering from drug addiction, alcoholism, or venereal disease. These teams are found in the outreach units of various neighborhood-based health and multiservice centers, storefront clinics, free clinics, and drug treatment programs, and their teamwork problems are likely to be complex.

5. *Management-oriented teams* are composed of top- and middle-level administrators who have set themselves the joint task of managing health-care facilities and operations. Here, too, issues and problems tend to be complex.

Although health teams have proved to be a practicable means of organizing personnel for better delivery of health services, their use has not been without problems. Such is the mystique surrounding the idea of teams, for example, that their effective functioning is sometimes assumed to be automatic, a misapprehension that frequently leads to expectations too great to be met. Further, as the review of types suggests, the closer a team works with life-and-death issues, the sharper the clarity of its mission and procedures; the farther from such issues, the likelier are vagueness and ambiguity to characterize team operations. Finally, as in the case of administrative and control issues, resistance to change in the delivery of services is great and will not easily be reduced.

Employee health

The effect of organizational life in general on employees' health is yet another problematic area. That the type of work people do plays a significant role in their susceptibility to certain disabilities and diseases is a well-documented clinical fact. In reducing these susceptibilities much organizational improvement has resulted from education, legislation, and organizational compliance with health and safety standards. In regard to the sociopsychological conditions under which people work, however, two factors continue to constitute major determinants of organizational problems:

(1) the norms or standards that govern employees' behavior and (2) whether an organization's membership is perceived as including more than its employees alone.

Although norms, or typical behavioral patterns, may differ from one organization to the next, there can be no disputing the fact that employees now want more from their work than just pay. They want the work to be interesting and meaningful as well, and, when it is not, organizations and employees alike develop neurotic symptoms.[3] Employees who feel that their skills are inadequately used, who grumble about worries, frustrations, a sense of impotence, or a loss of self-esteem, become inefficient, blame others for their work problems, and seek ways of avoiding the job—by taking sick leave, for example, or going on vacation.

As frustrations intensify, subgroups form on the basis of friendship ties, and members meet over coffee or lunch to exchange complaints, share rumors, or plan defensive strategies. Such meetings serve only to heighten anxiety, however, and, until problems are dealt with directly, this gradually deteriorating climate will conduce to a highly unpleasant working environment.

In addition to meeting the needs and interests of workers themselves, organizations should expand their view of membership to include others who are also of importance to overall organizational effectiveness. To accommodate the needs and interests of workers' families, for example, industrial organizations increasingly are providing services that are not directly related to the job, such as child-care services and recreational centers.

For human-service enterprises, this means that clients, too, should be regarded as organization members and treated with dignity and respect. In this view, students and their families are as much a part of a school system as are its teachers. The same applies to prisons and their inmates, welfare agencies and their clients, mental institutions and their patients, nursing homes and their residents.

Organizations that exhibit any or all of the problems described in this chapter must adopt strategies for change, either planning and shaping the change from within or allowing change to be imposed by an outside force. To initiate change efforts, many organizations have their own training-and-staff–development units or organization-development units, or they may employ personnel trained in the management sciences. Others make use of outside consultants; indeed, external consultants are increasingly being used to help hospitals, medical schools, and neighborhood health centers deal with issues of behavioral change. In order for such resources to be genuinely useful, however, they must be grounded in relevant theory and practice, the subjects of the two chapters that follow.

REFERENCES

1. I. Rubin, M. S. Plovnick, and R. E. Fry, "Initiating Planned Change in Health-Care Systems," *Journal of Applied Behavioral Science* 10, no. 1 (1974): 107–24.
2. R. Reiff, "The Control of Knowledge: The Power of the Helping Professions," *Journal of Applied Behavioral Science* 10, no. 3 (1974): 451–61.
3. J. B. Harvey and D. R. Albertson, "Neurotic Organizations: Symptoms, Causes, and Treatment," in *Contemporary Organization Development*, ed. W. W. Burke, pp. 16–19.

6
Theories of organizational behavior and change

A CONCEPT OF ORGANIZATION

Health educators who want to be instrumental in bringing about organizational change must begin by forming a concept of the organization as a whole. Recognizing that many theories have arisen as different disciplines and professions have applied their own unique perspectives to defining the concept, they must then attempt to integrate these various contributions into a coherent strategy for organizational change. Among the disciplines that have made important contributions to this field of study are psychology, sociology, political science, management science, systems analysis, computer science, and behavioral science.

Psychology Within the context of organizational structures, psychologists' interest in individual behavior has resulted in four branches of study: industrial, leadership, motivation, and personnel theory. *Industrial theory* arose out of the interest created by a series of studies undertaken at Western Electric's Hawthorne plant near Chicago between 1927 and 1932.[1] The Hawthorne studies demonstrated that employees' morale and production rose as efforts were made to improve their working environment, not because of any actual improvement in working conditions but because the attention alone gave them a greater sense of importance. Further studies have revealed the importance of involving employees themselves in their own change efforts.

Although research in *leadership theory* began in the early 1930s, it was stimulated by the Theory X and Theory Y leadership constructs developed by Douglas McGregor beginning in 1957.[2] Briefly, Theory X characterizes the autocratic leader; Theory Y, the democratic-participative leader; and McGregor promoted the Theory Y mode. The constructs moved from the stance of having only a few people making decisions in the organization to one in which more workers were included in decision-making processes, especially those to be affected by the decisions. It was believed that by involving workers in decision making, they would become more motivated, committed, and productive and would assist in carrying out the organization's goals.

During the 1940s and 1950s, motivation and personnel theories were explored by several researchers. Initially stimulated by the work of Kurt Goldstein, Abraham Maslow, and others, *motivation theory* was directly applied to organizational behavior by Frederick Herzberg's concept of hygiene factors,[3] which suggested that what employees perceive as rewards and punishments is important in solving problems pertaining to employee performance and organizational productivity.

Personnel theory, which grew out of the trend toward greater specialization of personnel roles and functions, brought about the development of various tests and measurements, particularly for screening job applicants on the basis of their knowledge, skills, aptitudes, and personality. Personnel psychologists also concern themselves with issues pertaining to interviewing, training, supervision, promotion, discipline, and personnel policies in general.

Sociology   The dynamics of roles and the structural interrelationships of various organizational groupings (including boards, unions, managers, and consumers) have long been of interest to sociologists, who have attempted to identify respective norms or standards, characterize interrelationships, and arrive at useful determinants for predicting or analyzing behavior. In helping organizations to develop health teams, especially, health educators must understand role theory, which helps to clarify the effect of roles and relationships on organizational change.

Political science   Adopting the tools for analyzing decision making, influence, and power from studies of social policy and governance and applying them to the study of related organizational processes has contributed greatly to furthering an understanding of organizations in general. In the health-care field, particularly, such tools are very important in influencing the resolution of critical issues that arise from interactions of governing boards, administrators, professional groups, and employee unions. In this regard, the health educator is at times an applied psychologist, sociologist, and political scientist in addition to adapting the roles made useful by other applied professions.

Management science Schools of business management specialize in the training and development of professional managers for national and international business and industry. Their fields of study include organizational behavior, financial management and forecasting, program budgeting, cost accounting, marketing, and the use of various management tools that are increasingly being used by health organizations.

Systems analysis A high-level technical assistance specialty, systems analysis—the design and study of systems—has roots in a variety of fields, including engineering, computer technology, and social planning. It employs people who are skilled in diagnosing systems-operations problems and in modifying or changing the systems to resolve the problems.

Technically, the term *system* denotes a rational arrangement of specially organized resources (units), each contributing in a prearranged way to the development of an organization's product or service. An automobile production line, for example, is a system arranged so that a sequence of trained workers (units) can administer special services to a car until the completed vehicle can be moved to a delivery area.

At a more complex level, the production line becomes a unit in itself, collaborating with other units (such as administration) in an even larger organizational system (such as the community). Further, the community can be regarded as a unit in a larger state or national system. The larger systems are usually termed *macrosystems;* the smaller, *microsystems.*

In health-care organizations, systems are composed of specialized groupings of people who perform specific management and support functions in the delivery of specific health services (e.g., inpatient, outpatient, social services, etc.). The functions of these various units are coordinated so that input materials and dollars are used to produce the best outputs (cured or otherwise satisfied patients) at the lowest cost. Systems analysis helps health educators determine whether an organizational problem is owing to a systems deficiency or to a human interactional issue, and makes them more aware of the effect of technology on organizational behavior in general.

Computer science Very much a part of business, industry, and human-services systems today, computers are being increasingly used for rapid storage and retrieval of data, as well as, in health care, for diagnosis of disease and monitoring of treatment. But the use of computers has introduced difficulties as well. As these and other complex machines take over tasks that were formerly carried out by people, changes occur in personnel roles and relationships as a result of role threat, intergroup conflict, and normative resistance to change. Often, too, if people believe that a new piece of equipment will not work, they consciously or subconsciously behave in ways that may cause the equipment to fail.

Behavioral science Applied behavioral scientists have also studied organizations, both to gain a better understanding of their behavior and to help them change. Their methodology of change is called *organization development* (OD), and, in devising it, specialists have had to integrate the contributions of many other professions and disciplines. Health educators who specialize in this area must therefore acquire the basic knowledge and skills employed by these specialists. As Richard Beckhard has observed, the need for creative collaboration between applied behavioral scientists and leaders of health-education and delivery systems is growing at an alarming rate.[4] In short, for health educators to be effective in assisting organizations to fulfill their missions and goals, they must understand the underlying psychological, sociological, behavioral, political, and technological theories that affect organizational dynamics.

BEHAVIORAL THEORIES

Open-system theories

Early theorists were divided between those who viewed organizations as closed systems, entirely self-contained, self-sustaining, and independent from other organizations, and those who saw them as living organisms containing vital forces that impelled them toward self-actualization.[5] Later theorists increasingly saw organizations as artificial structures that enabled groups of people to pursue common goals, and, as they became aware of the need for interdependence, the open-system concept came to dominate modern theories of organizational behavior. This concept holds that organizations are subsystems of larger macrosystems and as such cannot operate in isolation from their environment. Key proponents of this view include Daniel Katz and Robert Kahn, the Tavistock group, George Homans, Rensis Likert, and Edgar Schein.

Katz and Kahn model The Katz and Kahn model for the understanding of organizations postulates a cyclical system in which the energic return from the output becomes part of the next input, thus continuously reactivating the system[6] (*energic* refers to forces of power, influence, or action). The system is "open" in the sense that the cycle requires the organization to engage in recurring, interdependent, mutually complementary activities with its environment in pursuit of a common outcome.

In the case of business and industrial organizations, the environment consists of the setting in which consumers live, the consumers' needs and demands in the way of products, and the determination through market research of specifically what will motivate them to buy one brand of product instead of another. The environment also includes money received from product sales, which becomes a resource input for purchasing new materials and paying salaries; competition from products produced by other organizations; and such forces as strikes, energy shortages, or the rising cost of raw materials, all of which may affect the quantity and quality of the product.

In the case of health-services organizations, the environment consists of consumers (clients or patients); other agencies that provide related services; the policies and programs of federal, state, and local governments and their decisions regarding budgets and allocations; third-party health-insurance companies and their reimbursement rates; professional organizations and unions that speak for employees; and citizen advocate groups that push for better services. Because health educators often help their organizations to participate with others in the community in health planning, community education, or other programs, they tend to be more aware of open systems and their environments than most of their health-care colleagues.

Tavistock model The Tavistock model, which arose from studies conducted in the early 1950s by a group of social scientists associated with the Tavistock Institute of London, is based on observations of changing technology in the British coal-mining industry and the redesign of work in Indian textile mills. E. L. Trist and his associates are credited with developing the concept of sociotechnical systems; A. K. Rice, with formulating a more general definition of open-system organizations.[7]

The term *sociotechnical system* suggests that a productive organization, or any part thereof, is composed of both a technological system (equipment and procedures for producing a product) and a social system (interrelationships among those who perform tasks), and that these systems interact, each influencing or helping to shape the other. The sociotechnical system is "open" insofar as the organization imports various items from its environment, utilizes them in a conversion process, then exports the products and services that result from the conversion process. Imports include raw materials, money, equipment, people involved in the conversion process, and information that helps the organization determine its survival needs.

The Tavistock model is important in establishing that a relationship does, in fact, exist between people and technology. It will readily be seen, for example, that because the knowledge, skills, training, and equipment of a health-care organization differ from those of a school system, welfare department, or prison, the relationships between personnel and technology must differ as well. Indeed, important differences exist in this regard within the health-care field itself. The relationship between a health educator and his technology is flexible and contingent on existing conditions, while the relationship between a surgeon and the technology of surgery must of necessity be far more precisionistic.

Homans model   Formulated by George C. Homans, a sociologist, the Homans model preceded, but is somewhat more complex than, the Tavistock model. According to Homans, all social systems have three environments: physical (terrain, climate, layout), cultural (societal norms, values, and goals), and technological (state of knowledge and instrumentation available for task performance). The collective environment specifies certain activities and interactions for those involved in the social system, which in turn arouses certain feelings among them toward one another and toward the environment.[8]

These activities, interactions, and feelings, termed the *external system*, greatly affect the organization's *internal system* (or what most theorists call the *informal system*). In Homans's view, changes in the external and internal systems are interdependent; that is, changes in workers' attitudes, for example, will affect how equipment is used and work is done. For health education, the significance of this theory lies in illuminating the interdependencies between workers' attitudes and their technology.

Likert model   To the business and industrial sector, particularly, Rensis Likert has contributed two important theories: the linking-pin theory and the interrelated variables theory.[9] The linking-pin theory views the organization as a system of interlocking groups connected by individuals who occupy key positions in two or more of the groups. The management team of a health-care agency, for example, is composed of a variety of departmental heads who, in sharing information that is important to all and in making decisions that affect all, become linking pins between their departments and top management.

To Likert, the relevant environment for any group or system is likely to be a set of other groups or systems: (1) subsystems within the given system, such as formal and informal work groups within the organization; (2) systems that share common purposes, such as related organizations within a community; or (3) larger-scale systems, such as the complex of political, economic, and social organizations at national, state, and local levels that make up society as a whole.

Thus, Likert views the organization as being linked to its environment through people who occupy key positions in both the organization and its environmental system, and environmental segments as similarly linked through key people. In the community setting, for example, health educators often work with interagency councils composed of linking-pin representatives.

Likert's interrelated variables theory groups organizational variables into three interrelated classes: causal, intervening, and end-result (see figure 5). Causal variables determine what the organization is supposed to do and how it should operate; they include only those factors which the organization and its management can change, such as systemic structures, policies, and procedures. Intervening variables reflect the organization's internal health in terms of its members' loyalties, attitudes, perceptions, motivations, and performance goals, as well as in their collective capacity for effective interaction, communication, and decision making. End-result variables reflect the organization's achievements, such as productivity and the quality of services it provides.

The theory is that changes in the most influential causal variables will lead to systematic changes in related operating procedures, which will in turn bring about changes in end-result variables. According to Likert, attempting to induce a desired shift in a management system by concentrating directly on the intervening and end-result variables will result in disappointment, a concept of particular use to health educators in suggesting a strategy for organizational change.

Schein's redefinition Because of the growth of organizational theory, the concept of organization had eventually to be redefined, and this was undertaken by Edgar Schein, who offers the following six points as characterizing his view of product-producing organizations particularly.[10]

1. The organization is an open system that is in constant interaction with its environment, taking in raw materials, people, information, and energy, converting these into products or services, and exporting the latter back into the environment.

2. The organization's multiple purposes or functions involve multiple interactions with its environment through subsystem activity. A hospital, for example, is a complex organization each of whose many subsystems has special interactions with the community; hence, health educators who work in a hospital setting must know how these separate parts contribute to the hospital's overall activity.

3. The organization's subsystems interact dynamically with one another. Thus, instead of analyzing organizational phenomena in terms of in-

FIGURE 5
**Sequence of Organizational Change Based on Likert's
Interrelated Variables**

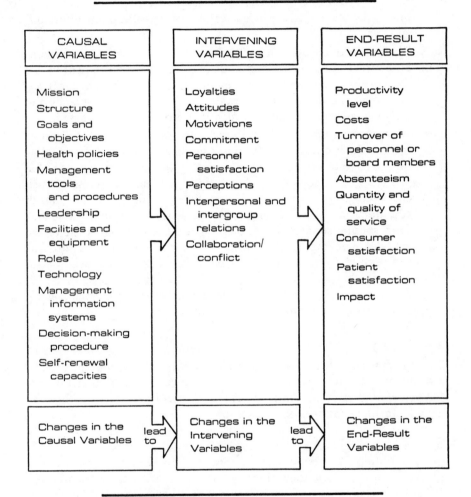

CAUSAL VARIABLES	INTERVENING VARIABLES	END-RESULT VARIABLES
Mission	Loyalties	Productivity level
Structure	Attitudes	Costs
Goals and objectives	Motivations	Turnover of personnel or board members
Health policies	Commitment	
Management tools and procedures	Personnel satisfaction	Absenteeism
Leadership	Perceptions	Quantity and quality of service
Facilities and equipment	Interpersonal and intergroup relations	Consumer satisfaction
Roles	Collaboration/ conflict	Patient satisfaction
Technology		Impact
Management information systems		
Decision-making procedure		
Self-renewal capacities		

Changes in the Causal Variables	lead to	Changes in the Intervening Variables	lead to	Changes in the End-Result Variables

SOURCE: Adapted from Rensis Likert, *The Human Organization: Its Management and Value* (New York: McGraw-Hill, 1967), pp. 136–45.

dividual behavior alone, it is important to analyze subsystem dynamics as well—a concept on which Part 2 of this book has been based.

4. Because subsystems are interdependent, changes in one are likely to affect behavior in others. Health educators must therefore determine how subsystem interdependencies in their organizations affect one another.

5. The organization exists in a dynamic environment of other systems, both larger and smaller than itself. Because the environment makes demands and places constraints on the organization, its total functioning cannot be understood without reference to these demands and constraints—the concept on which Part 3 of this book is based.

6. Because the multiple links between an organization and its environment make it difficult to clarify the boundaries of any one organization, a concept of organization is better expressed in terms of stable processes of import, conversion, and export than in terms of such characteristics as size, shape, structure, or function. For health educators, this means distinguishing general organizational functions from specific services. In the sense that a hospital makes use of the experience of employees, patients, or of anyone who comes into contact with it, for example, it can be said to engage in general health education throughout the organization. In contrast, hospital health education can be regarded as a specific limited service when it is directed toward a particular set of patients.

Role theory

To organizational theory, sociology has contributed the concept of role, which is vital in understanding a pervasive aspect of organizational behavior. A *role* is a set of standards, descriptions, norms, or concepts (held by anyone) for the behaviors of a person or a position.[11] Acting out those behaviors is called *role function* or *role performance*. Roles can relate to a variety of factors: physical (age, sex, health); cultural (race, ethnic background, religion, education); economic (rich or poor, employed or unemployed, employer or employee); or political (party member, candidate, elected official).

People are taught to perform roles when they begin the socialization process, and they continue to learn and change roles throughout their lives, at any given moment playing several roles at once (citizen, spouse, parent, wage earner, professional association officer, community leader, etc.). For roles provide a means by which individuals can interact in such social contexts as families, friendship groups, work groups, and community life.

A difference exists, however, between *role concept* and *person concept*. Role concept pertains to an individual's performance in a single role; that is, a generalization has been made about a population of persons who hold the same position, and there is intragroup consensus on the behavioral characteristics of that position.[12] Person concept pertains to an individual's performance in a variety of roles. Thus, a health educator who plans and conducts health-education activities as part of a set of expected behaviors performed by health educators exemplifies the role concept. That one health educator may perform some of the activities more or less effectively than others exemplifies the person concept.

Sociologists and psychologists have made many significant contributions to role theory, examining such issues as the phases and processes of socialization, interdependencies among individuals, the organization and characteristics of social positions, the processes of conformity and sanctioning, the specialization of performance and division of labor.[13] Only those topics having the greatest relevance for health education will here be discussed, however, and these include role consensus, conflict, and negotiation; role specialization, structuring, and exchange; role clarification and integration; and Transactional Analysis.

Consensus, conflict, and negotiation *Role consensus* exists when a particular view of a role is shared commonly by everyone concerned, including the one who is performing it. It also exists when several people who have the same role behave in the same way.[14] Health educators must use their skills to help individuals attain role consensus without relinquishing principles that are important to them.

When perceptions differ about a role and the role player experiences a sense of ambivalence, confusion, or anxiety, *role conflict* exists. Although role conflict can serve as a source of motivation for social change,[15] it can also endanger institutional stability. Health educators must therefore help committee or team members to resolve role conflicts in nondestructive ways. Avoiding the issue is not a satisfactory solution.

Studies have suggested that three factors may influence how role conflict is resolved: recognition of the legitimacy of role expectations, perception of the sanctions that others may apply, and the individual's ability to respond differentially to legitimacy and sanctions.[16] In any case, the strategy for resolving role conflict is to work toward consensus through the process of *role negotiation*, either by changing some aspect of the conflict-causing behavior or by helping team members to reach agreement on a common concept.

Specialization, structuring, and exchange Although working for common ends, all groups may exhibit some degree of behavioral differentiation. *Role specialization* occurs when increased knowledge, skills, and experience have the effect of limiting a role to its more complex functions, a process that has dramatically altered the health-care field in recent years. *Division of labor* occurs as particular complements of specializations arise.[17] As members of a health team, for example, the board trustee, administrator, physician, nurse, health educator, occupational therapist, and social worker all have specializations and contribute in different ways through sharing the common goal of resolving problems that confront the team.

When the introduction of a new technology makes a role obsolete, or when new roles must be created to accommodate needed functions, *role structuring* (or restructuring) often occurs. This may take the form of developing a new role for the operation of new equipment, of redesigning work for those whose normal job roles are dull, of extending through others the functions of a scarce and costly resource (as the functions of a physician may be extended through a physician assistant or nurse practitioner), or of designing careers for the disadvantaged and unemployed.

When the functions of one role are needed to support the functions of another, *role exchange* takes place. In this respect, teams may be seen as organized sets of role exchanges. According to Oscar Oeser and Frank Harary, the rules or norms laid down by the group take absolute precedence over an individual's idiosyncratic modes of behaving.[18] Thus, when a health educator who wants to develop pamphlets and posters learns that colleagues prefer other types of educational services, the decision will more often favor the position of the group than the position of the dissenting individual.

Clarification and integration   In a team setting, especially, confusion and conflict may result when an individual who must perform several different roles does not distinguish clearly among them—as when a physician who provides services at a clinic is also the clinic's administrator—and when other team members are uncertain about which role is dominant at any given time. In this situation, *role clarification*—letting others know which role is being performed—is essential, especially if role expectations are likely to be confused. Assisting in role clarification is an important function of a health educator in a team setting.

When an individual performs numerous roles, keeping the roles organized so as to reduce intrapersonal confusion and conflict is the task of *role integration*. People whose separate roles are integrated function effectively because they are able to contain their diversity within a unified self rather than acting as separate selves unable to manage the separateness well.

Transactional Analysis   In recent years a body of specialized theory and practice has been built upon understanding and analyzing individual personality development as it is expressed through role relationships. Conducted as part of a therapeutic treatment approach, Transactional Analysis (TA) is especially useful in patient education, family or group therapy, team building, and resolving interpersonal conflicts within organizational settings.[19]

TA focuses on the parent-adult-child states of personality development and their structural interrelationships. A healthy relationship is said to exist when two adults can interact at the adult ego level. When adults interact at the parent-child level, as in the boss-employee, teacher-student, or old-young relationships, transactions become distorted and conflicted. Treatment consists of helping persons to become aware of these states in their role concepts and behaviors in order to change them to constructive adult-adult transactions.

TA has heightened awareness of the "games people play," of the need for "strokes" (praise and reward), of "life scripts" and how they are sometimes compulsively acted out, of manipulative roles, time structuring, adult ethics, and other concepts. Within the context of education, not therapy, these concepts can greatly benefit health educators in their relationships with patients and consumers, students and leaders, and members of health teams.

Leadership theory

Leadership theory builds onto role theory, adding factors that are unique enough to merit scrutiny in their own right. Indeed, the role of the leader in various aspects of social interaction has probably been studied more extensively and defined in more ways than any other role concept. Health education must be acutely aware of leadership issues if it is to assist people in determining how their health needs can best be met. To this end, the following discussion will focus in turn on eight general characteristics of leadership, on styles of leadership, and on leadership training for organizational purposes.

Characteristics Launor Carter has identified five distinct characteristics that apply to organizational and social leadership as well as to group leadership, which was the subject of his study. According to Carter:

1. A leader is designated as such by other group members (a concept that says nothing about leadership characteristics, though it does indicate that members can identify their leader).
2. A leader is a focus of group behaviors around whom members polarize, who receives more communications and has more influence than the others on the group's decisions.
3. A leader is able to direct the group toward its goals by helping to

clarify these goals and by preventing the group from straying in other directions.

4. A leader engages in leadership behaviors that may differ according to the group's purposes.

5. A leader exercises the greatest influence on the group's performance. Insofar as each member may be able to influence performance to the extent of being perceived as a temporary leader, there may not be a single leader as such. In this sense, leadership is situational, changing as conditions change and providing the special leadership resources needed by the group at any given time.[20]

To Carter's five characteristics, Marvin Shaw has added two more.

6. A leader occupies a designated position of leadership that is recognized outside the group as well as within it (e.g., president of a company, administrator of a hospital, dean of a school, etc.).

7. A leader has the support of group members and is able to influence the group's direction, regardless of its goals, without recourse to external authority.[21]

A final characteristic that is highly evident in some aspects of health care, and in other systems as well, should also be noted.

8. A leader possesses special knowledge and skills that other members need in order to carry out their own tasks (e.g., the surgeon on the heart-transplant team, the physician in the diagnostic clinic, etc.).

Health educators generally perform facilitating roles in groups or teams. Helping to clarify leadership roles is among their most important functions.

Styles Although much early research reflected the view that people become leaders because of certain inherent traits, relationships between the two were eventually found to be inconsistent. In general, however, according to Shaw, leaders exemplify traits related to ability, sociability, and motivation more than do other members of the group.[22] *Ability* denotes intelligence and scholarship, verbal facility, situational insight, knowledge of how to get things done, and adaptability. *Sociability* means activity and social participation, cooperativeness, popularity, and dependability in exercising responsibility. *Motivation* means initiative and persistence.

Nevertheless, different leaders exhibit very different styles of leadership which can greatly affect the functioning of groups, organizations, and larger social systems. A pioneering study of autocratic, democratic, and laissez-faire styles of leadership conducted by Kurt Lewin and his associates in 1939 showed the democratic style to be the most effective in changing attitudes,[23] though it is easier to be a good autocratic leader because it is easier to issue orders than to utilize the resources of group members effectively.

Numerous studies have also been devoted to comparing directive and nondirective styles of leadership. Among their conclusions are two of importance to organizations. (1) Nondirective leadership arouses more affirmative reactions toward the group than does directive leadership, and (2) Directive-led groups are usually more productive than nondirective-led groups, although there is sometimes no significant difference between the two in relation to group productivity.[24]

Training   In recent years the behavioral and management sciences have given considerable attention to leadership training in an effort to improve the functioning of leaders. To this end, four strategies have been indicated: (1) changing the leader's position of power from one job to another, (2) changing the task structure to fit a leader's style, (3) changing the leader's style, or (4) helping members to understand and accommodate the leader's style.

Whereas such training once concentrated almost exclusively on helping leaders to identify and change their leadership styles, the current emphasis is on improving the relationships between leaders and members. For research and training alike indicate that leaders are as dependent on the group for help in leading as the group is dependent on its leader for leadership. Unless the needs of both are met, either or both will become unhappy with the relationship.

In corroboration, Robert Tannenbaum and Warren Schmidt have studied a range of organizational leadership behavior in which the "total area of freedom shared by manager and nonmanager is constantly redefined by interactions between them and the forces in the environment"[25] (see figure 6).

New modes of behavior indicate that: (1) both managers and nonmanagers can be governing forces in their group's environment, contributing to the definition of the total area of freedom; (2) a group can function with managerial functions shared by group members; and (3) a group as a unit can be delegated authority and assume responsibility within a larger organizational context.

A fairly high degree of subordinate-centered behavior is associated with improving the quality of managerial decisions, raising the level of employee motivation, enhancing organizational teamwork and morale, furthering the individual development of employees, and increasing subordinates' readiness to accept change. Managers can permit subordinates greater freedom if the latter have an understanding and sense of identification with the organization's goals coupled with relatively high needs for independence, an inter-

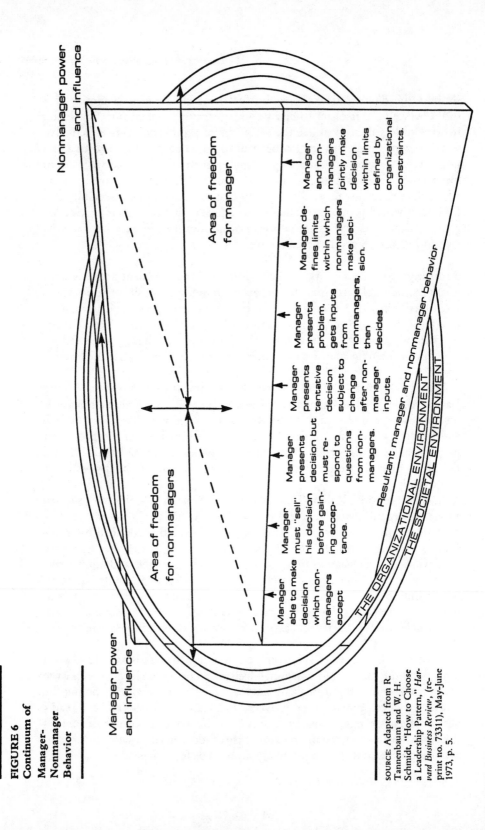

FIGURE 6
Continuum of Manager-Nonmanager Behavior

Manager power and influence

Nonmanager power and influence

Area of freedom for nonmanagers

Area of freedom for manager

Manager able to make decision which nonmanagers accept.

Manager must "sell" his decision before gaining acceptance.

Manager presents decision but must respond to questions from nonmanagers.

Manager presents tentative decision subject to change after nonmanager inputs.

Manager presents problem, gets inputs from nonmanagers, then decides.

Manager defines limits within which nonmanagers make decision.

Manager and nonmanagers jointly make decision within limits defined by organizational constraints.

Resultant manager and nonmanager behavior

THE ORGANIZATIONAL ENVIRONMENT

THE SOCIETAL ENVIRONMENT

SOURCE: Adapted from R. Tannenbaum and W. H. Schmidt, "How to Choose a Leadership Pattern," *Harvard Business Review*, (reprint no. 73311), May–June 1973, p. 5.

est or stake in the problem at hand, sufficient knowledge and experience to deal with the problem, an expectation of sharing in decision making, a readiness to assume responsibility for decision making, and a relatively high tolerance for ambiguity.

Domain theory

Business, industrial, and human-services organizations have a number of features in common. All, for example, have inputs, outputs, and environmental constraints; physical facilities and technologies; managers, nonmanagerial employees, and customers. But they also differ in significant ways, and these differences had to be recognized and studied before a body of theory could be developed that dealt with the unique features of the human-services organization.

Weisbord's Three-System Theory To the question of why standard organization development practices work better for industry than for medical school organizations, Marvin Weisbord answers, in essence, that medical centers have few of the formal organizational characteristics of industrial firms, where OD was originally developed and tested. Because scientists and especially physicians are socialized to autonomous, specialized, expert behavior which is antithetical to any but the narrowest industrialized pursuits, much important medical-center activity is unconnected to administrative machinery.

According to Weisbord, health professionals are enmeshed in three concurrent social systems: task, professional identity, and governance (see figure 7). The task system refers to a specific organization of work that seeks to coordinate research, education, and patient care. The professional identity system refers to the medical-science career track on which the status and self-esteem of health professionals depend. The governance system is the network of agencies, boards, and committees that sets standards for the profession.[26]

Each of these systems has its own membership requirements and ground rules; and though each is in some ways at odds with the others, each is nevertheless necessary to the others' functioning. Of the three, however, the governance system is the least influential, which is the reverse of the situation that obtains in industrial organizations; and for this reason alone standard OD theory is inadequate for health service organizations.

Medical schools are increasingly employing health educators for a variety of functions—among them, teaching health education to medical students and participating in curriculum development with regard to the health-education content of medical courses. For them, Weisbord's observations

FIGURE 7
Differences between Industrial and Health-Care Systems

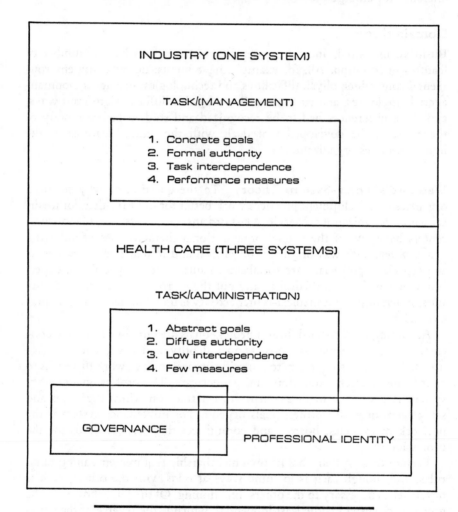

SOURCE: Adapted from M. R. Weisbord, "Why Organization Development Hasn't Worked (So Far) in Medical Centers," *Health Care Management Review*, Spring 1976, p. 20.

should be useful in fostering an understanding of how such organizations behave.

Kouzes-Mico's Domain Theory Domain theory evolved out of work done by Paul Mico and James Kouzes with a variety of human services organizations in the San Francisco Bay Area from 1977 to 1979.[27] Additional insights were provided by Daniel Bell's three-realm theory[28] and Weisbord's three-system theory. Domain theory advances the view that, unlike the traditional business or industrial organization, which can be regarded as a single domain characterized by management principles throughout, the health organization consists of three primary domains—policy, management, and service—each of which has a unique sphere of function or influence and is governed by principles of its own (see figure 8).

The policy domain is the organizational level at which basic policies are formulated. In health-care organizations this domain is occupied by trustees or by people who are either elected or appointed to boards of directors. Like the boards of industrial concerns, they are responsible for the overall direction and functioning of the organization, but there the similarity ends.

- Industrial directors hold ownership in their organizations; health directors do not.
- Industrial directors serve a self-interest; health directors serve the public good.
- Industrial directors earn board membership on the basis of ownership or special influence and can serve indefinitely; health directors are elected or appointed to represent a constituent group for a specified term.
- Industrial directors need only operate within the law and be responsive to it; health directors are usually sanctioned by law to carry out certain mandates.
- Industrial directors are bound by the principles that govern all levels of the organization; health directors are governed by principles different from those governing the management and service domains.
- Industrial directors are engaged in a relatively equitable interaction with the organization's environment; health directors are subject to high environmental impact (federal and state laws and policies, limited financial bases, consumer advocate groups, etc.).
- Industrial directors can operate in comparative anonymity; health directors must operate under public scrutiny.

Because of these factors, boards of directors of health-care organizations operate according to the principles of constituent representation, employing participation and negotiation processes and democratic decision making. The results of their efforts are measured in terms of fairness and equity toward their constituents.

FIGURE 8
The Three Domains of Human Service Organizations

THE ELECTORATE

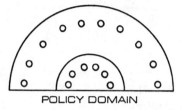

POLICY DOMAIN

Principles: Consent of the Governed
Success Measures: Equity
Structure: Representative
                 Participative
Work Modes: Voting
                   Bargaining
                   Negotiating

DISCORDANCE   DISJUNCTION   CONFLICTS

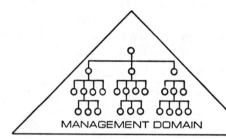

MANAGEMENT DOMAIN

Principles: Hierarchical Control and
                 Coordination
Success Measures: Cost Efficiency
                           Effectiveness
Structure: Bureaucratic
Work Modes: Use of Linear Tech-
                   niques and Tools

DISCORDANCE   DISJUNCTION   CONFLICTS

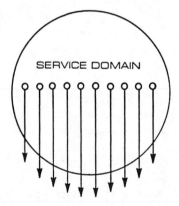

SERVICE DOMAIN

Principles: Autonomy
                 Self-regulation
Success Measures: Quality of Service
                           Good Standards
                           of Practice
Structure: Collegial
Work Modes: Client-specific
                   Problem-solving

SOURCE: Adapted from James M. Kouzes and Paul R. Mico, "Domain Theory: An Introduction to Organizational Behavior in Human Service Organizations," *Journal of Applied Behavioral Science* 15, no. 4 (1979): 458.

The management domain of the health organization operates on essentially the same principles as its business or industrial counterpart, exercising control and coordination from the top down, employing bureaucratic work structures and units as a means of organizing people according to specialized resources, using management tools, and measuring success on the bases of efficiency and productivity.

The service domain consists of professionals and support staff who provide direct services to the organization's patients, clients, or consumers. As previously noted, health professionals are highly specialized and expert in their training, highly identified with their disciplines or professions, highly differentiated in their roles, and highly subject to standards and regulations set by outside professional associations and boards. They operate with great autonomy as they work with their clients and are measured primarily on the basis of the quality of services they provide, although their effectiveness will depend to a considerable extent on patient compliance.

If the health-care organization is to discharge its public mandate, ways must be found to foster interdependent interactions among these three domains. Likert's linking-pin theory can help representatives of each domain to collaborate in keeping their areas linked. Boards should develop policy-making processes that involve the other two domains to a greater extent than is currently the case. Management tools should be modified to provide meaningful exchanges with the other domains. The service domain must develop better feedback mechanisms to keep the other domains informed of its activities. In short, all three domains must make more effective use of interdomain communication processes. Finally, health educators must understand domain theory because their work is likely to differ from one domain to another, and they should be able to bridge into the other domains when crossing over is of assistance.

CHANGING ORGANIZATIONS

General methods

There are many ways of changing organizations, though not all of them reflect the values associated with democratic decision making, participatory management, or planned change.

• In the case of *autocratic direction*, the organization's leader decides what changes are to be made; directives are issued downward, and employees must either comply or face supervisory action.

• *Changes in federal, state, or local laws and regulations* can also effect organizational changes, especially in health-care organizations. In 1975, for example, changes in federal law forced a nationwide disbandment of comprehensive health-planning agencies in favor of the current health-systems agencies.

• *Changes in funding* likewise have an immediate impact on organizations that depend upon external financial resources. The awarding of a federal or state grant can create new organizations or add new programs and staffs to existing ones, just as reducing or terminating grants can do away with new or existing programs. In 1978 California's Proposition 13 changed the structure of property taxation, thereby forcing a major reduction in funds for all public agencies in California that had depended on this source for money.

• *Reorganizing* generally means rearranging units or groupings of organizational personnel and resources. This often occurs when a new leader wants to reshape an organization to conform with a personal image or theory, and it may or may not be done autocratically.

• *Merging* separate organizations into one occurs in the private sector when one large company buys other companies and forms a conglomerate. In the public sector, the federal or state government may decide to merge separate agencies having similar functions into a single new agency. Just as mergers produce organizational change, so breaking a single organization into separate new ones will produce change as well.

• *Decentralization* occurs when agencies serving large geographical territories or widespread populations set up offices near the specific groups they serve, though retaining a central system of authority and resources. *Centralization* may occur when an operation is for some reason unable to manage widely spread components and decides to bring them together into a single location.

• *Mechanization,* or the introduction of new technology, can induce many planned or unplanned organizational changes, not only in personnel roles but in the way employees and clientele alike must use the system if it is to work efficiently.

The difficulty with these methods of change is that none of them draws from a body of organized doctrine; whether they are carried out constructively will depend upon on how they are used by those with the authority to use them. As the following section will demonstrate, organization development differs from these methods in requiring commitment to an applied body of principles and practices. While the methods enumerated here can be conducted with no consideration of OD, OD can include any of them as long as the method is appropriate to the problem at hand.

Organization Development

In organizational terms, *culture* denotes shared assumptions about the norms, standards, or rules that regulate members' behavior. Generally speaking, then, organization development is the application of a long-range planned-change technology to improve the problem-solving and renewal processes by means of which an organization changes its culture; that is, it is designed to strengthen the examination of such processes for the purpose of planning and implementing change efforts.[29] In addition to improving the health of organizations in general, OD can improve the services delivered by health-care organizations in particular. Health educators must collaborate with other members of their organizations as participants in their own OD processes.

History According to Wendell French and Cecil Bell, OD evolved from two primary experiences: (1) the application of laboratory-training insights to industrial organizations and (2) the use of survey research and feedback methodology in workshop settings.[30] From these early experiences came the recognition that external consultants and internal staff must work in collaboration to improve organizational problem solving. Robert Blake, Herbert Shepard, and Jane Mouton are credited with coining the term *organization development*.[31]

In the course of conducting a group dynamics workshop for Connecticut's State Interracial Commission in 1946, Kurt Lewin, Leland Bradford, Kenneth Benne, and Ronald Lippitt became fascinated by group dynamics and gradually expanded their findings into a methodology of sensitivity training. Over the next decade they and other trainers began to conduct T-group (training-group) programs in business, industry, school, and other organizational systems but experienced great frustration in attempting to adapt laboratory theories about individual growth to organizational problem solving.

In 1957 Douglas McGregor took a step toward bridging this gap by helping Union Carbide to establish a small internal consulting group (later called an organization development group) for assisting its line managers. In 1957, too, Herbert Shepard joined Esso's Employee Relations Department and during the next few years launched three experiments that resulted in the development of an action-planning method: an interview survey–diagnostic approach was discussed with top executives and followed by a series of three-day workshops for all members of management. Further experience firmly established the importance of two factors: the requirement of active involvement in planning by top management and the need for on-the-job application in the work setting.

The use of attitude-survey research and data feedback enabled workshop groups to deal with the organization's overall problems. Such action-research efforts began at the Research Center for Group Dynamics, founded by Kurt Lewin at the Massachusetts Institute of Technology (MIT) in 1945.

In addition to Lewin, prime movers included Marian Ladke, Leon Festinger, Ronald Lippitt, Douglas McGregor, John R. P. French, Jr., Dorwin Cartwright, and Morton Deutsch at MIT, and, later, Floyd Mann and Rensis Likert at the University of Michigan.

Character and methods OD is a form of applied behavioral science using both theoretical and practical doctrine derived from social psychology, social anthropology, sociology, psychiatry, economics, and political science for the purpose of initiating a strategy of normative reeducation leading to organizational change. It takes a systems approach to organizations, emphasizing the interrelatedness of organizational phenomena and dynamics. It takes a data-based approach to planned change, inculcating in organization members a conviction of the validity and desirability of data about the system's own culture and processes. It is experience-based, holding that people best learn how to do things by actually doing them.

An ongoing interactive process consisting of interventions in the client system and of clients' responses to the interventions, OD emphasizes the importance of goals and plans, as well as of structuring learning activities to improve goal-setting and planning skills. Its activities focus on intact work teams on the principle that most organizational work is done through such teams; hence, changing their culture, processes, relationships, and ways of performing tasks is a way of achieving lasting improvement in the organization.[32]

Finally, OD employs five basic intervention methods: team building, conflict management, technostructural, data feedback, and training. [33]

1. Team building, which includes team organization and agenda building, involves a continuing diagnosis of the effectiveness of a group's work procedures and interpersonal relationships.

2. Conflict management means examining the effectiveness of individual and group interrelationships, exposing unproductive conflict, and seeking ways of maintaining collaboration.

3. Technostructural interventions are based on the assumption that since organizational life and functioning are regulated by forms of organizational structure and by technological and environmental constraints, organizational change may be mediated by such factors as patterns of work flow, hierarchical relationships, formal communication systems, division of labor, and inventory systems.

4. Data feedback can be used as an effective intervention for change by feeding data back to those who generated them, thereby stimulating an action-planning follow-up.

5. Training is based on the assumption that organizations improve when members are trained to perform their work proficiently.

Two specific methods

Health educators can utilize several of the above methods either separately from or within the OD context, and the latter is clearly preferable. Because establishing conditions hospitable to an organization-wide OD effort is difficult, however, two methods in particular merit closer attention.

Team building Determining how to organize personnel resources for better delivery of increasingly complex and comprehensive services is often a problem for health organizations. Although forming health-care teams has been helpful, organizational change should focus on the organization as a whole rather than on groups alone, for groups or teams do not operate in a vacuum. The point of team building is to enable the encompassing organization to change in ways that will enable it to attain its overall goals.

Team building is primarily directed toward the maintenance of interdependent collaboration. Methods include changing organizational structure and procedures; changing team norms; introducing training to improve role performance and goal-setting, communication, decision-making, and problem-solving processes; attempting creative management of conflict, and using data feedback to clarify and facilitate all these efforts.

The modification of group dynamics should also be guided by concentration on the team's organizational context. This is likely to involve placing great emphasis on the maintenance of interpersonal relationships, on the team's task accomplishments, and on whatever technical assistance the team may need for restructuring sociotechnical and normative procedures in order to carry out its tasks. OD is an important technical specialty today, and much can be learned about its technology by those who are involved in team building.

Conflict management The process of change often creates conflicts between persons and their roles, between groups, and within or between organizations; for conflict is intrinsic to change, and effective management of the one is impossible without effective management of the other. Five general principles help to illuminate this interdependency.

1. Conflict occurs when persons or groups need one another to meet needs or attain goals because the interdependency produces expectations that are used to test mutual commitment and performance. These expectations may be assumed rather than stated; but once de-

veloped and perceived as unmet, they produce responses that can lead to conflict.

2. Conflict occurs among interdependent parties when the resources needed by some are inadequate to meet the needs of all and when this inadequacy is perceived as constituting a threat to any party's survival.

3. Conflict occurs when value differences are not mutually understood or mutually acceptable.

4. Conflict occurs when there are pressures to pursue multiple goals or to become more comprehensive in the performance of functions that were once regarded as basic and simple.

5. Conflict occurs where there is a major imbalance in the power and influence held and exercised by interdependent parties. For the desire to achieve power is invariably countered by the defense to hold it, and the resulting struggle frequently results in win-lose interactions.

Because conflict *is* inherent in change, it should be accepted and put to use in constructive problem solving. First, it should be recognized that many aspects of conflict are constructive and desirable. Among other things, conflict provides opportunities for differences to be aired, for solutions to be explored, and for individuals and groups to test themselves and make greater use of their resources. It helps to establish individual or group identity, to stabilize human relationships, and to build cohesiveness within groups. Certainly, it is at the root of all significant personal, group, organizational, and social change.

Second, the cause of the conflict must be understood so that an appropriate problem-solving approach can be developed. Third, the strategy employed for conflict resolution must be a win-win strategy, or one that is most constructive for all parties. Fourth, the ground rules for resolving the conflict must be understood and accepted by all parties. Negotiating ground rules is probably the most important single factor in creating conditions for a win-win approach. Fifth, a third-party resource should be available to assist in conflict resolution lest the parties to the conflict lose sight of rational management processes. Finally, the conflict-resolution learnings should be discussed, understood, and assimilated for future personal and organizational improvements.

Whether caught up in conflict processes as members of their own organizational teams or helping others to deal with conflict, health educators will find themselves increasingly involved in conflict management, which, properly conducted, can provide a health basis for personal growth and creative problem solving.

The health field has many ways of facilitating organizational change both outside and within its own confines. Health educators can help to enhance the overall humanness of health care, for example, by redirecting the values of health workers toward total care of the total patient, by helping patients to take better charge of their own health, and by facilitating greater citizen participation in health activities. Health-services delivery can be improved by focusing on primary care, family health, and patient education; by enlarging the roles and functions of ambulatory services and primary care centers, designing meaningful roles for new categories of health workers, and promoting interdisciplinary team building.

Finally, health-systems management can be improved by means of reorganization wherever necessary; by the introduction of more effective tools and processes, including training in management skills, role negotiation, and conflict management; and by making more effective domain exchanges as well as better linkages with other health organizations. For health-care organizations are open systems, interacting with their environment and highly susceptible to environmental impact. The health-care organization is but one unit of a larger community or social system which, as the next chapter will show, is itself a focus of behavioral study and change.

REFERENCES

1. For a good description of these studies, see R. L. Durbin and W. H. Springall, *Organization and Administration of Health Care*, pp. 11–14.
2. D. McGregor, *The Human Side of Enterprise*.
3. F. Herzberg, B. Mausner, and B. Snyderman, *The Motivation to Work*.
4. R. Beckhard, "ABS in Health-Care Systems: Who Needs It?" *Journal of Applied Behavioral Science* 10, no. 1 (1974): 93–106.
5. D. Katz and R. L. Kahn, *The Social Psychology of Organizations*, pp. 14–29.
6. Ibid., p. 16.
7. A. K. Rice, "Productivity and Social Organization in an Indian Weaving Shed: An Examination of Some Aspects of the Sociotechnical System of an Experimental Automatic Loom Shed," *Human Relations* 6 (1953): 297–329.
8. G. C. Homans, *The Human Group*, pp. 81–155.
9. R. Likert, *New Patterns of Management*; and idem, *The Human Organization*.
10. E. H. Schein, *Organizational Psychology*, pp. 115–16.
11. B. J. Biddle and E. J. Thomas, eds., *Role Theory*, pp. 11–12.
12. W. Emmerich, "Family Role Concepts of Children Ages Six to Ten," *Child Development* 32 (1961): 609–24.
13. Biddle and Thomas, *Role Theory*, p. 17.
14. Ibid., p. 12.

15. T. Parsons, "Role Conflicts and the Genesis of Deviance," in Biddle and Thomas, *Role Theory*, p. 276.

16. Ibid., p. 274.

17. Ibid., p. 40.

18. O. A. Oeser and F. Harary, "Role Structures: A Description in Terms of Graph Theory," in Biddle and Thomas, *Role Theory*, p. 95.

19. E. Berne, *Transactional Analysis in Psychotherapy;* idem, *The Structure ana Dynamics of Organizations and Groups;* idem, *Games People Play;* T. A. Harris, *I'm OK—You're OK;* and G. A. Holland, "Transactional Analysis," in *Current Psychotherapies,* ed. R. Corsini, pp. 353–99.

20. L. F. Carter, "On Defining Leadership," in *Group Relations at the Crossroads,* ed. M. Sherif and M. O. Wilson, pp. 262–65.

21. M. E. Shaw, *Group Dynamics,* pp. 272–79.

22. Ibid., pp. 274–75.

23. K. Lewin, R. Lippitt, and R. K. White, "Patterns of Aggressive Behavior in Experientially Created Social Climates," *Journal of Social Psychology* 10 (1939): 271–99; and R. Lippitt and R. K. White, "The 'Social Climate' of Children's Groups," in *Child Behavior and Development,* ed. R. G. Barker, J. Kownin, and H. Wright, pp. 485–508.

24. Shaw, *Group Dynamics,* pp. 278–79.

25. R. Tannenbaum and W. H. Schmidt, "How To Choose a Leadership Pattern," *Harvard Business Review* (reprint no. 73311), May–June 1973, pp. 1–10.

26. M. R. Weisbord, "Why Organization Development Hasn't Worked (So Far) in Medical Centers," *Health Care Management Review,* Spring 1976, pp. 17–28

27. J. M. Kouzes and P. R. Mico, "Domain Theory: An Introduction to Organizational Behavior in Human Services Organizations," *Journal of Applied Behavioral Science* 15, no. 4 (1979): 449–69. The work was done through the Joint Center for Human Services Development, School of Social Work, San Jose State University, in three separate but related one-year projects funded by the U.S. Department of Health, Education and Welfare's Social and Rehabilitation Service. The clients were the health and social services agencies of a twelve-county Bay Area/University Service Area, all of which were engaged in planning and implementing the integration of their human services and resources.

28. D. Bell, *The Cultural Contradictions of Capitalism.*

29. W. L. French and C. H. Bell, *Organization Development,* pp. 15–20.

30. Ibid., pp. 21–29.

31. Ibid., pp. 23–24.

32. Ibid., pp. 15–20.

33. W. W. Burke and H. A. Hornstein, eds., *The Social Technology of Organization Development,* p. 1.

7
Programs in organizational health education

Of a variety of health-education programs that are currently producing organizational change, three types have been selected for discussion here: occupational, school, and hospital health education, all of which have been established as program priorities by either the federal Bureau of Health Education[1] or the National Center for Health Education.[2]

OCCUPATIONAL HEALTH EDUCATION

There can no longer be any question that the workplace is responsible for a great many safety and health problems which contribute in turn to low industrial productivity, huge monetary costs, worker alienation, and labor-management disputes.[3] This section will focus on two factors that have direct bearing on the alleviation of these problems: the Occupational Safety and Health Act of 1970 and current organizational approaches to dealing with alcoholism.

Occupational Safety and Health Act

Much occupational health–education activity today is directly related to the 1970 Occupational Safety and Health Act (OSHA), which imposes on virtually all employers the duty of providing a place of employment that is free of recognized hazards to human health. Passage of this act has brought about a great increase in the dissemination of information to employers on recognizing, monitoring, and controlling occupational hazards, and the main providers of this information have been management groups, trade associations, and insurance carriers.

The Conference Board and the Industrial Health Foundation, two trade agencies that service industrial organizations, regularly disseminate their research findings among member companies. In 1971 the National Association of Manufacturers sponsored a nationwide closed-circuit teleconference on OSHA requirements that reached more than 10,000 executives through whom it was presumed indirectly to benefit employees as well.

Some unions and a few public-interest groups are also attempting to provide workers with vitally needed education concerning their legal rights under OSHA, with technical information on work-related disease, and with training in the identification and monitoring of workplace hazards. Worker self-help programs are being established along with regional and national training centers and programs.[4] Increasingly more companies and unions are employing health educators to assist in the organization and development of safety and health education.

The workplace is an ideal setting for health education, not only because workers are more willing to participate in such programs at the work site but because communication is easier, surveillance and follow-up are simplified, and travel costs are eliminated. For gathering data on which to develop health-education programs in the workplace, Clarence Pearson provides the following guidelines.

• Listen carefully to employees during group discussion, assessing their level of health awareness and knowledge to produce the baseline data necessary for the development of a health-education program. Analyze available data on accidents and absenteeism, and feed all data back to employees to increase both their knowledge and their participation in the educational program.

• Analyze employees' use of the company's medical-department services to discover whether utilization is cost-effective. Conduct a longitudinal survey of the medical department's reports to discover any trends that indicate change.

• Determine the degree of employee participation in community health projects. Study medical claims, evaluate the reports of local physicians and available morbidity and mortality data, to identify problem areas.

• Conduct research experiments to determine which intervention strategies will be most cost-effective for the company.[5]

Two approaches to alcoholism

Problem drinking costs U.S. industry from $10 billion to $20 billion annually, the cost of each problem drinker running an average of $3,000 per year in accidents, sick pay, lost production, and (especially in the case of executives) bad judgment.[6] Although many industries have programs dealing with alcoholism, the two selected for presentation here are especially useful in showing how threat can modify behavior.

The IAMAW program Members of the International Association of Machinists and Aerospace Workers range from unskilled floor sweepers to highly trained mechanics. Of nearly 1 million members, between 40,000 and 50,000 are regarded as problem drinkers or alcoholics whose abuse of alcohol harms not only their companies but the union as well. In response to this problem, the union has formulated a joint union-management policy toward alcohol abuse, urging its local and district units to encourage active participation in alcohol rehabilitation programs throughout the industry.

Four key clauses in the union's contract illustrate its position on the problem. The first clause states:

> The unions and company jointly recognize alcoholism as an illness which can be successfully treated. It is also recognized that it is for the best interests of the employee, the unions, and the company that this illness be treated and controlled under the existing collective bargaining contractual relationship. This policy relates to those instances of alcohol abuse causing poor attendance and unsatisfactory performance on the job.[7]

Alcohol abuse is thus seen as a medical, not a moral, problem and is dealt with only insofar as it affects the worker's job performance, a tangible basis for intervention upon which both union and management can agree. The clause reflects the view that a problem drinker can best be motivated to become rehabilitated by the threat of job loss. By agreeing to use this threat as a motivational tool, union and management avoid working at cross-purposes in the grievance and arbitration processes.

The results of the program demonstrate its effectiveness. The union reports that 70–75 percent of those referred to treatment through the program are rehabilitated, whereas only 30–35 percent of workers' family members who voluntarily enter treatment achieve recovery.[8] Although this approach might raise ethical questions for health educators, who prefer voluntary participation over the use of threat, what is significant about it from the viewpoint of organizational change is that union and management are required to agree on its use.

The second key clause states:

A joint labor-management program will be established for the purpose of helping the individual with this disease to recover. The program is to be designed for rehabilitation and not elimination of the employee. Any program administrators (by whatever title) will be selected with equal representation from management and the union, and will be allowed sufficient time at full pay to perform their program duties.[9]

This emphasizes that, although the threat to job security may be used, the program is not to be punitive unless the employee fails to cooperate, a stricture that may minimize ethical concerns for health educators. Further, in appointing specifically designated program administrators instead of using an advisory committee, it assures the kind of aggressive line implementation that a staff committee structure cannot provide. These administrators perform the tasks of training-shop stewards and foremen, setting up referral systems, investigating community resources, and developing inplant counselors if needed—in short, amply demonstrating the open-system concept of organization.

The third key clause deals with two vital elements, health-insurance coverage and confidentiality.

Any employee who participates in this program will be entitled to all of the rights and benefits provided to other employees who are sick, in addition to specific services and assistance which this program may provide. An individual's participation in an alcoholism program will remain confidential; medical records, if any, will be protected in the same confidential manner as other medical records, and will not be released by the doctor or medical department without written permission from the individual concerned.[10]

Alcoholics are far more prone to disease and death than are nonalcoholics: they are two to three times more susceptible to heart attacks, asthma, ulcers, cirrhosis of the liver, and hypertension, six times likelier to die of pneumonia or influenza, and ten times likelier to have fatal accidents. Because the cost of treatment for these secondary illnesses usually far exceeds the cost of treatment aimed specifically at the habituating disease, health-insurance coverage for the latter saves the company money.

Moreover, active participation by the union has the added benefit of reassuring white-collar problem drinkers. Afraid to reveal their difficulties to upper management, they will often voluntarily seek help from union counselors because they feel that this assures them greater anonymity and confidentiality.

The final key clause restates the need for insurance coverage for special treatment facilities: "Insurance coverage for employees and dependents will cover such facilities and programs as hospitals, detoxification centers, rehabilitation centers, and counseling programs when agreed upon by both parties of this agreement."[11]

The union has found that a program established along these lines, and having the full support of union and management, can achieve significant success. First, however, management must be convinced that rehabilitation programs are economically sound investments, while unions must overcome a tendency to downgrade the problem drinker. Health educators can be most useful in helping both organizations to establish and conduct such programs.

The INSIGHT program For another example of the open-system concept, a number of outside counseling and referral services make programs available to businesses that seek alternatives to setting up programs of their own. In one such instance, a division of the Kennecott Copper Company in Utah employed 8,000 workers of whom an estimated 7 percent suffered from problem drinking, at an annual cost to management of approximately $500,000.[12]

The company contracted an outside service to construct, staff, and administer a "troubled employee" program to help not only these workers but those having other problems as well. It was found that this broad-brush approach, by eluding the stigma attached to alcohol and drug problems specifically, enabled the program to reach problem cases earlier than do most alcohol programs.

Operating twenty-four hours a day, seven days a week, the program was built into the company's normal disciplinary procedure. At the first warning of diminished job performance the employee was advised to phone the program for referral to a staff person or to a community resource for discussion and counseling. This advice was repeated, and communicated to the program, at each further disciplinary step. If the problem persisted, the employee was threatened with dismissal unless he or she contacted and cooperated with the program. To follow-up on referrals, the program maintained working relationships with community social-service agencies. All calls and records were kept confidential.

In the meantime, the program provided the company with educational material and conducted seminars for supervisors and union personnel. Both management and the company's nineteen unions supported the program and believed that the confidentiality ensured by use of an outside resource contributed greatly to its success.

Conceptually uncomplicated and low in costs, this model can provide service in areas where unions and management are unwilling to establish their own programs. Indeed, according to the program description, the concept

> ... has applicability in any area where community organizations exist. We are convinced it can be effectively promulgated by any large organization or a consortium of smaller ones. The cost need not exceed fifty to seventy-five cents per month per employee. So long as the program embodies the concept of voluntarism, confidentiality, qualified administrators, and is service oriented, it should succeed and pay handsome dividends to all who participate.[13]

A detailed study showed that, as a result of the program, attendance improved by 52 percent, weekly indemnities decreased by 74.6 percent, and health, medical, and surgical costs decreased by 55.4 percent. In contrast, a control study of nonparticipants showed a 5.68 percent increase in absenteeism and a 1.46 percent increase in health, medical, and surgical costs.[14]

Such a program works because it creates awareness of a problem, educates, necessitates organization, refers, and follows-up. For health educators, who are trained to provide these essential services, the greatest remaining problem is to resolve their own ethical difficulties concerning the appropriate use of threat as a motivational tool.

SCHOOL HEALTH EDUCATION

At the state level

When the American School Health Association conducted a survey in 1976 to determine the current status of school health programs at the state level, only sixteen states legally required comprehensive school health education: Arkansas, Florida, Hawaii, Illinois, Maine, Maryland, Michigan, Nebraska, New Jersey, New York, Oregon, South Carolina, Tennessee, Texas, Virginia, and Wisconsin. In Alaska, California, Colorado, Delaware, Idaho, and New Mexico, school districts were given the option of deciding whether to provide comprehensive health-education programs. Kentucky, Massachusetts, Missouri, North Dakota, and Utah had mandated certain individual subject areas, with an overall result resembling comprehensive programs.[15] The subjects most frequently required by state legislation are listed in table 6.

In some states—among them, Arizona, Delaware, Georgia, New Mexico, and North Carolina—permissive state legislation made various

TABLE 6
State-mandated Subjects in School Health Education

Subject	Number of States
Use of Drugs, Alcohol, and Tobacco	35
Safety	16
Mental Health	13
Diseases and Disease Conditions	13
Nutrition	11
Community Health	10
Personal Health	10
Venereal Disease*	8
Environmental Health	8
Consumer Health Education	8
Family Life/Sex	7
Dental Health/Oral Hygiene	7
Growth and Development	6
First Aid	6
Anatomy and Physiology	5
Health Careers	4

SOURCE: A. S. Castile and S. J. Jerrick, *School Health in America: A Survey of State School Health Programs* (Kent, Ohio: American School Health Association, 1976), pp. 4–5.
*May be included in other states as part of instruction on community health, communicable disease, personal health, or family life/sex education.

subject offerings an option for local school-district officials; also, some local school districts had legislation that took precedence over state law. Ambiguity concerning what specifically constitutes health education caused some health-instruction content to be included as part of other courses, such as physical education, home economics, general science, or biology.

Finally, although various subjects may not be required in some states, this does not mean that they are prohibited from inclusion in the curriculum. Louisiana alone had a statute declaring that "no instruction is permitted dealing with the human reproductive system as it pertains to human sexual intercourse. Not only is instruction forbidden but no survey, test, or quiz may be given about personal beliefs in sex or religion."[16] Only three states made no provision at the state level for any area of health education whatsoever.

Thirty-two states had standards for the environmental quality of schools, and the state department of health was normally responsible for enforcing the standards, which ranged from minimal requirements for toilet facilities to specific requirements for all phases of the school environment. In most cases, however, there were no standards requiring schools to employ professional sanitarians, whose services were usually supplied instead by local health departments.

The American School Health Association survey revealed that a great deal of change is needed in American school systems. To this end, a unique program—the School Health Curriculum Project—has been developed and is currently having a great impact on local school districts throughout the nation. Although the project is in many respects a broad social-change endeavor, our primary interest here is in how it works within individual organizations.

School Health Curriculum Project

At a time when teenage smoking, drinking, drug abuse, pregnancy, venereal and dental disease, and poor nutritional habits were reaching crisis proportions, the School Health Curriculum Project arose in response to concern about the need for better health education in elementary schools especially. The project was to be carried out in three three-year phases:

1. Developing and testing a health curriculum model for grades five, six, and seven
2. Developing a teacher/administrator training model and establishing the health curriculum in ten distant school districts
3. Establishing regional training resources and testing community-support mechanisms. [17]

The health curriculum model consists of four intensive units of study, one at each grade-level.* Organized around a given system of the human body and all that impinges on its health, each unit (occupying eight to ten weeks per school year) is comprehensive in its coverage of health-education content and strives for maximal integration with other basic curricular areas.

Each grade-level unit is subdivided into the following six phases:

1. Introductory and motivational activities
2. Experiences leading to an appreciation of the body and its systems

---

*When combined with the Primary Grades Health Curriculum Project, a similar project initiated by the Bureau of Health Education and the American Lung Association, units exist for grades kindergarten through seven.

3. Intensive study of a particular system's structure and functioning
4. Study of diseases, disease conditions, and other problems of that system
5. Study of health protection and care and the prevention of systemic problems
6. Reinforcing activities.

Emphasis is placed, in short, on understanding and appreciating the body, developing disease-prevention skills, and encouraging young people to make their own decisions about factors that affect health. Recent revisions have placed less emphasis on a body-system approach than on total health.

The teacher/administrator training model involves about sixty hours of in-depth team training per unit. A team typically includes two classroom teachers and their principal plus one or two additional support personnel, such as nurses, health educators, curriculum supervisors, librarians, or educational materials specialists. Training methods and activities parallel those employed in the classroom curriculum model. Districts usually buy materials on their own, such as three-dimensional models, films, tapes, charts, and texts, and these are arranged in sequential sets that are applicable to pupil desk work, to group projects, or to parent and community participation. Trainees are regularly monitored at each site and are reconvened for a follow-up session about nine months after the initial training.

Next, two classroom examples of each grade-level unit are established in the school district. Following training, the team returns to these classrooms to develop two operating models and must plan further for the training and support of other teachers at the same grade-level within the year. During the following year a second unit is introduced to a different team from a different school; the process is repeated during the third year, and so on. Finally, each district is expected to conduct its own evaluative activity. Evaluation is based on assessing changes in students' attitudes and behaviors, changes in trainees' teaching and administrative practices, and indications of the program's impact on the district or community.

Success in extending this program into the larger community or state setting depends upon two conditions. First, one or several school districts (as represented by administration, curriculum directors, teachers, and health specialists) must evidence interest in it. Second, schools and community agencies must be made aware of the costs involved and have ways of gaining and sustaining financial support. Costs include training subsequent grade-level teams, spreading the training to other district teachers at each grade-level, and providing and supporting district supervision and monitoring teams. If these conditions exist, the project may be introduced at an informal meeting of school and community-agency people. The Bureau of

Health Education can send a qualified person to the district to describe the project further, and visits to a participating school can be arranged.

To date, the model has been introduced into more than 300 districts in thirty-three states. In some states, many districts have been involved; in others, only one. Sites have ranged from large urban to small rural districts, and from relatively wealthy to financially poor schools, with efforts focusing on minority or disadvantaged populations in many instances. Community agencies have offered substantial moral and financial support. Official health agencies, voluntary health organizations, professional societies, school districts, fire departments, and a host of other federal, state, and local organizations have all contributed greatly to the program's introduction and support.

Teacher-training institutions have recently begun to play an important part in participating with the teams, assisting in the spread of training to other district teachers, facilitating regional training, and introducing some of the program's basic concepts and approaches into preservice teacher-training. Graduate credit or salary increment is available to trainees in accord with local policy.

The success of the School Health Curriculum Project is believed to be attributable to its well-organized curriculum, its highly structured and intensive team building, its marshaling of administrative, curricular, and community support, and to the availability of essential resources. Above all, the project is successful in demonstrating the importance of involving those affected by a program in the program's planning.

HOSPITAL HEALTH EDUCATION

Presented earlier as a primary orientation for individual change, patient education presents a focal point for organizational change as well. Here the emphasis is not on providing services to patients but on the hospital's adopting an institution-wide program for patient education. Adopting such a program requires changing many organizational procedures, however. The following pages will offer examples of how these changes can be made, first by discussing organizational change in general and then by examining change in a specific hospital situation.

General organizational change

In early 1976 the Bureau of Health Education brought together administrators and health-education practitioners from a number of hospitals and health-care settings for the purpose of assessing the current state of patient education in the United States.[18] On the basis of studies of several patient-education programs already existing in locations represented at the workshop, a plan emerged for the initiation of such hospital-based programs in general.

It was found, first, that the idea of a patient-education program tends to arise with a concerned board member, administrator, or physician responding to such stimuli as the need for new patient-discharge planning, for professional communications follow-up with health educators, for federal funding, or as a result of the review criteria accompanying a medical-nursing audit by the Joint Commission on Accreditation of Hospitals.[19]

Initiating such a program required broadly based support from medical, nursing, and other staffs but from administrative staffs particularly. Generally, the time span from introducing the idea to starting the program was found to range from nine months to a year, depending upon the institution's size and on whether the chosen director was an inside or outside person. Planning efforts move faster with an inside person—a senior member of a medical or nursing staff, for example—who has a knowledge of existing organizational procedures, climate, and culture. Outside persons who are recruited as coordinators work more slowly because familiarizing themselves with these factors is important in providing continuity of effort, especially where changes in key personnel are involved.

Approaches to program implementation and personnel involvement are likewise variable, depending upon where responsibility for the program is located. If the program is to be the product of a single service, responsibility for it may be vested totally within that service, limiting planning, communications, and decision-making processes solely to those involved in program development. But if all health-care workers are to carry out a health-education function, a coordinated, multidisciplinary team approach is indicated, which means developing these processes throughout the entire hospital system.

In the latter situation, a coordinator, pressured to demonstrate that health education can work quickly, may be enticed into providing direct service to patients instead of assisting others in so doing. But this error can be avoided by establishing basic policies clearly defining health education's role in the institution, specifying the precise mode of its delivery, and involving deliverers in the planning process. The support of top administrative and medical staffs remains necessary in any case.

At first it was generally agreed that a patient-education program should be based on the medical model; that is, professional staff should agree on the educational needs of each patient-service category before attempts are made to adapt resources and procedures or to delegate responsibilities to meet those needs. It has been recognized, however, that the educational approach differs from the medical model in requiring existing staff to change from a treatment to a teaching orientation. Outside ideas may here be useful, although most coordinators prefer having educational material adapted specifically to their situations.

Private physicians are the key figures in referring patients for educational services. In small hospitals, referral tends to arise from a relationship of mutual trust between physicians and educational staff; in larger hospitals it is usually necessary to gain the involvement and support of medical-staff opinion leaders so that they in turn will encourage others to participate. Not everyone involved in patient education is highly trained in educational principles and methods, however, and for this reason staff development must be treated as a separate though related program.

Coordinators must become keenly sensitive to trainees' real needs and concerns because to make hasty assumptions about these is to risk bypassing matters that may later be counterproductive to the program. At the outset of training, for example, it should be clearly determined which methods and skills can be learned through study alone, which require observation and practice, which require intensive training and consultation, and to what extent evaluative measures should be incorporated into program development.

Monitoring and evaluation of patient education are important in enhancing program quality and effectiveness, and methods have ranged from accepting informal subjective judgments to exploring formal, objective data analyses. In general, evaluation requires answering four questions:

1. When is the ongoing education considered to be part of routine care (e.g., knowledge of drugs, dosage, administration, and precautions)?
2. When does the educational content (e.g., the exchange concept for diabetics) considerably exceed requirements for immediate care?
3. When is requiring a continuing practice (e.g., the preparation and administration of insulin) considered to be part of a therapeutic regimen?
4. When does the educational content need social support (e.g., meal preparation, smoking behavior by peers)?[20]

Institutions that utilize problem-oriented medical records can address these questions directly; others may utilize the educational planning and discharge notes that are part of their medical and nursing audits. Conducting experimental studies of educational effectiveness in practice settings has been found to yield ambiguous results because of the difficulty of controlling variables. Experience has shown that programs lasting from three to five years are needed for purposes of accurate measurement.

The competencies required of a patient-education coordinator may vary according to an institution's size and experience with such programs. Generally speaking, the larger or more sophisticated the setting, the more a coordinator must be an effective manager of personnel and resources, capable of participating with other top-level managers in planning, decision-making, and problem-solving functions.

In addition to knowing how to apply the theory and practice of health education to a hospital setting, coordinators must have a knowledge of organizational behavior in order to recruit and supervise staff, to facilitate committee meetings and other group interactions, to interrelate with other health-education resources within the community, and to function as an individual within organizational settings. Finally, to relate well with persons from many different disciplines, they must be able to communicate clearly in both spoken and written forms.

A patient-education program benefits the hospital in several ways. As staff-patient relationships become less hierarchical and more collaborative, patient satisfaction increases, which is important to a hospital in a competitive market. Staff morale improves; the increase in interdisciplinary contacts provides for broader understanding and relationship building between departments; while greater concern for the education of inpatients leads to a similarly increased concern for outpatient and community health education in general.

Budgets have ranged from those supporting only one coordinator and one secretary to those providing large staffs for inpatient, outpatient, and community health-education programs. Although third-party fee reimbursements have made specially organized educational activities possible, such fees have not yet been sufficiently standardized to meet the needs of sound planning and budgeting.

A hospital project

One hospital project initiated in the mid-1960s systematically assessed the educational needs of patients and their families and attempted to determine whether the hospital could meet their needs by developing formalized patient and family education programs using both staff and community resources.[21] For the purpose of obtaining federal funding, a series of meetings was held with the Public Health Service, at which time an important change in perception occurred.

The hospital administrator had originally perceived the program as a mass communication activity to be enacted within a hospital setting, while Public Health Service personnel had viewed it as a patient-oriented educational program. At this juncture, the proposed program became a composite of both. Agreeing on common goals and engaging key personnel from both the hospital and community took eighteen months; additional time was needed to find a qualified, experienced health-education coordinator.

Once on the job, the coordinator took the following seven steps:

1. Formation of an advisory committee composed of representatives of key hospital departments and community agencies
2. Selection of administrative and medical staffs for program legitimacy and support
3. Preliminary assessment of patient-education needs and of existing in-hospital educational programs
4. Development and testing of educational tools, techniques, and a prescription for use by physicians in ordering educational services for their patients
5. Development of direct working relationships with nursing, respiratory therapy, physical therapy, personnel, and public relations staffs
6. Development of collaborative relationships with key community agencies in preparing educational materials for specific programs
7. Development of a strategy for bringing together official and voluntary community agencies to focus jointly on broader health-education needs and opportunities.

The last step came to be known as the Annual Health Education Workshop.

Federal participation in the project was extended for a total of six years and covered two phases, the second phase existing to resolve problems encountered during the first phase. Problems included the need for time to allow for program development, to obtain greater staff involvement and reduce dependency on the coordinator's efforts, to make objectives more specific, and to enable administration to assume financial responsibility for the project. Three programs were initiated in the first, and continued through the second phase: a stroke program, a mastectomy program, and the Annual Health Education Workshop.

The stroke program was designed to provide comprehensive, coordinated care to selected stroke patients under the primary medical supervision of the attending physician but utilizing both hospital and community resources and involving the patient's family as well. After establishing a program framework, an interdisciplinary team was developed and given in-service education. Patient and family education was conducted. Team case conferences were held to discuss team management and educational problems, and activities in community education and relationship building were conducted with other agencies.

An inpatient program under physician referral, the mastectomy program had three purposes: to develop a standardized program for teaching patients about exercises and prosthetic devices, to develop a means of handling referrals to appropriate outside agencies, and to stimulate the formation of educationally oriented self-help groups. A medical advisory committee helped to revise the form and content of the educational prescription for this program. The program itself, developed initially for patients with radical mastectomies, was later expanded to include those having simple mastectomies. Volunteers were eventually recruited and trained to help in the program.

The Annual Health Education Workshop differed from the others in being a community-based nonpatient program. Its planning committee was composed of community health leaders, and, under the coordinator's direction, its focus shifted gradually from education for hospital patients to comprehensive health planning and urban health services.

While these were not the only health-education activities conducted by the project, they were the ones most directly related to organizational behavior and change. For occupational, school, and hospital health-education programs alike have the potential for making a great impact on preventive health behavior if these organizations change their structure and functions to accommodate new programs. Trained in both health education and organizational development, health-education specialists can contribute significantly toward bringing about such change.

REFERENCES

1. U.S., Department of Health, Education and Welfare, Public Health Service, Center for Disease Control, *The Priorities of Section 1502: Papers on the National Health Guidelines. Health Education and Public Law 93–641,* prepared for the Bureau of Health Education by H. G. Ogden, HEW Publication no. 77–641, 1977.

2. D. J. Merwin, "The National Center for Health Education," (Speech presented at National Conference on Hospital-based Patient Education, Chicago, 9–10 August 1976).

3. N. A. Ashford, *Summary of Crisis in the Workplace.*

4. Ibid., pp. 28–29.

5. C. Pearson, "Education for Health in the Workplace" (Paper presented at Tenth International Conference on Health Education, London, England, 2–7 September 1979).

6. S. Cline, *Alcohol and Drugs and Work,* p. 6.

7. Ibid., p. 21.

8. Ibid., p. 22.

9. Ibid.

10. Ibid., pp. 22–23.

11. Ibid., p. 23.

12. Ibid., pp. 32–34.

13. Ibid., pp. 32–33.

14. Ibid., p. 33.
15. A. S. Castile and S. J. Jerrick, *School Health in America*, pp. 3–5.
16. Ibid.
17. Based on a summary prepared by R. L. Davis, U.S., Department of Health, Education and Welfare, Bureau of Health Education, *Focal Points*, February 1976.
18. U.S., Department of Health, Education and Welfare, *Patient Education Workshop* (Atlanta, Ga.: Center for Disease Control, 1976).
19. Ibid., p. 1.
20. Ibid., p. 7.
21. F. B. Fiori, M. de la Vega, and M. J. Vaccaro, "Health Education in a Hospital Setting: Report of a Public Health Service Project in Newark, New Jersey," *Health Education Monographs* 2, no. 1 (Spring 1974): 11–29.

PART THREE
HEALTH EDUCATION AND SOCIAL BEHAVIOR

Having explored the delivery of health-education services from the perspective of the individual and the organization, attention will now be focused on a third target, social behavior. The forces that shape social behavior, and the work that health educators do in helping to change it, are distinctive enough to require examination in their own right. To this end, chapter 8 will enumerate problems in social health behavior; chapter 9 will present various theories of social behavior; and chapter 10 will describe selected programs in social health education.

In these chapters the adjective *social* has reference primarily to the community and the social system. Although *community* is sometimes used in a very general sense—to designate a community of health educators, for example—for the most part it denotes a geographical grouping of people who share similar interests or concerns. *Social system* denotes a larger grouping of people who share similar relationships or beliefs in regard to matters of culture, value, or governance; in this sense, its implications are more spatial than geographical. Finally, the term *macrosystem* implies relationships among many organizations, in this sense more nearly defining the environment with which open-system organizations interact.

8

Problems in social health behavior

SOCIAL FORMS AND FORCES

In the context of social health, the term *social* encompasses both the forms and the forces that affect human behavior. *Forms* denotes the structural groupings of a society—political jurisdictions, communities, trade areas, and macrosystems—all of which identify their populations as sharing certain common needs and interests. *Forces* are the behavioral influences exerted on such populations by a variety of political, economic, and cultural factors.

Political jurisdictions are land areas that have been divided into functional districts for purposes of general or specific governance or taxation. Towns, cities, counties, states, territories, and the nation as a whole are all in some respects general-purpose districts. Special-purpose districts, though they often overlap general-purpose boundaries, are organized around such specific services as water, sewage, air, health, transportation, public utilities, law enforcement, schools, and so forth.

Communities are relatively self-contained populations that live and work in a common setting, sharing common needs, interests, and resources. These groupings are manifested in the form of urban centers or neighborhoods, rural towns, mountain villages, seaports, or other forms not necessarily defined by formal jurisdictional boundaries. Communities may also be so designated because their populations are related on the basis of race, ethnicity, religious or political affiliation, or professional pursuit. *Trade areas,* in contrast, are assemblies of people who identify with broader socioeconomic needs and interests.

Finally, *macrosystems* are networks of organizations that are linked together to accomplish a purpose which the member organizations cannot accomplish by working separately. A national voluntary health association, for example, is a *vertical macrosystem* in which state and local chapters are bound together by common aims and legal charters. An interagency council is a *horizontal macrosystem* in which local special-interest organizations have agreed to cooperate for a fixed period in order to achieve a specific objective.

In one way or another, all these structural groupings influence the social behavior of their member populations, who are also influenced by a number of social forces as well. History, geography, religious beliefs and values shape basic cultural patterns. Public opinion and mass communications are instrumental in shaping political patterns. Basic demographic factors, such as age, sex, race, education, and socioeconomic status, have direct bearing on human needs and how they are likely to be met. Disease or health, hunger or nourishment, poverty or affluence, illiteracy or education, crime or safety, racism or pluralism, apathy or participation—all have a part in determining a population's social behavior because all have some effect upon the overall quality of human life.

An example of a complex economic force is to be found in the current energy crisis. The severe shortage and increasing cost of energy supplies, coupled with problems of rising inflation, have spurred a search for alternative sources of energy but have also caused environmental protection groups to compromise some of their earlier strictures on blocking proposed developmental plans. For a similarly complex example of a political force, in 1978 California's Proposition 13 succeeded in reducing taxes but also reduced financial support of local health, education, social, and other governmental services, resulting in reduced public services throughout the state.

In the area of social health, especially, problems are inseparable from their causes. To confront malnutrition and hunger is inevitably to confront poverty, unemployment, substandard housing, illiteracy, and isolation as well. Environmental pollution is likewise inseparable from its sources in industrial wastes, commercial and domestic chemicals, automobile-exhaust emissions, uncontrolled land use, the high cost of pollution control, and self-serving liaisons among interest groups. To none of these problems can a simple solution be found.

Most health workers who participate in social problem-solving processes would agree, for example, that overpopulation is one of the gravest problems confronting the world today. Despite its gravity, however, few countries have made great progress in reducing their annual birthrate. In many parts of the world, cultural patterns forbid the use of family-planning practices and support the raising of large families to assist as farm labor or to care for parents in their later years. In these countries, merely informing people of the availability of family planning services is inadequate; more and better strategies and methods are needed to bring about attitudinal and behavioral change.

Industrialized societies, on the other hand, show a high incidence of mental illness coupled with a negative community attitude toward coping with it realistically. While much public education is required to create a greater awareness of its symptoms so that treatment can begin before the patient is beyond help, merely creating public awareness, even by means of mass communications media, is not enough. To stimulate a more positive public attitude toward mental disorders, community organization strategies must first deal with the public's deep-seated fear of mental disease.

There are estimated to be several million seriously malnourished people in the United States today, especially among the urban poor, among migrant workers in the rural South, and among Indians and Eskimos. Few will argue that malnutrition is associated with conditions of poverty, and it is evident that malnutrition will remain a serious health problem until these conditions are changed. But changing the conditions of poverty means bringing social, economic, political, health, and consumer resources together in imaginative ways, and the technologies for doing this effectively have yet to be demonstrated.

Bringing about changes in environmental pollution is complicated by a number of factors. First, it is often difficult for contiguous city and county governments to collaborate voluntarily in environmental problem solving because metropolitan governments are reluctant to yield authority and control to regionally organized bodies. Authority yielded is not easily reclaimed; yet regional bodies need such authority if they are to control their problems. Second, many conservative communities and neighborhoods are reluctant to participate in public housing programs for fear of opening residential areas to what they perceive as people of undesirable background.

Finally, the pressures of ecology groups to prevent oil spills by restricting offshore drilling, to force environmental-impact studies on developmental projects that threaten an area's ecological balance, or to support standards requiring automobile-exhaust emission devices create counterpressures of increased costs and economic threat. Again, in the case of oil, the economic consequences of embargoes to this country are so serious as to overshadow legitimate concerns for a healthy environment. Indeed, in all these social areas health educators are involved in economic and political processes that many leaders consider to outweigh considerations of health.

Though social problems affect a great many individuals and organizations, such is their complexity that few can be resolved by individuals or organizations working alone. Experience has proved that resources are generally inadequate; problem-solving approaches are often arbitrary and ineffective, and their impact on broad social, economic, political, and environmental systems, negligible. In the authors' judgment, the best problem-solving approach is a coordinated approach which first examines those problems having special implications for health education, then builds problem-solving macrosystems for action-planning purposes.

MACROSYSTEMS FOR SOCIAL CHANGE

Bringing together key organizational leaders and representatives does not in itself produce coordinated responses to a problem, however. Across the interagency table certain dynamics occur that contribute to the success or failure of collaborative efforts, and these dynamics arise from conditions within the various organizations, as well as from conditions existing in the joint setting itself. Like other agents of social change, health educators must familiarize themselves with these dynamics if they are to develop action-planning tools that will produce conditions more conducive to change.

Interfacing and interlocking

Several basic needs motivate organizations to enter into macrosystemic settings: (1) the need for identity and policy space, which requires the establishment and acceptance of mutual boundaries to minimize inter-organizational conflict; (2) the need for security or safety against a threat of potential conflict with competing organizations; (3) the need for survival when input resources, such as finances, become scarce and a better means must be devised for their collection and allocation; and (4) the need for life enhancement in general, as when joining forces alone can make community problem solving possible.

Interfacing denotes the interactions between organizations that result in the establishment of mutual boundaries. Interactions may be direct, in the form of oral communication in a face-to-face setting, or indirect, as in the form of a written communication. Boundaries may center around the organizations' goals, the nature and source of their inputs, or the nature and mode of providing outputs. Organizations can be said to have interfaced successfully when they are able to relate to one another harmoniously while still maintaining their mutual independence, for in this situation there is little or no need for crossing boundaries.

When basic needs require organizations to become interlocked, however, boundary-bridging methods are essential. For the purposes of this discussion, *interlocking* denotes that process which causes organizations to make and honor mutual commitments to attaining a common goal that cannot be attained by separate efforts. Effective macrosystemic efforts require organizational units to be interlocked, and for this reason it is instructive to examine the forces that constrain or inhibit interlocking.

Organizational alignment Organizations that serve, and are brought together from, the same geographical area can be viewed as occupying positions along a horizontal continuum. But those having vertical alignments as well differ significantly from these, and the differences between them may constitute barriers to interlocking. For example, many voluntary health and welfare agencies at the local level have binding legal commitments to their counterparts at state and national levels, and their charters or franchises can be revoked if violated. Many local-government welfare services are directly regulated by state and federal policies; likewise, many local social action agencies operate in direct relationship to their federal counterparts or through intermediate state or regional offices.

These vertical alignments of authority are important in determining the degree to which local organizations can participate in macrosystemic efforts. While top levels sometimes support collaborative efforts at lower levels, more often there are legal and policy limitations on the extent to which input resources can be shared, production processes exchanged or altered, and individual organizational goals modified to accommodate interorganizational problem solving.

Differing alignments in the source, nature, extent, and control of organizational input resources present collaborative social-action efforts with especially complex problems in joint financing as well.

• Official health agencies obtain most of their financial resources from federal, state, and local tax revenues. Their budgets are generally controlled by legislative bodies or by councils and boards, and significant portions of their budgets are allocated to prespecified programs.

• Voluntary health agencies are usually controlled by their own boards of directors. Some derive their financial support in prorated shares from the combined fund-raising activities of local United Way or United Fund councils; others conduct their own fund-raising activities.

• Hospitals and neighborhood health centers derive much of their funding from service fees and third-party insurance payments.

• Some local antipoverty organizations were once funded more or less directly by federal sources, though federal budgetary allocations may be decreasing at present.

Socially-oriented business organizations, controlled by corporate boards of directors, sometimes offer financial support and managerial talent to community-service causes, while local trusts and foundations, usually controlled by small groups of trustees, are constantly approached for financial support by many service organizations. Whatever the source of income, however, this diversity can produce constraint in matters of resource sharing, control, and competition and often results in interagency conflict.

Operational differences How organizations use their input resources in working toward goals is termed *production process,* and one of the primary survival concerns of a new organization is to demonstrate that it possesses the technical know-how to produce something that is either unavailable, in short supply, or not produced competently enough elsewhere. Hence, developing a unique core technology or functional specialty is essential to such organizations before they can begin to collaborate with others in pursuing a common goal.

In most health-care organizations, too, production processes are highly diffuse. Health educators, medical social workers, and family-health outreach workers work in very different ways, all of which differ from the ways of their staff physicians, who may themselves work in different ways. This diffusiveness can constrain the attempt to develop an interagency macrosystem because the constant negotiating that it requires can produce threats to an organization's autonomy.

There is often great variance as well in the individual operational effectiveness of participating organizational units. While some are managed well enough to devote constructive energy to external collaborative efforts, others must expend their most productive energy in dealing with internal conflicts, and this imbalance will diminish the potential effectiveness of any joint effort.

Finally, in an ideal macrosystemic situation no organization could achieve its own objectives unless the goal of the whole macrosystem were attained as well. Often, however, the objectives of some organizations are unrelated to the overall goal, thereby minimizing their motivation to pursue that goal. Often, too, the objectives of different organizations conflict with one another, with the result that energy is diverted to defensive interactions.

Even when motivations for interlocking are powerful, organizations and their representatives tend to approach one another with an eye to defending the purposes and programs of their own turf, which often produces attack-defend interactions that inhibit boundary bridging. When ground rules for working together either do not exist or exhibit a lack of consensus, dissension over untested assumptions and unmet expectations may not only minimize the productivity of a joint effort but disrupt it altogether.

Power manipulation In the macrosystemic context, power can derive from a number of conditions:

1. the ability to exercise legal or governmental sanctions in support of, or in opposition to, the macrogoal
2. significant control over the financial resources needed for problem solving
3. a macrosystemic administrative or management structure that requires the support of all key organizational units
4. control of technical know-how that is at once so vital and so limited that its presence or withdrawal can be manipulated for purposes of persuasion
5. the coalitioning or subgrouping of units within the macrosystem for pursuit of a course of action that differs from the overall proposed course
6. the ability to organize those who suffer from the social problem, or who are disenfranchised from macrosystemic decision making, for purposes of confrontation or negotiation
7. the ability to mobilize public opinion in support of one point of view, especially when those advocating that view have ready access to mass media.

Clearly, the ability of one or more parties to take control of the forces that facilitate or inhibit attainment of a macrogoal is a highly significant factor in macrosystemic problem solving.

Interpersonal problems Because many community-action programs in the past have evinced little felt success among participants, proposed new efforts are often viewed with skepticism, which means that considerable energy must be expended in such cases merely to create the conditions supportive of a new effort. Further, in an attempt to gain citizens' acceptance and participation, initiators sometimes oversell their programs, which produces distrust if the programs fail to deliver fully on their promises.

Within the macrosystemic setting, individual interactions may also leave much to be desired, for individuals who represent their organizations at joint meetings often lack the interpersonal skills necessary to make joint efforts succeed. Poor verbal communication skills may convey misinformation about, or result in misinterpretation of, organizational positions. Insensitivity may arouse interpersonal animosities that inhibit organizational cooperation. Poor coping skills may cause defensive reactions to confrontations, precipitating win-lose vendettas. Ineffective group problem-solving skills can cause joint efforts to fail because of frustration and disenchantment with the group's working processes.

Distrust can also arise from social-distancing tendencies. Social distancing is expressed, on the one hand, in the conscious or unconscious tendency of social agency professionals of middle-class background to develop a clientele of similar background. It is expressed, on the other hand, in the tendency of those excluded from this clientele to feel that they can be helped only by one who is either like themselves or at least living among them.

Social-distance barriers may arise from geographical, racial, ethnic, religious, political, or class differences, with their related differences in customs and values, and such barriers constitute a great impediment to interlocking. Mutual trust can be developed, however, if the desire for it is strong enough. Whatever degree of mutual trust that already exists can be enhanced through intergroup activities that foster open and honest inquiry and confrontation.

EXPANDING LATITUDES

Our current knowledge of social behavior derives from a number of sciences and professions, among them anthropology, social psychology, sociology, economics, political science, public administration, communications, and planning.

Anthropology, the study of man's origin and development, provides an understanding of the sociocultural forces that shape human behavior and of how these forces are integrated in society. Social psychology studies the behavioral forces that affect individual participation in group and other social settings. Sociology advances the view that variations in individual and group behavior are attributable to social positioning and to the clustering of such factors as age, sex, occupation, religion, and location, so that such phenomena as health or voting behavior, buying habits, or child rearing tends to show predictable variation along class or status lines.

Economics is the study of the development and operation of the interdependent market system and of the production, distribution, and consumption of commodities. Its relevance to social theory arises from the interrelated nature of comprehensive social problems, for, as noted earlier, to confront malnutrition or disease, for example, is inevitably to confront economic problems as well.

Political science provides an understanding of public participation in political processes, of power and influence, of policy and the forces that shape it, and of public decision making. Public administration, the study of the management of public institutions, illuminates policy analysis, governance processes, and the management of public services.

In dealing with the uses of the mass media, the communication sciences contribute to an understanding of communication processes, including the flow of communications and the forces affecting message transmittal and reception. Finally, planning contributes to an understanding of such linear procedural tools and techniques as measurement indicators, needs assessment, goal setting, strategizing, feasibility testing, monitoring, and evaluation, all of which are important in developing and implementing programs and services.

Because health education has traditionally been characterized by a direct-service relationship with clients or communities, health-care workers have tended to regard it as a strategy exclusively for organizing or motivating people to overcome specific health problems. In this respect, health education has heretofore been seriously limited in its scope and application; but this must change because behavior affecting health encompasses human interaction in every conceivable form. Health education's scope must be expanded so that its resources can be put to use wherever a potential exists for constructively influencing health behavior, and an important step can be taken in this direction if health educators familiarize themselves with the elements of social theory reviewed in chapter 9.

9

Theories of social behavior

Although all health educators to some extent plan and act on the basis of hunches or pet strategies developed through trial and error, practical theorists should be able to identify and explain the theories on which their programs are based. To illuminate this area, the opening section of chapter 9 will review the theoretical background of, and several general strategies for, social change, while the concluding section will focus on seven specific methods and their applications.

INTRODUCTION TO SOCIAL BEHAVIOR

Theoretical background

In general, social change can be approached theoretically at the broad societal level, at the narrower community level, or at the level of public opinion and attitude. At the top level, for example, Daniel Bell believes that much current turmoil and strife is owing directly to disjunctions between society's political, economic, and cultural realms and that this disjunctiveness needs greater research and study.[1]

Alfred Kuhn, however, believes that chaos is the natural state of social life and that it is therefore order, not chaos, that needs further study. Kuhn sees social change occurring as the result of a human desire for change in the way things are done. In his view, people do what is advantageous to themselves and represent this behavior as being advantageous to all. From the sum of these behaviors social norms are formed, and societal decisions are made from within the normative context.[2]

Finally, Alvin Gouldner observes that most people live in groups throughout their lives and believe that social-change behavior is influenced by their interactions. Agreeing that norms are a central force in shaping human behavior, he contends that the shaping is done through cultural values, symbols, and signs.[3]

At another level of approach, Roland Warren holds that communities change their structure and functions in order to accommodate various social, political, and economic developments and that this change can be viewed in terms of either a horizontal (local) or vertical (specialized) axis.[4] The horizontal axis emphasizes individual-to-individual or group-to-group relationships within the community (e.g., a health-consumer coalition at the state level). The vertical axis involves the relationship of the individual to a local interest group, and the relationship of the latter to a state, regional, or national organization (e.g., a national voluntary health agency). The principal task of the vertical axis is to accomplish a specific objective; its principal leadership role is that of the problem-area specialist.

As communities grow, however, roles and functions become increasingly more specialized. There are greater needs both for further division of labor and for better functional coordination, and this increasing complexity may present a problem when respect for the principle of self-determination outweighs the value placed on a proposed improvement. For communities, like individuals, have a right to self-determination, and though health educators can help them to develop their own policies, plans, and programs, these should not be imposed upon them by health educators or anyone else.

Public opinion is a powerful force for social change because it reflects people's deepest convictions and values. According to Robert Nisbet, however, *public* opinion should be clearly distinguished from *popular* opinion, especially insofar as the legitimacy of modern democracy is at least theoretically proportional to its roots in public opinion or the people's will.[5] Vested in the organized community, public opinion gains its character from genuine consensus and unifying tradition and spirit. Popular opinion, in contrast, is rooted in fashion or fad, is easily formed around a single issue or person, is subject to caprice, and lacks the binding quality that time, tradition, and convention alone can bestow. Deliberately or not, so-called public opinion polls and surveys often confuse the two.

An opinion is a personal belief held with conviction; an attitude is a relatively enduring organization of beliefs predisposing one toward some preferential response.[6] Attitudes have both cognitive and evaluative components; they are a state of mind or feeling about a certain subject, matter, or concern. Unlike a conditioned response, however, an attitude does not in itself necessarily change behavior; a change in attitude produces only a change of predisposition to act in a particular way. Action can be brought about either through a change in the organization of beliefs or through a change in the content of one or more of the beliefs composing the organization.

One of the principal vehicles of attitudinal change is communication, by means of which a sender transmits a message to a receiver in such a way as to persuade the latter to alter a previously held attitude. Elihu Katz and Paul F. Lazarsfeld have shown that a message transmitted to a general public by a mass medium tends to be received first by a "gatekeeper" or "opinion leader," who in turn transmits it on an impersonal basis to members of his own social group.[7] This process is important in the development of public opinion and attitudes alike and is also helpful in determining the advantages and disadvantages of using mass media for health-education purposes.

Of the communication process, research has also revealed three prominent components: credibility, attractiveness, and power. By *credibility* is meant that sources perceived as having a high degree of expertise and trustworthiness are generally the more effective persuaders. Similarly, the greater the source's personal *attractiveness,* or likableness, the more effective the persuasion. *Power* denotes the source's ability to administer reward or punishment to gain the receiver's compliance.[8]

In regard to the message itself, it is important to recognize the existence of opposition in order to defuse counterarguments. If an audience knows that there is another side to an issue, for example, the message must deal with this other side, for if people lack effective counterarguments their position can be weakened at some later date.[9] A message's fear-arousal content may also be important to its persuasiveness, depending upon the message's content, source, and audience.[10]

General strategies

Determinants of change According to N. J. Smelzer, all social change depends upon four factors: structural setting, social controls, mobilization, and impetus.[11] First, organizational and macrosystemic settings must either be already structured to facilitate change or be restructured by means of existing legal controls or new legislation. Second, cultural forces, aided by mass communications, must be disposed to push rather than to repress issues for change. Third, forces for change must be marshaled around either a charismatic leader or a critical social issue. Fourth, impetus for change must exhibit energy and direction. Henrik L. Blum believes impetus to be the prime ingredient in social change. In his view, impetus arises from a desire to reduce dissonance created by discrepancies between value-derived goals, expectations, and accomplishments. [12]

Assumptions for change Further, all approaches to planned change make certain assumptions about how patterns and institutions of practice can best be modified. Robert Chin and Kenneth D. Benne stylize these assumptions in three types of strategy: empirical-rational, normative-reeducative, and power-coercive. [13]

The empirical-rational strategy, which is most frequently employed in the United States and Western Europe, assumes that insofar as man is a creature of rational self-interest, people who are to be changed will adopt the desired changes if these are shown to be rationally justified. Normative-reeducative strategies posit the existence of sociocultural norms that support patterns of practice, the norms themselves supported by people's attitudes and values. In this view, a pattern of practice will change only if people develop new normative commitments, and this requires not only changes in information, knowledge, and rationale but a reeducation of values, attitudes, and significant relationships as well. Finally, power-coercive strategies proceed on the assumption that the less powerful will accede to the leadership of the more powerful.

Models for community change Jack Rothman has described three models of community-organization practice based on change attempts in international communities as well as in the United States. [14] An overview of these models, together with selected practice variables, is given in table 7. The health educator may utilize all or only parts of these approaches depending upon the community's needs and level of development, both of which can be established by means of a community diagnosis process.

Model A features a locality-development approach and suggests that change will occur at the community level when a broad spectrum of people participates in pursuing common goal-setting and action needs. The model emphasizes full reliance on community initiative, development of indigenous leadership, active participation, democratic cooperation, and educational objectives.

Model B, featuring the social-planning approach, emphasizes technical problem solving and the professional expertise required for conducting needs assessments, setting short-range and long-range priorities and goals, devising alternative strategies for action, and designing monitoring and data-feedback systems to facilitate implementation. By and large, the con-

TABLE 7
Rothman's Three Models of Community Organization Practice

	Model A (Locality Development)	Model B (Social Planning)	Model C (Social Action)
1. Goal categories of community action	Self-help, community capacity and integration (process goals)	Problem-solving with regard to substantive community problems (task goals)	Shifting of power relationships and resources; basic institutional change (task or process goals)
2. Assumptions concerning community structure and problem conditions	Community eclipsed, anomie; lack of relationships and democratic problem-solving capacities; static traditional community	Substantive social problems: mental and physical health, housing, recreation	Disadvantaged populations, social injustice, deprivation, inequity
3. Basic change strategy	Broad cross section of people involved in determining and solving their own problems	Fact-gathering about problems and decisions on the most rational course of action	Crystallization of issues and organization of people to take action against enemy targets
4. Characteristic change tactics and techniques	Consensus: communication among community groups and interests; group discussion	Consensus or conflict	Conflict or contest: confrontation, direct action, negotiation
5. Salient practitioner roles	Enabler-catalyst, coordinator; teacher of problem-solving skills and ethical values	Fact-gatherer and analyst, program implementer, facilitator	Activist-advocate: agitator, broker, negotiator, partisan
6. Medium of change	Manipulation of small task-oriented groups	Manipulation of formal organizations and of data	Manipulation of mass organizations and political processes
7. Orientation toward power structure(s)	Members of power structure as collaborators in a common venture	Power structure as employers and sponsors	Power structure as external target of action: oppressors to be coerced or over-turned
8. Boundary definition of the community client or constituency	Total geographic community	Total community or community segment (including "functional" community)	Community segment

TABLE 7 (continued)

	Model A (Locality Development)	Model B (Social Planning)	Model C (Social Action)
9. Assumptions regarding interests of community subparts	Common interests or reconcilable differences	Interests reconcilable or in conflict	Conflicting interests which are not easily reconcilable: scarce resources
10. Conception of the public interest	Rationalist-unitary	Idealist-unitary	Realist-individualist
11. Conception of the client population or constituency	Citizens	Consumers	Victims
12. Conception of client role	Participants in interactional problem-solving process	Consumers or recipients	Employers, constituents, members

Some Personnel Aspects of Community Organization Models

Agency Type	Settlement houses, overseas community development: Peace Corps, Friends Service Committee	Welfare council, city planning board, federal bureaucracy	Alinsky, civil rights, black power, New Left, welfare rights, cause and social movement groups, trade unions
Practice Positions	Village worker, neighborhood worker, consultant to community development team, agricultural extension worker	Planning division head, planner	Local organizer
Professional Analogues	Adult educator, nonclinical group worker, group dynamics professional, agricultural extension worker	Demographer, social survey specialist, public administrator, hospital planning specialist	Labor organizer, civil rights worker, welfare rights organizer

SOURCE: G. Zaltman, P. Kotler, and I. Kaufman, eds., *Creating Social Change* (New York: Holt, Rinehart & Winston, 1972), pp. 477–78.

cern here is with delivering services to those who need them. The nature and extent of community participation varies, depending upon type of planning and rationale for participation.

Model C posits a disadvantaged subpopulation that needs to be organized so that it can make demands on the larger community for increased resources or for treatment in better accord with social justice. In seeking redistribution of power, resources, or decision making, this model aims at making basic changes in formal institutional or community practices.

Planned and unplanned change Gerald Zaltman, Philip Kotler, and Ira Kaufman suggest that long-term planned change can be precipitated within a given social system by the consequences of short-term unplanned change originating outside the system, as when new ideas or techniques are introduced from one system into another.[15] Studying unplanned change is therefore an important first step in preparing for planned change. As table 8 demonstrates, six types of social change can be identified by distinguishing between short-term and long-term levels of individual, group, and societal change. For purposes of illustration, each type will here be related to the discovery and use of the oral contraceptive pill.

Initially reflecting a short-term individual change in attitude and behavior (Type 1), adoption of the Pill may lead over the long term to intergenerational upward mobility (Type 2) as people with fewer children have more

TABLE 8
Zaltman's Six Types of Social Change

Time Dimension	Level of Society		
	Micro (Individual)	*Intermediate (Group)*	*Macro (Society)*
Short-term	*Type 1* 1) Attitude change 2) Behavior change	*Type 3* 1) Normative change 2) Administrative change	*Type 5* 1) Invention-Innovation 2) Revolution
Long-term	*Type 2* Life-cycle change	*Type 4* Organizational change	*Type 6* Sociocultural evolution

SOURCE: G. Zaltman, P. Kotler, and I. Kaufman, eds., *Creating Social Change* (New York: Holt, Rinehart & Winston, 1972), p. 3.

money to spend on educating them. Similarly, short-term changes in group sexual norms and values (Type 3) may lead to long-term changes in family structure and function (Type 4). Finally, the discovery and widespread use of the Pill, which revolutionized contemporary life styles (Type 5), may have long-term ramifications that range from changing female occupational behavior to accelerating the modernization of underdeveloped countries (Type 6).

This is not to suggest that the six types are sequential, so that a change in Type 3, for example, automatically precipitates a change in Type 4. Rather, the theory offers an insight into the points of juncture between technology and behavior. Thus, in the health-care field, the impact of rapid technological developments in medicine, equipment, facilities, and treatment (Type 5) forced immediate long-term organizational change (Type 4), with slower but significant short- and long-term sociocultural change (Type 6), but having only minimal direct impact at the level of individual or group behavior (Types 1–3).

Typology of social change James E. Crowfoot and Mark A. Chesler have developed a typology of planned social change based on professional-technical, political, and countercultural perspectives (see table 9).[16] Health educators who cannot identify these perspectives and apprehend their implications cannot explore the full range of effective strategies for change. Though no one approach can apply to all situations, a community-diagnosis process can help to determine which aspects of the three are most appropriate to a given situation.

From the professional-technical perspective, society is composed of numerous subsystems which have complex interrelationships as well as discrete internal structures and processes. Though basically sound, all subsystems need to cope better with processes of change, which should be systematically planned and directed by professionals working with small groups, organizations, or communities. To facilitate change, rational and collective problem-solving systems should be created for establishing new norms, defining roles, and designing operating procedures. Emphasis on open, informal interpersonal communication will help reduce resistance to change.

From the political perspective, society is composed of numerous groups, each defined by its members' shared interests. Whether a group is loosely organized or well integrated, planned change is likely to originate in discontent with its resources, while attempts to change the distribution of scarce resources will inevitably evoke resistance from those who will have to relinquish some of their share. Moreover, as power is usually concentrated among a few key interest groups, these elites will seek to maintain their

TABLE 9
Crowfoot-Chesler Approaches to Planned Social Change

Key Questions	Professional-Technical	Political	Countercultural
What are its general images of society?	Complex system with functionally specialized structure Organizations and communities based on technical rationality and bureaucratic authority Made up of consensually minded persons having interdependent economic relationships and moral obligations Conflict is dysfunctional; harmony and natural order of consensus and cooperation preferred	Society consists of many different groups, each defined by the shared interests or values of its members Competition and conflict over resources are basic processes Distribution of power among groups with different interests determinative of societal functioning	Society consists of organizations which are uniformly over-technocratic and overbureaucratic Organizations result in individual conformity and dehumanization Basic trend of social change is more of the same
What are its general images of the individual?	Normatively committed role occupants Information processors and problem-solvers Responsive to system-controlled rewards	Powerless to meet needs by himself or herself Interdependence and group membership required to satisfy needs False consciousness frequently prevents individual from satisfying his or her needs	Innately good—capable of love, joy, and creativity More emotional and intuitive than cognitive and rational Goodness is distorted and suppressed
What are its diagnoses of contemporary society?	Society, as managed by and represented by legitimate officials, is basically all right, although adjustments are needed.	State has failed in some of its regulatory functions Power is concentrated in relatively small number of persons or organizations	Individual is alienated—evaluated in terms of material possessions and ability to produce

TABLE 9 (continued)

Key Questions	Professional-Technical	Political	Countercultural
	Change is inevitable. It arises from developing technology, larger scales of production, and administrative complexity Maintenance of old bureaucratic patterns prevent adaptation to change	Oppressed see resource allocation as unfair, and elites see it as just but difficult to maintain Laws, norms, intelligence systems, and socialization are seen as maintaining elite control: the powerless see them as oppressing them, and elites see them as not being effective enough	Society's institutions are repressive: antihumanistic, racist, sexist, etc. Institutions operate to destroy people, land, and natural resources
What are its priorities with regard to change?	Professionals need to plan and manage functional adaptations to change Ongoing, incremental planned change Target of change is small groups, organizations, and social roles, attitudes, and skills of individuals Social planning at societal level Create rational problem-solving systems	For oppressed it is altering consciousness and mobilization to achieve greater power and resources For elites it is making their control more effective and more satisfying to exercise	Individual change in self and life style, identity, and intimate relations Life styles centered on individuality, openness, and full acceptance of and participation in a community Alternative organizations based fully on humanistic values and new life styles

SOURCE: J. E. Crowfoot and M. A. Chesler, "Contemporary Perspectives on Planned Social Change: A Comparison," *Journal of Applied Behavioral Science* 10, no. 3 (1974): p. 288–89.

control, while oppressed groups, by making known their oppression, will seek a redistribution of power.

From the countercultural perspective, contemporary society is excessively technocratic and bureaucratic, its institutions no longer meeting basic human needs for freedom, affection, and wholeness. As most conventional social change is viewed as only further diminishing social tolerance for individuality, nonconformity, and creativity, it is believed that change must begin with the self and result in new personal values and life styles that support acceptance of, and full participation in, a community of others. These changes must be extended through humanistic alternative organizations, such as communes, which are characterized by racial and sexual equality, interpersonal cooperation, and consensual decision making.

SEVEN METHODS AND APPLICATIONS

The remainder of this chapter is devoted to analyses of seven methods for planned social change, ranging from low-resistance to high-resistance modes (see table 10). The first five methods can be applied to the practice of health education wherever conditions are appropriate; the sixth could be applied as a last resort where other methods have failed to resolve the problem. Although it is impossible to envisage a health-education situation that would necessitate use of the seventh method, violent disruption is nevertheless included here as an example whose symptoms should be recognized and avoided.

Diffusion and adoption

The method here termed diffusion and adoption (D&A) arose in part from studies of the two-step flow of communication conducted during the 1950s by Katz and Lazarsfeld.[17] These studies suggested that an idea, in its outward flow from its source, tends to be picked up first by those who have some personal interest in it ("gatekeepers" or "opinion leaders"), who then convey it to others in an attempt to influence or change their opinions, attitudes, or behaviors. Opinion leaders, then, constitute the first step in the communication process, and those influenced by them constitute the second step. In health education, for example, a nurse who conveys health information to a patient is an opinion leader.

Within the health field particularly, and with specific reference to heart disease, David V. McQueen has found three sets of related variables—independent, dependent, and outcome—to be at work in the D&A process.[18] Independent variables include the social-psychological and physiological risk factors associated with heart disease, ranging from hypertension,

TABLE 10
Seven Methods of Planned Social Change

Methods	Examples	Theories	Strategies	Conditions
1. Diffusion and adoption	Smoking Cancer Heart disease Fluoridation Immunization	Communication process Opinion leadership	Mass communications Personal contact Small groups	Threatening situation Limited time Widespread response Involvement of opinion leaders
2. Consensus organizing	Communes Voluntary health agencies Professional health associations Coalitions Councils	Empirical/ Rational Individual rights Shared interests	Rational idea Personal contact Group formation Common interests Consensual decision making	Lack of organized resistance Shared self-interests
3. Social planning	Health-systems agencies Special interest planning Human resources planning	Normative-reeducative Linear-rational progression	Implementation of planning steps Citizen participation	Unknown needs Limited resources Competition for resources Citizen participation
4. Political action	President's Committee on Health Education National health insurance Equal Rights Amendment	Power and influence Democratic decision making	Legislation Lobbying Elections Legal suits Regulations	Organized resistance Policies must be changed Availability of resources Limited time
5. Confrontive negotiation	City-agency/ neighborhood Health team/ community Social problem-solving project	Power-negotiative Normative reeducative Policy development Social growth	Problem orientation Third-party intervention Constructive confrontation MOAs	Organized resistance Possibility of violence Desire for win-win
6. Nonviolent disruption	Civil rights Migrant farm workers Save environment Strikes Boycotts	Power-coercive Change requires conflict Power to the people	Cohesive minority Strategizing Power building Systems disruption	When above methods are not given a chance to be used
7. Violent disruption	Revolutions Riots Terrorism	Power control Change requires reconstruction of society	Cohesive minority Military plan Attack Win-lose or lose-lose	None Should not be used by health educators

diet, and blood lipids to geographical and social mobility, role confusion, and such coronary-prone behavioral patterns as high excitability, smoking, and workaholism. The types of health professionals involved in the D&A process form another set of independent variables. These include physicians, nurses, health-education specialists, nutritionists, occupational and physical therapists, and social workers, all with their various categorical specialties.

Within this population of health professionals, dependent variables include such factors as accepting the validity of the risk factors, believing that the risk factors can be altered, having the desire and ability to precipitate change in others, and having a strong interest in communicating a health message. Accepting the validity of the risk factors is especially crucial to the D&A process, which will clearly not be enhanced, for example, by health professionals who do not accept as conclusive the data linking smoking with lung cancer or by physicians whose orientation to physiological risk factors causes them to disregard social-psychological factors.

Clearly important, too, is belief that risk factors can be changed, although this will depend upon the types of risk factors involved, the professional's specialty and skills, and whether the professional relates well enough to clients' values and norms to communicate the risks effectively. If a strong desire exists to help others change, the professional will make special efforts toward that end, choosing the strategies that will best meet the purpose. Having the ability to alter others will actually produce a change in the status of the disease or in the individual's health.

Finally, professionals who exhibit acceptance, belief, desire, and ability are likely to want strongly to communicate their message. To increase their ability to produce change, then, the function of the health educator is to involve them in either in-service training or continuing education both to foster these qualities and to increase their communication skills.

To the outcome variable Lawrence W. Green has linked four factors: system effects, attribution effects, discontinuance of adopted practices, and communication effects.[19] System effects are those produced by a system change that either hinders or helps D&A. As an example of the latter, airlines now have in-flight smoking and nonsmoking sections, a system change whose cumulative effect has been to influence wider acceptance of such an innovation.

Attribution effects are those produced by the qualities of an innovation that make it seem desirable—e.g., its advantages over an old idea; its compatibility with past experience, existing needs and values; its flexibility for division into less venturesome parts; and its degree of visibility to others. In attempting to quit smoking, for example, some smokers prefer low-visibility individual methods to the high-visibility methods frequently suggested by health professionals. In weight reduction, on the other hand, high-visibility group methods seem to have greater success.

Discontinuance of adopted practices means simply that some people will revert to their previous behaviors. Studies in this area, however, have yielded two generalizations—that late adopters of an idea are likelier than early adopters to discontinue a new behavior and that innovations with a high rate of adoption have a low rate of discontinuance.

Last, communication effects are those that best link the health profession with a wider audience that is still to be influenced. Indigenous health workers and specially designed educational materials, for example, may enhance communication with people whose social, cultural, or economic backgrounds differ from those of designated health professionals.

D&A is applicable in almost every field that has social change as a goal. In health education generally, it has been the basis for the production of films, pamphlets, posters, television programs, and other mass-education efforts to promote immunization, fluoridation, disease-screening and detection, driving safety, antipollution and antismoking programs. Figure 9 shows a D&A program strategy developed by the U.S. Public Health Service's Center for Disease Control. To achieve public response to a community-wide influenza campaign in 1976–77, twenty-two activities were organized ranging from personal contact to the use of mass media, with health educators involved in every phase of the program's planning, evolution, and implementation.

For health-education purposes, D&A should be the primary method of planned social change when:

1. a great many people are to be affected by a problem and time allows development of a program to effect a gradual shift in public perception and attitude
2. a required behavioral response is general enough for individuals to help themselves or obtain services from a nearby clinic
3. needed health professionals can be mobilized to provide program services.

Consensus organizing

Among other modes of structural classification, community organization can also be viewed in terms of degree of resistance or conflict on the part of those to be organized. Consensus organizing is a method that encounters little or no resistance because it arises from the assumption, discussed earlier in relation to Chin and Benne,[20] that people will pursue a proposed change if it is shown to be beneficial to their rational self-interest. It is based further

FIGURE 9
A Community-wide Influenza Campaign

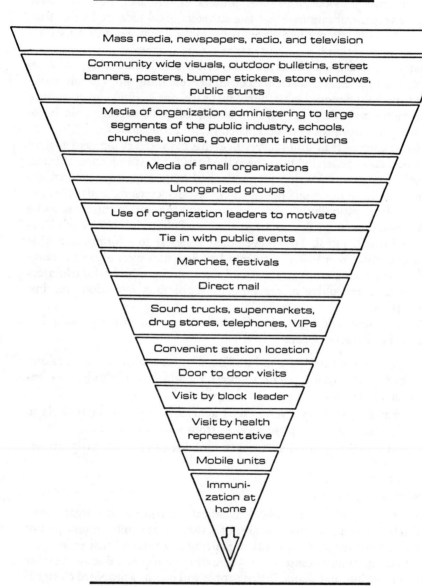

Mass media, newspapers, radio, and television

Community wide visuals, outdoor bulletins, street banners, posters, bumper stickers, store windows, public stunts

Media of organization administering to large segments of the public industry, schools, churches, unions, government institutions

Media of small organizations

Unorganized groups

Use of organization leaders to motivate

Tie in with public events

Marches, festivals

Direct mail

Sound trucks, supermarkets, drug stores, telephones, VIPs

Convenient station location

Door to door visits

Visit by block leader

Visit by health representative

Mobile units

Immunization at home

SOURCE: Adapted from U.S. Department of Health, Education and Welfare, Public Health Service, Center for Disease Control, Atlanta, GA.

on the conviction that those who share common interests and goals can successfully pool their efforts in a shared activity.

People may join forces, for example, to develop a voluntary health agency, such as the American Cancer Society, whose widespread chapters and numerous programs are financed by voluntary contributions. Others may join forces to organize a professional membership association, such as the Society for Public Health Education, dedicated to improving standards for professional preparation and practice. Other examples of consensus organizing include communes, consumer cooperatives, credit unions, and consumer advocate groups.

The initial focus of consensus organizing is on engaging enough people for the project to be meaningfully realized. This means, first, appealing to human rationality, which may require the preparation of educational background materials and counterarguments. Next, opinion leaders must be contacted, and possibly trained, to introduce the idea to others and gain their participation. The next step usually involves planning and conducting group meetings in which common interests, needs, and objectives begin to be formulated.

As an organizational structure evolves to provide leadership and direction, the process becomes essentially one of organizational refinement: seeking financial resources and maintaining a balance between income and expenditures; developing guidelines for the provision of services; improving membership participation, communication, and decision-making procedures, measuring the effectiveness of group efforts; and developing collaborative relationships with other agencies and groups.

Consensus organizing can only work when there is little or no resistance among those to be organized and when the latter are numerically few enough to permit effective use of personal contacts and small-group or conference methods. Those brought together must be cohesive enough to help the initial organizers move from merely discussing the idea to securing the commitment of others to action.

Social planning

As a strategy for change, social planning has been adopted throughout the health-care field. For the improvement of general health-care resources, health-systems agencies have introduced the planning process at regional levels throughout the nation. At state and local levels, planning has also been utilized for such special-interest purposes as aging and mental retardation. In many parts of the country, municipal and United Way organizations are applying social-planning approaches to human resources development. Communities, too, have engaged in planning for economic development, neighborhood development, community action, and many other purposes.

The basic assumption behind social planning is that public health will improve as a result of effective health services, and that health services will become effective as a result of a rational sequence of planned efforts toward what Chin and Benne call "normative reeducation."[21] According to this view, patterns of health practice arise from individual commitments to sociocultural norms which are themselves supported by individual attitudes and values. Hence, changes in patterns of health practice will occur only as people develop commitments to new normative orientations.

Henrik Blum suggests that planning for ordered change should consist of defining the desired improvements, achieving them, and measuring the achievement.[22] More particularly, the basic components of planning models include: present and future needs assessment, problem definition, systems analysis, goal setting, alternative interventions, cost-benefit analysis, implementation, and evaluation.*

Social planning, then, is the primary model to apply when:

1. the problem is so little understood as to require illumination for rational decision making
2. resolving the problem requires a strategy ensuring ongoing continuity of effort
3. a scarcity of available resources requires a strategy for determining their most effective use
4. conflict over scarce resources requires a strategy promoting collaborative use and commitment to whatever allocation decisions are made
5. organizational or systemic change will be so extensive as to require a strategy that engages all involved units in planning change
6. a strategy is needed to link policy determination and problem solving in order to maintain needed services or to prevent recurrence of the problem in the future.

Political action

The 1973 report of President Nixon's Committee on Health Education contributed to the creation of a public-sector Bureau of Health Education (1974), a private-sector National Center for Health Education (1974–75), and to the passage of a number of important laws affecting health education in the United States. Clearly, political action can be a potent force for social change depending upon the relationship between the change agent

*For an in-depth description of planning steps and procedures for health education, see chapter 11.

and the change population (i.e., the greater the dependency on the change agent, the greater the agent's influence in creating change). Clearly, too, as a method of social change, political action relies less on persuasive education than on authority, influence, and power as these are exercised through democratic public processes.

For the purposes of health education, political action is almost always directed toward attaining new or improved policies affecting public health or the social environment. Though in the final analysis all political-action outcomes require either majority and minority support or some enforcement procedure to assure compliance, the action may take any of several forms:

• Persuading a legislator to introduce a bill into Congress, then promoting support of the bill through lobbying activities or community contact with legislators

• Placing a referendum or initiative issue on the ballot and campaigning for majority support

• Persuading a city council or county board of supervisors to enact a regulation or ordinance governing some aspect of the existing health system or requiring someone's compliance in eliminating a health hazard

• Filing a legal suit to contest an action or to test the validity of a new law in a higher court of appeal.

In general, political action is the preferred method when:

1. the change population has low recognition of a need for change (hence the federal requirement that automobile manufacturers install seat belts in cars)

2. the change population has the capacity and resources to adopt the proposed change (e.g., to install equipment and establish procedures necessary to meet the requirements of a Grade A milk program)

3. the change agent has available resources (money, volunteers) to conduct the activity

4. one group obstructs a change desired by many others (e.g., school desegregation)

5. the strategy for countering anticipated high resistance is to introduce a change quickly and firmly (e.g., school desegregation)

6. a change population is unlikely to make needed concessions voluntarily (e.g., land claims)

7. time pressures prohibit the lengthy procedures involved in planning or other essentially educational approaches

8. those involved in a political-action method understand and believe in the political process.

Confrontive negotiation

Social problems arise from many complex forces—among them, primal disjunctions between society's political, economic, and cultural realms,[24] the pursuit of self-interests and of win-lose strategies among competitors for power and resources, and haphazard processes of change in general. This overall condition, whose primary ingredients are an admixture of poor communication and power conflicts,[25] can be termed *social decline,* and its symptoms are reflected in racism, depersonalization, fear, a sense of power-lessness, and apathy.

These negative behavioral forces are still behavioral forces, however, and are therefore presumably susceptible to behavioral problem-solving efforts. Problem solving consists of developing policy to bridge societal disjunctions, creating common goals and win-win strategies, and planning creative conflict to reduce dissonance. The development of positive, constructive social-behavioral forces constitutes *social growth,* and it is reflected in the conversion of racism to pluralism, of depersonalization to a recognition of individual dignity, of fear to security, of powerlessness to potency, and of apathy to energy.

The method known as confrontive negotiation employs elements of both power (confrontation) and communication (negotiation) to set the stage for equitable social negotiations. Problem-Oriented Applied Behavioral Science (PO-ABS), a specific method for confrontive negotiation, is based on the hypothesis that social growth can result only from comprehensive long-term programs of change focused on the problems causing the behavioral difficulties.

PO-ABS is a problem-solving intervention whose goal is to produce changes in social policy leading to overall social growth. In this method, haves and have-nots are alike aided in organizing themselves for effective participation. Great emphasis is placed on confrontation and negotiation strategies, which are assisted by third-party facilitators and based on the commitment of all parties to an equitable win-win problem-solving process. As figure 10 indicates, the entire process is accompanied by planning, training, and technical assistance.

PO-ABS was conceived by Paul Mico while working with others under contract to clients in community and social-change projects that aimed at applying a behavioral-based change strategy to a community problem-solving situation.[26] The approach has been used in the following instances:

1. Assisting a large federal agency in placing health professionals in rural areas where many issues had to be confronted and resolved between health teams and community representatives

FIGURE 10
PO-ABS Model

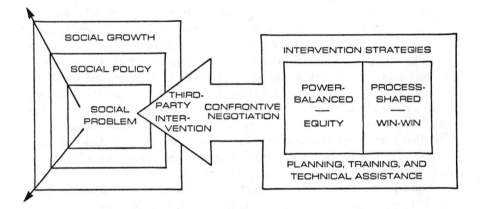

2. Assisting three city-government departments (police, welfare, and recreation) in reducing problems and improving relationships and services in three problem neighborhoods
3. Negotiating new agreements on child-health disability programs between local health and welfare departments
4. Intervening where a minority group was confronting political, economic, and social institutions to correct historical inequities, and assisting both the haves and have-nots in the process.

PO-ABS A problem-solving approach to social change, PO-ABS requires, first, a systematic diagnosis ascertaining the problem's causes and effects, the organizations that must work together for necessary resources to be marshaled, the forces that will help or hinder problem solving, and the direction in which comprehensive action-planning efforts should move. Because social growth is related to constructive changes in social policy, analyzing policy is a major step in diagnosis and planning. Top-level policy teams can be useful in identifying the policy spaces and systems involved in the problem, diagnosing their weight in contributing to or alleviating the problem, and planning any needed policy changes.

Building a network of collaborating organizations is another critical step in planning because this gives planners access to key resource units that span governmental-political jurisdictions at the horizontal level and national-state-local linkages along the vertical dimension. Though there are many complexities to be considered in designing an effective macrosystem, PO-ABS focuses on two. First, an equitable balance of power must be negotiated between organizational units, particularly between those constituting the *first party* (who are affected by the problem but lack the resources to resolve it) and those constituting the *second party* (who are also affected by the problem but possess the resources needed by the first party).

Second, the macrosystemic process must be collaborative so that all parties ultimately feel satisfied in respect to matters of mutual commitment, responsibility, involvement, influence, usefulness, learning, and effectiveness. In general, social change strategies fall into three categories: win-win, win-lose, and lose-lose. Behavioral science values hold that the only acceptable macrosystemic strategy is win-win, in which all participating parties feel that they have contributed to a solution to which all feel mutually committed. But problems nevertheless arise in the macrosystemic setting, and these may be approached by several means.

Third-party intervention is essential for problem-oriented action, particularly where a win-win strategy is employed. In a third-party intervention, the third party's role is to facilitate the processes by which the first and second parties resolve the problems between them. The *third party* consists of a change-oriented outside resource plus an inside group that has been specially organized to sanction the intervention. This group, which is composed of representatives of both the have-nots and the haves, must have credibility in the eyes of the parties they represent and must willingly make itself accountable for the intervention's consequences.

Ongoing open negotiations among the parties and units of a macrosystem are also essential to a vital problem-solving process. When success is minimized because of tenuous working relationships among them, units can be linked into collaborative change efforts by the Memorandum of Agreement (MOA). The MOA is a written agreement between the parties involved, detailing their objectives, responsibilities, and ground rules for working together and also specifying the planning, training, and technical-assistance services to be provided (see figure 11). MOAs should be negotiated between third and first parties, between third and second parties, between first and second parties, and between units within each party.

In the social problem-solving context, a crisis is a disruption that breaks relations between two or more vital units. Such disruptions can be prevented, or at least their consequences minimized, by a Crisis-Prevention Intervention System (CPIS). CPIS is a data-based collection-and-response system which identifies clues that a crisis may be brewing, thereby enabling problem-solving responses to be developed at stages early enough to prevent serious disruption from occurring.

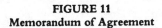

FIGURE 11
Memorandum of Agreement

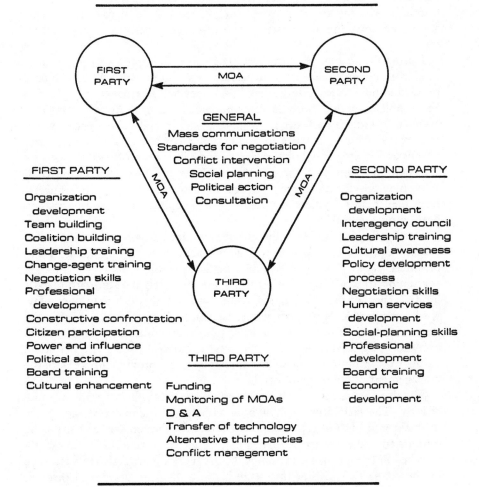

NOTE: Three-party planning, training, and technical assistance services.

Third-party intervention Bringing separate parties together to work on common problems does not entail a loss of respective identities; neither does it necessarily mean the development of consensus on all issues and procedures. Rather, the PO-ABS approach recognizes that since most social problems must be worked out over a long period of time, it is important to work them out on the basis of priorities. Beginning with a problem that is both substantial and manageable, certain benefits accrue as each is dealt with successfully. Leadership is trained, strengthened, and made more visible to each party; each learns to what extent the other will respond to its needs and priorities; working arrangements are negotiated and clarified; disagreements are worked out; morale is raised. The approach usually proceeds in three stages.

During the first stage, third-party facilitators help the two primary parties, working independently, to perform a twofold task: (1) to diagnose problems and develop priorities and (2) to develop internal communication and problem-solving skills to meet potential tensions. At this point it is essential to build a high degree of understanding and cohesiveness within each party, which generally means building coalitions among first-party groups and interagency linkages for second-party groups. Facilitators offer consultation about party working procedures and interpersonal relationships, may provide training experiences for better functioning, and, if necessary, may help to collect attitudinal, demographic, or other information bearing on the problem.

During the second stage the two parties are assisted in making initial contact, under carefully designed circumstances, to share appraisals and priorities, as well as to determine whether a viable basis exists for their continuing to work together. At this stage they seek an important but delimited aspect of the problem that can be successfully dealt with over a few weeks or months. Now very active, facilitators help to design cross-party confrontations; serve as consultants or moderators during joint meetings in order to bring disagreements to the surface and deal with them; help both parties to communicate openly and intelligibly; and provide supports for the management of tension and conflict.

The third stage centers on a joint effort to deal with the problem more directly. The facilitators' role is now to help the members of each party maintain good intraparty communication and cohesion while at the same time assisting the two parties in negotiating and managing their increasingly specific joint working relationships. MOA working arrangements are very important to PO-ABS at this stage because they are developed through open negotiation. Indeed, the very process of making time-limited agreements that are open to renegotiation both emphasizes and augments each party's autonomy.

At this point, too, facilitators must negotiate explicit agreements about their own responsibilities toward each of the parties and toward the problem-solving effort as a whole. Negotiations may be undertaken to limit the facilitators' role, and ways must be established for each party to influence third-party interventions.

Problem resolution can be said to have occurred when policies exist establishing the nature, extent, and means of delivery of second-party resources to first-party people. In successful situations, the role of the third party will gradually reduce as the first and second parties are better able to continue their joint working with diminished need for outside help. Problems and actors change, however, and because the knowledge, skills, and experience of one generation are not automatically transferred to the next, a third-party capability should always be available.

In general, confrontive negotiation should be used as a primary method when:

1. a serious imbalance of power exists between first- and second-party groups
2. second-party groups believe that problems either do not exist or that first-party groups have no legitimate claim to their demands
3. first-party groups lack the knowledge, sophistication, power, or resources to engage in political action
4. the potential for violence is great and responsible leadership in any or all parties prefers a win-win resolution
5. conditions for social planning or political action do not exist.

Nonviolent disruption

Peaceful resistance—the term applied to the social-change method employed by Mahatma Gandhi, Martin Luther King, and César Chávez among others—is in fact a nonviolent disruption of second-party systems by first-party groups to prevent them from functioning effectively so that their leadership can be forced either to negotiate or to accede to first-party demands. During the vast social upheavals of the 1960s, when peaceful resistance was practiced by groups ranging from city employees and labor unions to antinuclear and conservationist groups, the views of no person aroused more impassioned controversy than those of Saul Alinsky.

According to Robert Pruger and Harry Specht, Alinsky was basically concerned with alienation among the socially disadvantaged, believing that societal arrangements were deliberately such as to enable some people to reap society's rewards while causing others to feel unworthy of sharing in them. The rewards would therefore have to be seized, and to do so the disadvantaged would have to organize their numbers. As they became oriented to the uses of power, they would eventually gain their desired structural reforms as well as the sense of self-worth that accompanies full social participation.[27]

Nonviolent disruption is based on the view that the power of a ruler is dependent upon the acquiescence of his followers. When they do not acquiesce, new understandings between ruler and ruled must be worked out.

Its basic strategy is therefore power-coercive,[28] and its processes focus on the development and use of power.

To build power is to use any means necessary for the creation of a group (presumably representative of the community to be organized) whose major property is power. The organizer's aim is to recruit and train a cadre of leaders, to build its influence as quickly as possible, and to maneuver for power to be yielded to it as soon as it is able to seize it. To maintain its own power, the group must secure high levels of committed participation, win conflicts, and either outlast or co-opt competitors for its local power base. Organizing activities differ from others only in placing greater emphasis on power, gaining members' commitment to its pursuit even at the risk of inflammatory confrontation.

To use power is essentially to undertake a series of campaigns designed to keep the opposition (generally, the second-party resources of the community) off balance. Once victory has been experienced, the strategy is to take on increasingly larger issues and to get more people committed to carrying out activities. Nonviolent disruption may be an appropriate course of action when every effort to apply confrontive negotiation has failed to cause second parties to participate in problem-solving issues in which they are believed to be legitimately involved.

Violent disruption

Violent disruption is mentioned here, not because it constitutes an acceptable alternative for health education, but because it is a form of planned social change that has been used throughout history in forms ranging from revolution and civil war to political terrorism, riots, and extortion. Its basic theory is that change will occur only when conflict succeeds in destroying an old social system and replacing it with a new one. It is an all-out win-lose attempt to gain control of power.

Generally, a deviant minority group will adopt a specific issue as a basis for developing commitment and cohesion. The group will then develop a military plan of action, arm and train itself to engage in open violence or combat, select a strategy designed to surprise the enemy, and attempt to wrest the greatest perceived source of power into its control. Thereafter it will manipulate all forms of power and influence in order to achieve its goals. As our democratic society is now constituted, there are no conditions that call for the use of violent disruption.

The seven methods for social change presented here do not constitute a united sequential strategy; each is a separate method and should be regarded as such even when used in conjunction with two or more others. The skill of health educators lies in their ability to assist in diagnosing community problems at the level of citizens' needs, in involving citizens in planning and implementing their change programs, in recognizing that no one approach to community action works for all situations, and in applying the methods that are best suited to the given situation. Finally, not all health-education programs reveal clearly which methods have been applied. In those selected for discussion in chapter 10, for example, some methods will be obvious and others only implied.

REFERENCES

1. D. Bell, *The Cultural Contradictions of Capitalism*, pp. 3–30.
2. A. Kuhn, *The Logic of Social Systems*, pp. 427–56.
3. A. Gouldner, "Some Observations on Systematic Theory, 1945–1955," in *Modern Social Theories*, ed. C. P. Loomis and B. I. Loomis, p. 583.
4. R. Warren, *Perspectives on the American Community*, pp. 70–76.
5. R. Nisbet, "Public Opinion versus Popular Opinion," in *The American Commonwealth, 1976*, ed. N. Glazer and I. Kristol, pp. 166–92.
6. M. Rokeach, "Attitude Change and Behavior Change," *Public Opinion Quarterly* 30 (1966–67): 529–50.
7. E. Katz and P. F. Lazarsfeld, *Personal Influence*, p. 32.
8. W. J. McGuire, "The Nature of Attitudes and Attitude Change," in *The Handbook of Social Psychology*, ed. G. Lindzey and E. Aronson, 3:182–98.
9. Ibid.
10. G. Lindzey, C. S. Hall, and R. F. Thompson, *Psychology*. pp. 622–23.
11. N. J. Smelzer, *Essays in Sociological Explanation*, p. 205.
12. H. L. Blum, *Planning for Health*, p. 20.
13. R. Chin and K. D. Benne, "General Strategies for Effecting Change in Human Systems," in *Creating Social Change*, ed. G. Zaltman, P. Kotler, and I. Kaufman, pp. 233–54.
14. J. Rothman, "Three Models of Community Organization Practice," in Zaltman, Kotler, and Kaufman, *Creating Social Change*, pp. 472–501.
15. Zaltman, Kotler, and Kaufman, *Creating Social Change*, pp. 1–7.
16. J. E. Crowfoot and M. A. Chesler, "Contemporary Perspectives on Planned Social Change: A Comparison," *Journal of Applied Behavioral Science* 10, no. 3 (1974): 278–303.
17. Katz and Lazarsfeld, *Personal Influence*, pp. 32, 309–20.
18. D. V. McQueen, "Diffusion of Heart Disease Risk Factors to Health Professionals," in *Applying Behavioral Science to Cardiovascular Risk*, ed. A. J. Enelow and J. B. Henderson, pp. 71–80.
19. L. W. Green, "Diffusion and Adoption of Innovations Related to Cardiovascular Risk Behavior in the Public," in Enelow and Henderson, *Applying Behavioral Science to Cardiovascular Risk*, pp. 84–100.
20. Chin and Benne, "General Strategies," pp. 233–54.
21. Ibid.

22. Blum, *Planning for Health*, p. 8.
23. Adapted from G. Zaltman and R. Duncan, *Strategies for Planned Change*, pp. 152–65.
24. Bell, *Cultural Contradictions of Capitalism*, pp. 3–30.
25. A. Etzioni, *The Active Society*, pp. 350–86.
26. P. R. Mico, *Problem-Oriented Applied Behavioral Science*.
27. R. Pruger and H. Specht, "Assessing Theoretical Models of Community Organization Practice: Alinksy as a Case in Point," in Zaltman, Kotler, and Kaufman, *Creating Social Change*, pp. 491–501.
28. Chin and Benne, "General Strategies," pp. 233–54.

10
Programs in social health education

This chapter will observe health education at work at national, state, and local levels, in urban centers and isolated rural areas, among broad social systems, organizations, and individuals. Many health professionals, including health-education specialists, will be seen at their work, some of it successful, some less so though still hopeful of success. Our purpose here is to reflect some of the diversity of health-education practice in the social area while at the same time showing the relationship of practice to theory. As will be seen, no two situations are identical. The health educator's task is always to assure that the appropriate theory is being applied and that the program is flexible enough to allow theory to be translated into effective practice.

NATIONAL PROGRAMS

National Center for Health Education   A private nonprofit organization that has been instrumental in developing national strategies for health education, the National Center for Health Education was brought into being in 1974–75 by efforts of the President's Committee on Health Education and the National Health Council.[1] Attributing the relative ineffectiveness of many current efforts to the absence of unified national agreement on matters of health education, the center established three sets of major objectives and related priorities.

Its first objective was to attempt to close the gap between current health problems and resources by assessing the problems and the programs designed to address them. Its second objective was to speak for the overall field of health education at the national level and to obtain for it a greater share of the resources allocated to health-care systems in general. Its third objective was to improve the art of health education by finding better approaches, developing more objective means of evaluation, and seeing to it that learning is better disseminated throughout the nation to reduce unevennesses in practice.

A source of consultation and technical assistance to the field, the center's major priorities have also been three. First, it has made increasing use of the workplace as a focus for health education, not only in connection with work-related problems but in relation to the health of workers and of their families as well. Second, in connection with the 1974 Health Planning and Health Resources Development Act, it has been exploring the community responsibilities of health-systems agencies and the role of health education in enhancing their work. Third, it has encouraged the development of a financing mechanism that will equate quality patient education with all the other components of good health care.

All these priorities are essentially centered on prevention: primary prevention, particularly in the workplace; secondary prevention, both in the workplace and in terms of patient education; and tertiary prevention, with particular emphasis on patient education. The center regards prevention as among the most important of health education's many functions, and its basic methods toward that end have included diffusion and adoption, consensus organizing, and political action.

Bureau of Health Education   In the Department of Health, Education and Welfare (HEW),* health-education activities are carried out under the general headings of health communication, promotion, and information. The Center for Disease Control is HEW's chief preventive arm; the National Institute for Health, its primary biomedical-research arm; the Health Services Administration is concerned primarily with the delivery of health services.

All Public Health Service agencies have an educational mission along with their other tasks, as do HEW's Social Security Administration, Office of Human Development, and Office of Education. All categorical-disease

*Reorganized in 1980 as the Department of Health and Human Services (HHS).

programs (e.g., alcoholism and drug abuse, venereal disease, family planning) and health-service programs (e.g., the Indian Health Service, neighborhood health center programs, or early screening, diagnosis, and treatment programs) are likewise required to provide educational services as well as health care.

The Bureau of Health Education was brought into being in 1974 by the President's Committee on Health Education and a governmental decision to act on two of its 1973 recommendations: (1) to establish a focal point within HEW for coordinating the health-education activities conducted by its many agencies, and (2) to consider whether a similar focal point should be created in the private sector. Both recommendations were approved and implemented by an HEW task force.[2]

The bureau's concerns include school health education, patient education, community health education, health education in the workplace, education through the health-care system, and making better use of mass media for health-education purposes. It is engaged in developing health-education model programs, applying theories, testing ideas, and demonstrating methods. To improve the art of health education, it is documenting the success of various methods in various settings and widely publicizing their results. It has also examined the programs of HEW and other government agencies, awarding a key contract to the American Heart Association to examine the state of patient education in hospitals around the nation. A bureau contract awarded to the National Health Council resulted in a feasibility study leading to development of the National Center for Health Education.

Public Law 94–317 In P. L. 94–317 (1976), the term *health education* encompasses health information and promotion, preventive health services, and education in the use of the health-care system. Title 1, the National Health Information and Promotion Act of 1976, represents a set of compromises between highly disparate earlier bills.

• Section 1701 creates a new Title 17 to the Public Health Service Act giving the HEW Secretary broad authority for setting national goals and priorities for health information and promotion and for education in the use of the health-care system.

• Section 1702 provides authority for organizations or persons to carry out research and evaluation projects related to the act's purposes.

• Section 1703 calls for state and community programs to demonstrate methodologies related to education in the school and health-care system setting.

• Section 1704 calls for more effective use of mass and internally produced media to inform the public in plain language on the appropriate use of the health-care system. This includes telling people how to shop for health insurance, and it emphasizes the development of model projects allowing states to publish comparative studies of the type of health insurance money can buy.

• Section 1705 calls for reports to the president for transmission to Congress. The first report was due in 1978, two years after the date of enactment. Thereafter reports were to be made annually covering goals and strategies, progress being made, and recommendations for legislative modification of the act or for new legislation.

• Section 1706 created an Office of Health Information and Health Promotion to be located in the office of the Assistant Secretary for Health. All these activities came about through political action.

National immunization program Recent studies have revealed not only a national decline in immunization levels, most notably for poliomyelitis, but that motivating and organizing people for immunization has lagged far behind the development of new vaccines.[3] Further, an inverse correlation has been found to exist between socioeconomic status and immunization levels: the lower the socioeconomic status, the lower the levels of immunization.[4] Finally, Robert E. Marklund and Douglas E. Durand have found that inadequately immunized populations do not constitute a homogeneous group but are composed of several subpopulations with substantial differences among them.[5]

As a result of these findings, a National Work Group on Health Information and Public Awareness proposed in 1977 that a national immunization policy should take into consideration a target population differentiated into "high-risk" and "hard-to-reach" people. It recommended further that a significant portion of the scarce resources expended in reaching the undifferentiated target population should be diverted toward the hard-to-reach by means of intensive community/neighborhood health-education efforts, for experience had shown that local immunization programs were most successful when those receiving immunization were involved in the programs' planning and implementation.

Nationwide immunization programs require three components, each with its own special imperatives:

1. Broadly based national programs of public information and health education utilizing the combined efforts and resources of federal and state agencies together with those of professional and voluntary health associations. National drives alone, however, are unlikely to reach more than two-thirds of those who need immunization.
2. State-initiated and state-focused campaigns that mobilize state and

local resources, including professional and voluntary health associations. This effort can raise immunizations to a level approaching 80 to 90 percent.

3. Specially tailored programs planned and operated at the local level by local citizens, volunteer groups, health agencies, and other health professionals to reach the most elusive subpopulations.[6]

The work group was concerned in addition with levels of public acceptance. Hence, the program was implemented primarily by means of diffusion and adoption, while the educational process employed a variety of behavioral, social science, and learning methodologies, making use of public relations, mass communications, community organization, group decision-making processes, and counseling in face-to-face settings. This full range of methodologies was aimed toward reaching a 90 percent level of immunization for children, the generally accepted U.S. standard for epidemic prevention.

A STATE PROGRAM

Introduced in Hawaii in 1973, VISTA Bilingual Health Aides, a state-level health-education program, was sponsored by the Health Education Office of the Hawaii State Department of Health and funded by ACTION, a federal agency formed to coordinate six federal volunteer-service programs of which VISTA (Volunteers in Service to America) was one. Directed at newly arriving immigrants with tuberculosis, the program's purpose was to use bilingual health aides to help them cope with disease-related problems and to make use of community health services. The immigrants of particular concern were from China, Korea, the Philippines, and Samoa.[7]

Believing that volunteers might be effective in extending the Health Education Office's work with Hawaii's disadvantaged, an ACTION consultant and a health-education officer began to gather information by making informal calls on several program managers within the State Department of Health. From the Communicable Disease Division they learned of Hawaii's rising tuberculosis rates caused by new immigrants. Another resource was a subprogram for immigrants that provided much information about the pressing health problems of immigrants from Southeast Asia and the South Pacific especially.

To involve them without delay in problem identification, goal setting, objectives development, work plans, and evaluation measures, the health-education officer convened interested governmental and private groups that served the areas in which newly arriving immigrants were settling. VISTA assisted in writing the program proposal, and the Health Education Office provided supporting services guided by the local ACTION office.

Immigrants are often reluctant to use state services for fear of becoming public charges and risking deportation. In addition, they are generally less concerned about their health than about matters of employment, income, and housing. To communicate with them, to gain their confidence, and to help them meet their own priority needs, health aides were selected who were themselves bilingual immigrants with training in health or in health-related fields. Residents of the same living areas were involved in contacting them through door-to-door visits; a referral and follow-up system was established through the collaboration of schools, churches, public and private agencies, and hospitals; and the mass media were likewise involved in the program.

Aides were trained in matters pertaining to Hawaii's immigration laws and amendments; its health-care system, including public laws and community or individual responsibilities; and in community facilities and services, with emphasis on how to utilize agency resources and what to expect of physicians, public health nurses, social workers, and teachers. They learned about tuberculosis and other communicable diseases, the epidemiology of parasites, basic nutrition and hygiene, maternal and child health, as well as the basics of medical regimens including how to follow medical instructions and how to give medication.

Trained also in such communication skills as interviewing, interpreting interviews, and writing reports, aides were then placed in clinics and immigrant centers, participating in community and neighborhood meetings, workshops, and health fairs, throughout these activities developing health information records and other materials. Basic approaches included diffusion and adoption, consensus organizing, and social planning.

As a result of these efforts, 2,757 immigrants were contacted and approximately 65 percent assisted in obtaining medical and other needed services.[8] The project was evaluated by studying the aides' monthly reports, by checking health assessment forms, by interviewing immigrant families and talking with health professionals, social workers, and school personnel about the aides' services. Evaluations yielded the following learnings.

1. All persons interested in such a program should be actively involved in its early stages.
2. Governmental clearances must be obtained without delay. Because of a tight financial situation in Hawaii, clearance had to be obtained from the governor, the State Department of Budget and Finance, the Director of Health, and the Department of Health's business office.

3. Sufficient time must be allowed to meet unanticipated obstacles. In this case, aides had not only to meet VISTA training requirements but to be specially oriented toward the Hawaiian system as well, so that supervising them consumed from 40 to 60 percent of the staff's time, far more than had been expected.
4. In any enterprise involving several agencies, certain built-in problems must be anticipated. New federal-agency goals and guidelines, for example, were confusing to volunteers who staffed the local VISTA office, and their attempts to interpret or clarify them caused delays in the project.
5. Expert help should be sought in developing evaluation instruments. Though the overall goal here was to assist in tuberculosis control, important helping relationships were not evaluated well enough to demonstrate their importance.

COMMUNITY PROGRAMS

This section focuses on such community-level efforts as health maintenance organizations (HMOs), community outreach programs, cardiovascular disease-prevention programs, and rural health education, and concludes with an example of a health-education program conducted outside the United States. Through the efforts of the World Health Organization and other agencies, health educators have participated for at least twenty-five years in the development of health-education programs in other countries. Our example was chosen because it demonstrates that U.S. methods can be successfully undertaken elsewhere and because it is a typical program that can be replicated in other parts of the world.

Health Maintenance Organizations

As Irving S. Shapiro suggests, HMOs are uniquely suited for testing health education's effectiveness.[9] Because they provide a full range of medical-care services to a defined population in return for a prepaid fixed annual fee, providing the best possible care to their members at the least possible cost is vital. If health education is to be an integral part of this program, it must help HMO members change their health behaviors in significant ways at reasonable costs. To what extent health education is cost-effective will be demonstrated in the three examples that follow, in all of which the basic approaches employed were diffusion and adoption, consensus organizing, and, to some extent, social planning.

Health Insurance Plan of Greater New York The Health Insurance Plan (HIP) of Greater New York has had a health-education program since its beginning in 1945. Serving 750,000 people, HIP provides comprehensive health services through a network of twenty-seven medical groups with a total of about 1,000 physicians. Each medical-group office contracts with HIP to provide these services in return for a yearly capitation fee based on the number of enrollees served; HIP in turn must use these monies to pay the costs of its services.

Of interest to health education are the following HIP organizational features:

1. Broad orientation toward health as expressed in the staffing of nutritionists, social workers, mental-health workers, and health-education specialists
2. Necessary care rendered only by qualified physicians
3. Close working relationships between physicians and allied health professionals
4. Provision of unit medical records
5. Team service to an identifiable group of members, allowing educational responsibilities to be shared
6. Physicians' agreement to endorse, sponsor, or participate in educational efforts for their members
7. Separation of finance management from services management, facilitating allocation of funds for health education.

Over the years HIP has developed a great variety of health-education activities that range from providing orientation for visitors and letters of welcome, from consultation, guidance, and evaluation activities, to in-service training courses and field and residency programs for students. In addition to offering regularly mailed bulletins, newsletters, and interpretive booklets, it screens and distributes material produced elsewhere. Subscriber committees are formed; large and small meetings, classes, and continuing group discussions are held. Health-education activities arose in connection with HIP's first hospital, establishment of a new Multiphasic Health Testing Center, and interest in the problem-oriented medical record.

These activities, whose listing could be considerably expanded, have embraced a far-reaching content:

1. Health maintenance (human biology, mental health, nutrition, health hazards, preventive medicine)
2. Special subjects (health problems of groups particularized according

to age and sex, chronic illness, diabetes, allergy, headaches, meno-
pause, addictions, food fads, child care, radiation hazards)

3. Medical care (historical and national trends, the nature of medical
practice, the nature of group practice, doctors' instruments and procedures)

4. Use of available services (how to recognize need, the value of prompt
action, specific steps to take, the reasons for various medical and administrative procedures)

5. Development of special clinics and services (adolescent clinics, family
planning and counseling services, cooperation with nutritionists and
social workers, consultation with students and outreach workers)

6. Special campaigns (polio and measles immunization, tonometry
screening for glaucoma, expectant-parent group education)

7. Staff-patient contact (in-service training sessions in interpersonal relations, how well the patient understands the doctor, how Spanish-
speaking members view health, illness, medical treatment, etc.).

Evaluation of achievement has been based on close observation of program activities and reactions to them as discovered through responses to
bulletin articles, questionnaires, and personal interviews with subscribers
and physicians alike. Among the things observed are subscribers' attendance, questions, and comments at meetings; the number of physicians and
administrators participating and their response to subscribers' comments
and suggestions; subscribers' reactions to medical-group information or directives; and community response to the whole.

Group Health Cooperative of Puget Sound Seattle's Group Health
Cooperative of Puget Sound is a prepaid group-practice plan owned and
operated by a consumer cooperative whose health-education unit has been
carrying out activities involving its membership, medical and other staff,
and the community for at least fifteen years. Activities include large meetings and small-group discussions; consultation, guidance, in-service training
conferences and workshops for staff; and the development of questionnaires, audiovisual materials, newsletters, leaflets, and reports. All these efforts focus on orienting members to the plan, on health maintenance and
preventive procedures, and on enhancing understanding between patients
and staff, among staff units, and with community organizations.

In response to the recent enrollment of poverty groups, the health-
education unit has trained outreach workers recruited from this population
to function as auxiliary health educators, nurses, and social workers. In addition, a health educator has organized and guided a task force of staff nurses,

social workers, physicians, and administrators to study and install family-planning services for members.

Kaiser-Permanente Medical Group   In 1967 the Kaiser-Permanente Medical Group in Oakland, California, initiated the use of nurse-instructors in an ambulatory-care unit to achieve two objectives. The first objective was to improve care by influencing patient motivation and compliance. With health-education staff members as resource people, the nurse-educators use many teaching methods and tools to allay patients' anxiety and confusion and to guide them in proper self-care and use of services.

The second objective was to increase the efficiency of medical-care delivery while at the same time conserving physicians' time. To this end a system was developed for regulating the flow of patients on the basis of their identification as either "well," "worried well," "early sick," or "sick," each category of patient following a different route to receive the necessary services. Thus, "with health testing as the heart of the system, the entry mix is sorted into its components, which fan out to each of three distinct divisions of service: a health-education service, a preventive maintenance service, and a sick-care service."[10]

In Oakland, too, a Health Education Research Center has been established which contains a popular Exhibit Theater with displays on a variety of subjects. Here open-house programs are conducted, and a health-education library has been established for patients. Classes are offered in maternal and baby care, family planning, nutrition, sex education, adult immunization, hypertension, back pain, and diabetes, among other subjects, and patients are referred to the center for advice and counseling in many areas of health.

These three organizations demonstrate that health education is a highly efficient mechanism for providing HMO patients with scientifically accurate information and with reassurance about illness, for enhancing their cooperation during treatment and recovery, and for encouraging health maintenance thereafter. Such programs reduce misunderstanding, friction, and delay by illuminating medical-group practice, administrative functions, and specific medical care procedures. Health educators can establish, maintain, and extend communication channels between patient and doctor, as well as between the HMO and its members. They can also help to build greater good will between patients and staff, and between the HMO and the community.[11]

Community outreach programs

Though not new at the time, community outreach programs received great impetus as a result of the federal social-action programs of the middle and late 1960s. Multiservice and neighborhood health centers developed special facilities and programs to reach the disadvantaged, and one of these became the model for the Office of Economic Opportunity's Neighborhood Health Center Act, which resulted in the establishment of many such centers around the nation.

Located in a public housing development, Boston's Columbia Point Neighborhood Health Center was the first center to establish its own health-education unit, which trained residents of the development as health aides to participate in outreach educational efforts. It was also the first center to have a board of directors composed of residents of the development, in both these efforts involving participants directly in program planning and implementation. The outreach concept was also adopted by a number of community-based hospitals, and one of these, financed by a federal grant, will here be discussed in detail.

Griffin Hospital Community Health-Education Program   A 260-bed general facility in Connecticut, Griffin Hospital served a community of five cities and towns which until 1974 lacked a full-time health department, a lack that forced the hospital to take a broader look at its services and responsibilities toward the community's 75,000 residents.[12] At this point, two needs were identified. First, a strategy was needed for reducing unnecessary, inappropriate, and inefficient use of the hospital's resources. Second, realistic communication links were needed to enhance the community's ability to share responsibility for health problems, especially for special-risk groups, and to provide the hospital with a continuing basis for scientifically and socially responsible interventions.

In 1967, as the result of a proposal written by a planning consultant in collaboration with the head of the health-education section of the Yale School of Medicine's Department of Epidemiology and Public Health, Griffin Hospital obtained a three-year grant from the U.S. Public Health Service to fund a project in health education. The purpose of the project was to demonstrate methods of stimulating and organizing joint planning between hospital and personnel and community groups for the early detection, treatment, and rehabilitation of the chronically ill.

Recruited to carry out the project were program planners, nurses, social workers, and a health-education specialist. A needs-assessment activity undertaken to establish priorities involved staff, patients, and community residents. The priorities were community health activities, patient discharge planning, health education, and program development.

The health-education project, in particular, became involved in a great many activities:

• Planning in behalf of patients; screening all patients for discharge planning; establishing a community council for health and welfare planning

- Producing a directory of health, welfare, educational, and recreational resources; studying health, housing, and job needs in a depressed area; assisting a child day-care center
- Conducting educational programs for diabetic patients and for those requiring colostomy or catheter care; acting as a catalyst for a patient-education committee of the Connecticut Hospital Association; conducting drug education programs for local school systems; assisting a self-help community of ex-addicts; assisting Alcoholics Anonymous in a hospital program for alcoholism
- Cooperating in annual influenza immunization programs for the elderly; proposing and planning a transportation system to bring the elderly and ill to medical facilities
- Reorienting the hospital's emergency services to give primary care in addition to accident care; bringing together a committee of representatives from extended-care facilities.

Two of these activities will be described in greater detail: the development of a coordinating health-planning force to push for broad community change and the development of a transportation system to bring the ill and elderly to medical facilities.

During its third year, discussions initiated by the health-education project with the hospital, the United Fund, and South-Central Connecticut's Comprehensive Health Planning Agency (CHPA) resulted in the establishment of a community council staffed through CHPA funds and supervised by CHPA's director and the project's director. The goal in establishing this entity was twofold: (1) to create a health planning council that would represent the five-town area in a larger twenty-town area that was funded under the then current Comprehensive Health Planning Act; and (2) to create for the Connecticut Valley area a community council that would organize and coordinate citizen participation in study, planning, and action to achieve high standards of community health, recreation, and general welfare.

Consolidating these functions in a community council enabled the hospital to work with a single, well-coordinated community agency and also reduced community dependence on the hospital for all matters pertaining to health policy and programs. The hospital came to be seen as only one, rather than the sole, resource for meeting community-wide health needs. Under the council's leadership, efforts were made to establish in the five-town area a regional health department to replace five inadequate part-time services, and a study of area-wide home health services was initiated. Previously, the hospital had been unsuccessful in establishing these programs because, working alone, it had lacked the power to influence community decision making.

Concerned, too, about a lack of transportation for the ill and elderly, the project staff spent much time designing grant proposals for that purpose. After three years of failure, however, the regional planning agency reviewed these proposals, and its action resulted in a grant from the U.S. Department of Transportation. Under government contract, the Rensselaer Research Corporation conducted research on minibus carriers, and the local demonstration—the only one of its kind in the nation—tested not only vehicle design but a system for transportation that met health needs.

The resultant program was operated by the Valley Transit District, an agency created by the Connecticut legislature and controlled by representatives from the towns, and the Griffin Hospital offered facilities for its administration. The Department of Community Health and the community council cooperated with the regional planning agency in getting the transportation project under way.

Cardiovascular disease-prevention programs

Epidemic within the United States and other industrialized countries as well, cardiovascular diseases are associated with several behavioral risk-factors whose early identification and modification could prevent much disability and death. Described here are two widely differing preventive efforts: a controlled action-research project called the Stanford Heart Disease-Prevention Program and a community promotional effort conducted as part of a National High Blood-Pressure Education Program.[13-15]

Stanford Heart Disease–Prevention Program　The Stanford field experiment in the early 1970s involved three small communities in Northern California with populations of 15,000 each. One of these received no educational services; the other two were exposed to a year-long mass media campaign, and one had the additional input of intensive face-to-face instruction and group discussions.

Six behavioral recommendations were made for reducing cardiovascular risk-factors: (1) reduce intake of saturated fats, cholesterol, sugar, and salt; (2) restrict caloric intake to attain and maintain optimal body weight; (3) engage in regular physical activity to improve health and avoid overweight; (4) do not smoke; (5) acquire relaxation and stress-management skills; and (6) adhere to regimens of self-medication to control hypertension and hyperlipidemia.

The proposed intervention strategies were as follows: (1) external monitoring or self-observation of target behaviors; (2) self-control of environmental influences on behavior; (3) modeling and guided practice in the establishment of new behaviors; (4) social reinforcement for gradual attainment of desired habits; (5) contingency contracts specifying external or self-presented rewards for desired behaviors; (6) counterconditioning procedures to establish new positive or negative associations; and (7) stress-management training in deep-muscle relaxation, meditation and biofeedback.

According to Donald F. Roberts, the California study assumed that a successful campaign would depend upon the creation of a cognitive structure that was clear, comprehensible, and attractive enough to assure acceptance of the message.[16] It would have to have an effective means of motivation, such as clearly outlining the path to the goal, and would have also to create conditions or situations that triggered the desired behavior. To help create this cognitive structure, all the media and various types of appeals were used. The intent, however, was not to test whether one type of appeal was better than another but rather to create the needed cognitive structure by any means at hand.

Thus, some of the attitudinal and behavioral change may not have been directly engendered by the project message at all. It may be that A saw a television spot and said something about it to B, who in turn spoke with C, who changed because his aunt had just died of a heart attack. Although the change may in this way have been the result of a number of variables coinciding at the right instant, the campaign may nevertheless have set the agenda making the change much likelier to occur.

Agenda setting by means of the mass media began to receive greater attention from researchers, who held that, though the media cannot tell people how to think, they can have a significant effect in telling them what to think about. Compared with the control community in the Stanford program, the two other communities demonstrated significant attitudinal and behavioral change toward such issues as the importance of regular exercise and the dangers of cholesterol intake.

The community that received both mass-media and interpersonal treatment showed a marked decrease in its weekly consumption of eggs (one indicator of cholesterol intake). There were also tentative indications of decreased retail sales of whole milk and eggs in the communities that received intensive instruction in the dangers of cholesterol and the foods in which it is found. The program is still conducting long-range follow-up research.

Community workshop program for hypertension control As part of a National High Blood-Pressure Education Program, a community program-development workshop was conducted in 1974 in New Orleans.[17] First, a planning committee was formed whose primary tasks were to bring together community leaders who could make direct contributions to community control of high blood pressure and to determine and recommend how this work could best be accomplished.

Leaders in the city's health-care delivery system, planning committee members represented medical schools, hospitals, city and state health departments, voluntary health agencies, community social-service agencies, the local medical society, and other organizations. Other vested-interest participants included insurance firms, pharmacies and pharmaceutical companies, and consumer representation groups such as the Urban League, Chamber of Commerce, labor groups, the housing authority, the financial community, and mass communications personnel.

Once a workshop format had been decided upon, four workshop goals were established: (1) emphasis on hypertension as a major community health factor; (2) development of a strategy for a coordinated community-wide effort to control hypertension; (3) development of a procedure for collecting action-recommendations and organizing task forces for program planning; and (4) formation of a coordinating committee to direct the program.

The workshop was structured around six task forces which developed the six basic components of the community control program: (1) public awareness and education, (2) professional education, (3) screening and referral, (4) community resources for diagnosis and therapy, (5) data coordination, and (6) financial needs and resources. Each work group had a moderator and resource consultant, and each was provided with educational materials and guidelines for initiating discussions, sharing experiences and concerns, and eliciting commitments for follow-up action. The work groups reported to one another in a brief wrap-up session, and all agreed to continue planning activities on a coordinated ongoing basis.

As a result of this workshop, the Lousiana legislature approved and funded a permanent blood-pressure control program. In addition, nurses in city health clinics were trained in hypertension-screening procedures; other screening programs adopted hypertension screening as part of their ongoing procedures; and the city's tuberculosis clinic expanded its services to include hypertension screening and therapy.

Hypertension was included in the city's sickle cell screening program for high school populations; blood-pressure screening was included in the parish school board's detection and therapy program; and Charity Hospital added an adolescent hypertension clinic to its adult clinic. Finally, plans were made for similar workshops to be conducted in other parts of the state.

Rural programs

Health education was originally rooted in rural health, working through agricultural extension services and community programs to promote clean water, grade A milk, community and home health services, and the like. Rural health needs remain great, however. Many communities today either have no physicians at all or have only elderly physicians with a limited practice, and efforts by community leaders to recruit young physicians are not always successful.

As Claudia Galiher suggests, rural populations must learn to think in terms of a comprehensive area system that links the resources of a number of communities, provides primary, secondary, and tertiary levels of care, and makes creative use of nurse practitioners and physician assistants.[18] How health education can help to meet rural needs, both domestic and foreign, is the subject of this concluding section.

Meeting domestic needs Health education can be a vital ingredient in improving rural health care, especially in primary and emergency care and their financing and in personal health maintenance as well. Primary care can be improved by three means: (1) orienting rural populations toward primary care and the actions they can take to initiate its development in their communities; (2) cultivating among them a better understanding of the options for health-care delivery; and (3) substituting small rural systems for private medical practice.

In building a comprehensive health-care system, community leaders must first identify sources of advice and help. This means drawing on state resources, finding nurses who will undergo the additional training necessary to become family nurse-practitioners, and finding a physician who will supervise the latter and help to arrange for specialty consultation.

Next, a site for a rural primary-care center must be found and renovated; community leaders must organize themselves into a corporate entity that is capable of administering and managing the center; and negotiations must be undertaken with hospitals and universities for the linkages that will make a complete range of services possible. Because farm accidents have always been a rural occupational hazard, community attention should be focused on an emergency system as back-up support for primary care.

Financing can be assisted (1) by helping local organizations to take leadership in negotiating group health-insurance plans to reduce individual costs, and (2) by helping individuals to become more sophisticated in purchasing health insurance so that they get the best buy for their money. Because of the high incidence of rural accidents, the federal Emergency Medical Services Program has assigned priority to the funding of emergency services for rural areas.

Finally, health education can greatly assist health maintenance by motivating individuals to become more adept at preventing illness and practicing self-care, and by helping community leaders to identify and maximize the potential for improved maintenance by individuals and families. Particularly where the nurse practitioner is to be the primary source of care, patient education is likely to improve, since nurses have traditionally been trained in consultation education and in encouraging patients toward self-maintenance skills.

A foreign program In 1974 a health-education program was undertaken to eradicate scabies—an infectious disease affecting schoolchildren particularly—in an Arab village of some 3,000 people in western Galilee.[19] For five years previously, repeated attempts to seek out and treat infected patients and family contacts had been unsuccessful; during one winter alone the number of reported cases among schoolchildren had risen by 24 percent.

The local health office had responded to this increase by assigning five nurses the task of visiting all the schools in the village, screening all students, and giving talks to all classes above the fourth grade. Pamphlets in Arabic were distributed, homes were visited, two physicians lectured at a special meeting of men, and parents were invited to clinics for free supplies and instructions. The turnout at clinics was disappointing, however, and within a few months the incidence of scabies had jumped from a 24 percent increase to a 31 percent increase of cases.

At about this time a special health-education team was organized consisting of nine nurses, a sanitary inspector, and a health educator who was the team leader. The group engaged in a series of training sessions to learn how to conduct health education and to develop a plan for responding to health problems at a community-wide level. Reviewing past experience and consulting with a dermatologist, entomologist, and professional exterminator, the team developed a four-phase program designed to eradicate scabies within six months.

• Phase 1 consisted of a three-month house-to-house demographic survey eliciting the prevailing beliefs about, and attitudes toward, scabies.

• Phase 2 consisted of a major informational campaign employing a variety of approaches:

1. Forming a committee of community leaders to join the team in helping the community understand the problem and what it should do to eradicate it
2. Obtaining direct support of village elders, religious leaders, and heads of clans by meeting in their homes
3. Arranging visits by the district health physician to local physicians and nurses to elicit their support and involvement
4. Holding separate meetings with schoolteachers, women's clubs, parent's council, village education committee, high school and college students, and village water-supply committee

5. Holding thirty-six informal coffee meetings in private homes, result-ing in the participation of 346 adults

6. Distributing carefully prepared pamphlets imparting clear messages about the problem and how to eradicate it and changing derogatory terms for scabies to more acceptable terms

7. Presenting health-education programs to all classes above the fourth grade

8. Having students take educational messages to their parents and en-couraging the latter to participate in educational discussions at home.

• Phase 3 consisted of the treatment program itself conducted over a period of one week. Except for two families who were out of the village at the time, the entire village appeared at the clinics, and 22 percent of the population (66 percent of the households) was found to have clinical symptoms of scabies. Those with the disease were given medication to be administered by the head of the household, and their homes were visited and treated by the exterminator.

• Phase 4 consisted of the program wrap-up and follow-up checks and treatment. A postprogram meeting was held for all interested people, and volunteers were presented with citations. During the following year only one case of scabies was reported and promptly treated. The program was regarded as highly successful.

We have thus seen, in Parts 1–3, health-education theory and practice at work with individuals, organizations, and social systems; at foreign, na-tional, state, and local levels, in urban centers and isolated rural areas; within the context of community health services and in relation to numerous sepa-rate problems as well. It has been shown that while health educators must employ a variety of methods and skills in any given program, no program can be applied to two different situations in exactly the same way. Numer-ous methods and techniques have here been alluded to, but few have been described in detail. Part 4 is devoted to describing the most basic of these at greater length.

REFERENCES

1. D. J. Merwin, "The National Center for Health Education" (Speech presented at National Conference on Hospital-based Patient Education, Chicago, 9–10 August 1976).

2. H. G. Ogden, "The Bureau of Health Education" (Speech presented at National Conference on Hospital-based Patient Education, Chicago, 9–10 August 1976).

3. J. J. Witte, "Recent Advances in Public Health," *American Journal of Public Health*

64, no. 10 (October 1974): 939–44; and H. M. Scmeck, "Too Few Americans Found Immunized," *New York Times*, 15 June 1974, p. 11.

4. C. N. D'Onofrio, *Reaching Our "Hard to Reach,"* pp. 11–15; L. W. Green, *Status Identity and Prevention Health Behavior;* and *Pacific Health Education Reports*, no. 1 (1970), pp. 107–19.

5. R. E. Marklund and D. E. Durand, "An Investigation of Sociopsychological Factors Affecting Infant Immunization," *American Journal of Public Health* 66, no. 2 (February 1976): 168–72.

6. JRB Associates, Inc., "Reports and Recommendations of the National Immunization Work Groups" (Submitted to the Office of the Assistant Secretary for Health, Contract no. 263–77–e–0076, 15 March 1977).

7. J. Simmons, ed., "Making Health Education Work," *American Journal of Public Health* 65 (supp.) (October 1975): 40–42.

8. Ibid.

9. I. S. Shapiro, "HMOs and Health Education," *American Journal of Public Health* 65, no. 5 (May 1975): 469–73.

10. Ibid., p. 471.

11. Ibid., pp. 472–73.

12. R. K. Conant, A. J DeLucca, and L. S. Levin, "Health Education: A Bridge to the Community," *American Journal of Public Health* 62, no. 9 (September 1972): 1239–44.

13. A. L. McAlister et al., "Behavioral Science Applied to Cardiovascular Health: Progress and Research Needs in the Modification of Risk-taking Habits in Adult Populations," *Health Education Monographs* 4, no. 1 (Spring 1976): 45–74.

14. J. W. Farquhar, "Research in Attitude Change and Motivation of Health Practices," in *Applying Behavioral Science to Cardiovascular Risk*, ed. A. J. Enelow and J. B. Henderson, pp. 58–62.

15. D. F. Roberts, "Attitude-Change Research and the Motivation of Health Practices," in Enelow and Henderson, *Applying Behavioral Science to Cardiovascular Risk*, pp. 42–57.

16. Ibid., pp. 52–53.

17. S. B. Garbus, T. R. Donohue, and G. Wilson, "The Community Workshop as a Stimulus for Hypertension-Control Programs," *American Journal of Public Health* 66, no. 7 (July 1976): 682–83.

18. C. Galiher, "Rural Initiatives and Health-Education Needs," *Health Education Monographs* 3, no. 1 (Spring 1975): 109–14.

19. H. A. K. Kanaaneh, S. A. Rabi, and S. M. Badarneh, "The Eradication of a Large Scabies Outbreak Using Community-wide Health Education," *American Journal of Public Health* 66, no. 6 (June 1976): 564–67.

PART FOUR
HEALTH-
EDUCATION
PRACTICE

11

*Planning for
health education*

12

*Methods for
health education*

13

*Evaluation of
health education*

Not only health-education specialists but anyone who employs a planned strategy for changing the health behavior of others may be said to be engaged in health education. Unlike the nonprofessional, however, who tends to concentrate on a particular activity to bring about a particular desired change, professional health educators concern themselves with a larger structure whose main components are planning, a broad range of methodology, and evaluation.

Planning gives health education its overall program direction. Methods, based on a considerable body of knowledge and skills, are the means by which the program is carried out. Evaluation helps to ascertain health education's ultimate effectiveness. Part 4 is devoted to exploring these important tools in greater detail than was either possible or practical in earlier chapters.

11
Planning for health education

There are many forms of planning, and different professions approach it in different ways. The highly mathematical computerized form has enabled NASA to send and return men from the moon. The technical-mechanized form enables engineers to reshape the environment. The systems form identifies the precise relationships among various parts of a complex structure. The social form endeavors to change disadvantageous social conditions, and the health form attempts to improve the delivery and use of health services.

Although primarily concerned with health planning, health education can contribute meaningfully to social planning by clarifying and facilitating the planning process for others, as well as by improving planning methodology to meet its own purposes. Of great social importance, the 1974 National Health Planning and Resources Development Act (P.L. 93–641) established health education as one of ten national priorities pertaining to the formulation of national health-planning goals and the development and operation of federal, state, and area health-planning and resources-development programs.[1] Since nearly all the other priorities have implications for health education as well, this chapter will begin by reviewing some general approaches to health planning and will then describe a specific model in detail.

GENERAL APPROACHES TO PLANNING

Reference to three sources meets the needs of a general review: Lawrence Green's PRECEDE framework for health-education planning, Darwin Palmiere's three types of planning, and Daniel Sullivan's comprehensive health-education model. Other valuable sources are the American Public Health Association's "Making Health Education Work," a 1975 supplement to the *American Journal of Public Health*,[2] and Henrik Blum's *Planning for Health* (1974), a methodological analysis of planning technologies as they relate to health.[3] In his more recent *Expanding Health Care Horizons* (1976), Blum describes a role for health educators in health governance and planning.[4]

PRECEDE framework   Green's PRECEDE framework (figure 12) identifies seven phases of health-education planning.[5] Phase 1 assesses quality of life by focusing on general social problems of concern to individuals or communities. Phase 2 identifies specific health problems that appear to be contributing to these social problems. Phase 3 identifies specific behaviors that appear to be linked with the health problems. Phase 4 identifies predisposing, enabling, and reinforcing factors that have a potential for affecting health behavior. Phase 5 locates the focus for intervention. Phase 6 encompasses the program's development and implementation, and Phase 7 (not pictured) includes evaluation as an integral and continuing part of program planning.

The PRECEDE framework is especially helpful in indicating the variety of factors that impinge on health and health behavior. Successful completion of phases 1, 2, and parts of 3, for example, requires the use of epidemiological methods; phases 3 and 4 require familiarity with social-behavioral concepts; phases 5 and 6 require knowledge and experience of administrative and educational theory. (Green does not cite a discipline for phase 7, which requires all disciplines.) The model thus emphasizes that because health is affected by multiple factors, health-education efforts must be multidimensional as well.

Three types of planning   Palmiere views health-care planning as a developmental process encompassing three types of activities: dispersed health planning, focused health planning, and central health planning.[6]

Dispersed health planning denotes the many decisions made by all individuals and organizations within the health-care system. Decisions may be divided into four groups: (1) definition and selection of health problems, goals, and standards; (2) establishment of priorities and acquisition or allocation of resources in accord with priorities; (3) establishment of coordinative and integrative activities with other health-system personnel and organizations; and (4) choice of day-to-day activities in the use, performance, or financing of health-care services.

Focused health planning denotes a voluntary association of persons and organizations to resolve common problems or to attain goals that cannot be resolved or attained independently. Unlike dispersed planning, which involves only a few persons and organizations at a time, focused planning brings the attention and efforts of a relatively large number of persons and organizations together simultaneously.

In dispersed planning, the scope of power encompasses only a narrow segment of health-care activity—e.g., a physician organizing a private practice or a family determining what care its members need. In focused planning, the planning agency is part of a larger association, such as a voluntary interagency council, and lacks the power to implement its plans alone. Central health planning, however, denotes power controlled by an individual or organization that forces others to use their resources in accord with its plans. Examples include the Medicare program, which is controlled by the Social Security Administration, and health-systems agencies, which are controlled by P.L. 93–641.

Comprehensive health-education model Sullivan's model for the comprehensive, systematic development of health education programs shows (1) planning components and their relationships, (2) steps in health-education planning, operation, and evaluation (figure 13), and (3) dynamic linkages in health education (see table 11 and figure 14).[7]

The basic components are: health status, personal actions, health-education practices, and health-education resources, each area requiring identification and study of affected population groups, facts about current status, and decisions about goals. Analysis of forces will indicate the causes of barriers that may hinder movement from current status toward goals and the factors that may facilitate such movement.

The steps for organizing these components are shown in a logical sequence: involving people, setting goals, defining problems, designing plans, conducting activities, and evaluating results. Although planning does not proceed this neatly, each phase brings insights that may lead to changes in previous decisions. Appropriate persons should be involved at each step, and the effort should be coordinated with health education at other levels and with related community programs as well.

FIGURE 12
The PRECEDE Framework

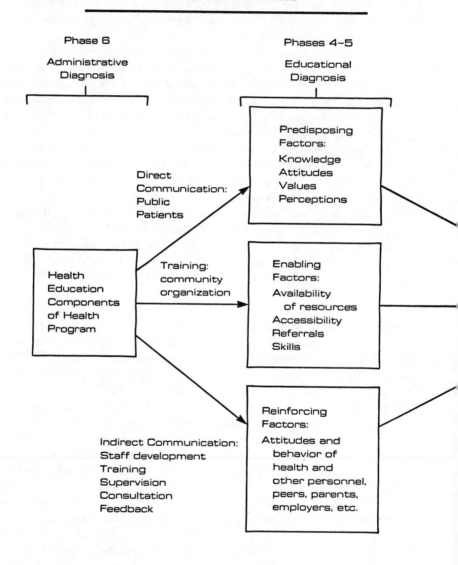

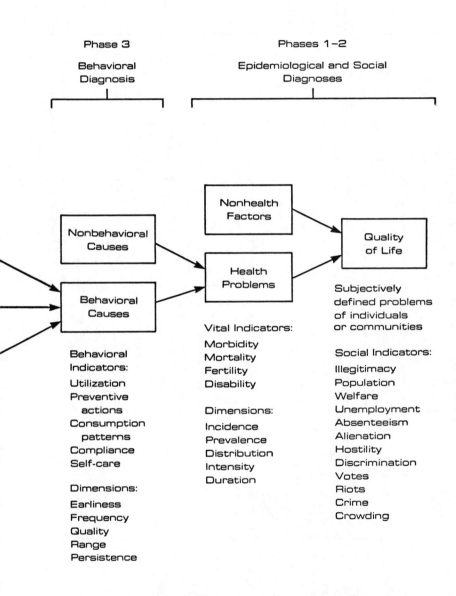

Phase 3

Behavioral
Diagnosis

Phases 1–2

Epidemiological and Social
Diagnoses

Nonbehavioral
Causes

Nonhealth
Factors

Quality
of Life

Behavioral
Causes

Health
Problems

Subjectively
defined problems
of individuals
or communities

Behavioral
Indicators:

Utilization
Preventive
    actions
Consumption
    patterns
Compliance
Self-care

Dimensions:

Earliness
Frequency
Quality
Range
Persistence

Vital Indicators:

Morbidity
Mortality
Fertility
Disability

Dimensions:

Incidence
Prevalence
Distribution
Intensity
Duration

Social Indicators:

Illegitimacy
Population
Welfare
Unemployment
Absenteeism
Alienation
Hostility
Discrimination
Votes
Riots
Crime
Crowding

SOURCE: Adapted from L. Green, *Health Education Today and the PRECEDE Framework* (Palo Alto, Calif.·
Mayfield Publishing Co., 1979), p. 15.

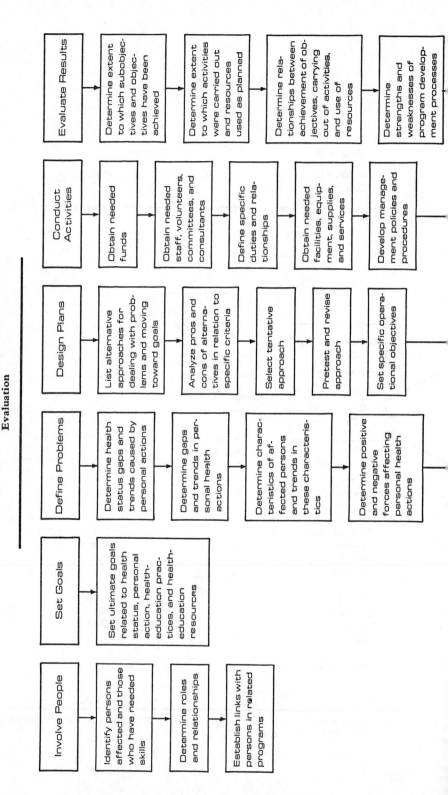

FIGURE 13
Steps in Health-Education Planning, Operation, and Evaluation

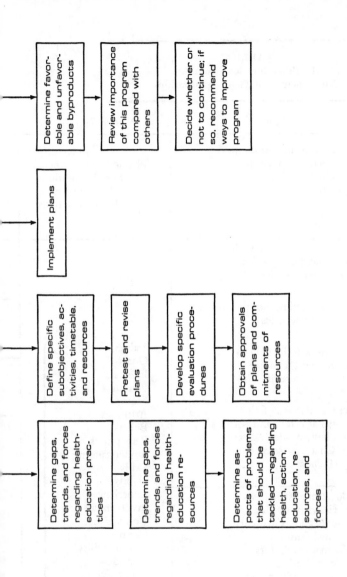

Boxes in the flowchart:

- Determine favorable and unfavorable byproducts
- Review importance of this program compared with others
- Decide whether or not to continue; if so, recommend ways to improve program

- Implement plans

- Define specific subobjectives, activities, timetable, and resources
- Pretest and revise plans
- Develop specific evaluation procedures
- Obtain approvals of plans and commitments of resources

- Determine gaps, trends, and forces regarding health-education practices
- Determine gaps, trends, and forces regarding health-education resources
- Determine aspects of problems that should be tackled—regarding health, action, education, resources, and forces

SOURCE: Adapted from D. Sullivan, "Model for Comprehensive, Systematic Program Development in Health Education," *Health Education Report* 1, no. 1 (November–December 1973):4–5.

TABLE 11
Health-Education Planning
Components and Their Relationships

	People	*Positive Forces*
Health	All persons in community or selected population • Characteristics • Trends	Heredity Physical environment Social conditions Health services Personal actions
Action	All persons but especially those having high risk • Characteristics • Trends Persons needing health services • Characteristics • Trends Persons who have been given medical advice • Characteristics • Trends Representatives of all groups affected, and persons who have needed skills • Characteristics • Trends	Values Goals Interests Pleasures Fears Attitudes Beliefs Perceptions Understanding Skills Habits
Education	Educational specialists Providers of service Patients and ex-patients Patients' families Informal counselors Opinion leaders Communications media • Characteristics • Trends	Experiences Involvement Convenience Comfort Compatibility Confidence Complexity Cost Timing
Resources	Agency administrators Advisory committees Community leaders Business, industry, labor Civic organizations Legislators Foundations Education consultants Behavioral scientists • Characteristics • Trends	Availability Policies Laws Technology Environment

Current Status	Negative Forces	Goals
Current health status: Degree of well-being Preventable disability and premature death caused by personal actions • Costs • Trends	Heredity Physical environment Social conditions Health services Personal actions	Vigorous well-being Reduction in preventable disability Reduction or delay in premature death
Current personal health practices • Gaps • Trends		Personal practices that promote vigorous well-being and prevent unnecessary disability and death
Current use of health services • Gaps • Trends	Values Goals Interests	Prompt use of appropriate health services when needed
Current following of medical advice • Gaps • Trends	Pleasures Fears Attitudes Beliefs	Carrying out of prescribed diagnostic, treatment, and rehabilitation procedures
Current participation in health program development • Gaps • Trends	Perceptions Understanding Skills Habits Experiences Involvement	Broad, effective participation in health program development
Current health education practices • Costs • Gaps • Trends	Convenience Comfort Compatability Confidence Complexity Cost Timing Availability Policies	Effective, efficient, appropriate application of what is known about how people learn
Current health-education financing, manpower, facilities, equipment, supplies, technical assistance, legislation • Costs • Gaps • Trends	Laws Technology Environment	Availability of needed health education resources: Adequate financing Appropriate quantity, preparation, distribution, and use of needed manpower Adequate facilities, equipment, and supplies Adequate technical assistance Adequate legislation

SOURCE: D. Sullivan, "Model for Comprehensive Systematic Program Development in Health Education," *Health Education Report* 1, no. 1 (November-December 1973): 4–5.

FIGURE 14
Dynamic Linkages in Health Education

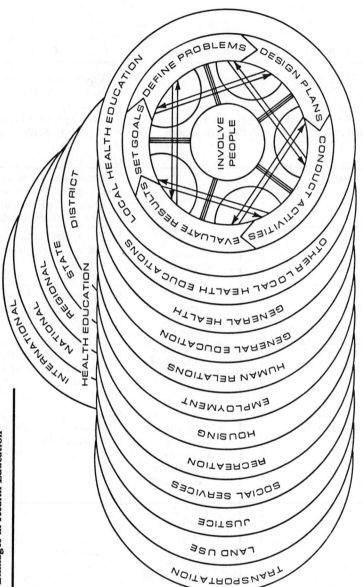

SOURCE: Adapted from D. Sullivan, "Model for Comprehensive, Systematic Program Development in Health Education," *Health Education Reports* 1, no. 1 (November–December 1973):4–5.

MODEL FOR HEALTH-EDUCATION PLANNING

The planning model to be examined here consists of two dimensions. Six horizontal phases, arranged hierarchically from the bottom upward, identify programmatic steps: (1) initiation of planning activity, (2) needs assessment, (3) goal setting, (4) planning or programming the activity to be carried out, (5) implementing the activity, and (6) evaluating the activity's effectiveness. The three vertical dimensions identify the activity's content or subject matter, the steps and techniques associated with each phase, and the process (or interactions) involved throughout (see table 12).

The following discussion posits the undertaking of a new activity beginning at phase 1. Health educators who have an activity currently under way can use the model by determining which phase they have reached and then either developing the activity throughout the remaining phases or reviewing past phases to see whether any overlooked steps can still be made up. While not all parts of the model will fit all situations, most parts will fit a given activity in some way.

Phase 1: Initiation

Phase 1 is in many respects the most critical phase of planning, for the activity's success or failure often depends upon what does or does not happen here. The key elements with regard to *content* are understanding the client's problem and something about the client's system. The key elements of *method* are entry or intervention strategy, developing an initial contract, and organizing the parties concerned. The key element of *process* is making the client aware that a problem exists to induce a readiness to work on it and to reduce the threat of the intervention.

Entry or intervention strategy is of great importance at this stage, the approach used depending upon the activity's intent. If the activity is to organize a patient-education program in diabetes control, the health educator may either directly inform patients of the opportunity to participate or ask doctors and nurses to help motivate their patients to participate. If team building is to be the activity, the approach may be either to meet with the team's leader alone or with the whole team together. To help a neighborhood conduct a sickle cell-screening program, the choice may be either to meet with a neighborhood health board or with key neighborhood leaders.

Many entry-level problems are diminished if the health educator is invited to meet with the client. But if the client is unaware that an approach is being employed, the health educator is conducting an intervention, and this must be done with careful attention to issues of content and process alike. Conducting a force-field analysis is a good way of diagnosing entry problems, and good interviewing skills are helpful as well. Finally, the greater

TABLE 12
Model for Health-Education Planning

	Content Dimension
Phase 6 *Evaluation*	4. Knowledge of problem and client system 3. Technology of feedback systems 2. Language and systems 1. Nature of evaluation
Phase 5 *Implementation*	4. Writing skills 3. Dynamics of problem solving 2. Knowledge of subject and content T&TA being provided for 1. Knowledge of plan, how it is to work
Phase 4 *Planning/Programming*	3. Nature of political process 2. Systems analysis and management science 1. Techniques of planning
Phase 3 *Goal Setting*	5. Theory of change 4. MBO technology 3. Forecasting 2. Nature of policy 1. Role of goals, how to set them, measure
Phase 2 *Needs Assessment*	4. Relevance of data 3. Language and systems 2. Data sources 1. Standards and criteria
Phase 1 *Initiate*	3. Power and influence structures, community organization, culture 2. Contract terminology and resources 1. Knowledge of problem and client system

Method Dimension	Process Dimension
4. Redefine problem and standards 3. Feedback to activity, reporting, accountability 2. Data collection and analysis 1. Clarify evaluation measures	4. Consensus of new definitions 3. Communication, threat reduction 2. Learning assimilation 1. Agreement
4. Reporting 3. Problem solving 2. Training and technical assistance, consultation 1. Initiate activity	4. Communications 3. Creativity conflict resolution, win-win 2. Skill development, helping 1. Communications, orientations
3. Negotiate commitments, MOAs 2. Design management systems and tools 1. Develop implementation plan	3. Negotiation 2. Role clarification, communications 1. Understanding and commitment
5. Determine strategies for implementation 4. Select goals and objectives 3. Alternative goals statement, force-field analysis 2. Link to policy development 1. Establish criteria for goals	5. Consensus 4. Decision making, consensus 3. Reality testing, creative problem solving 2. Understanding of process and roles 1. Agreement
4. Describe nature and extent of problem 3. Data collection and analysis 2. Determine data to be collected 1. Identify and review present criteria	4. Reduce fantasy by fact 3. Open communications, sensitivity to data sources 2. Agreement 1. Agreement on starting point
3. Organize concerned 2. Develop initial contract 1. Entry or intervention strategy, force-field analysis, interviewing	3. Involvement, leadership, values clarification 2. Legitimacy, commitment, trust, readiness 1. Unfreezing, threat reduction, credibility, awareness of need

NOTE: First developed by Paul Mico in 1966, this model has been periodically updated as continuing application and experience have made further refinements possible.

the health educator's perceived credibility, the lower will be the threat of the intervention and the easier the "unfreezing" process for the client.

Even more important than entry or intervention strategy is development of the initial contract with its concomitant process issues of gaining legitimacy and support for the activity, eliciting an initial commitment from the client, beginning the building of trust, and developing in the client an even greater readiness to participate. Although in some circumstances (such as when the client is paying for the health-education activity) a legal contract may be necessary, the term *contract* is used here in a psychosocial rather than a legal sense. It need not be written if both parties are in verbal agreement about what is to be done, although a written agreement does force a clarification of untested mutual assumptions.

In the final analysis, the activity will be only as good as the contract, which should cover the following elements:

1. The identity of the parties to the contract and of any others involved
2. The scope of the activity, identifying objectives, tasks, outcomes, and means of evaluation insofar as these can be determined at this early stage
3. The conditions or ground rules for the activity, covering how work should be done, what can or cannot be done, and how often client and educator should meet to review progress
4. The resources needed to carry out the work, including a consideration of time, costs, facilities, equipment, mutual authority and responsibilities, outside assistance, and the membership to be involved as the activity progresses
5. Mutual expectations about the activity and the client-educator relationship
6. Provision for renegotiating the contract to accommodate a changing situation.

In a patient-education group, a contract may consist of agreements on purposes, the frequency and duration of meetings, the educator's plans for each session, and the patients' overall expectations. A school situation may call for a learning contract between the health educator and the class. In the training of a community health board, the contract may focus on problems to be discussed, skills to be acquired, the number of sessions to be conducted, and at what time of day the sessions will be held.

Generally speaking, a healthy client-educator relationship can be said to exist when (1) it is expressed in writing, (2) it is periodically reviewed to see that agreements are still being honored, (3) it can be characterized as adult-

adult, (4) mutual communications are mutually understood, (5) it is supported by the top echelon of the client system, (6) it has the participation of those who are to be involved in the change effort, and (7) both parties have learned the value of the contract in the planning process.

Organizing all the parties concerned in a health-education effort sometimes, but not always, occurs at the entry or contractual stages, for on occasion the initial client-educator agreement opens the door to still another party (technically, the client's client). If, for example, a neighborhood health board agrees to support a community-wide immunization program, that community will have to be organized. If a health-care management team agrees that its service-delivery staff should be trained in health-education techniques, that staff will likewise have to be organized. In such cases, the health educator may become involved in another round of intervention and contracting.

At whatever stage organizing occurs, however, in the content dimension it requires knowledge of how the organization or community is structured, who its gatekeepers or opinion leaders are and how they can be reached, and the basic cultures of the people with whom they will be working. If the activity involves working with a very large client system, such as the entire population of a city, organizing requires a knowledge of the effective use of communications media as well. From the process standpoint, the key issue is involvment. Whoever is to be involved in the activity's implementation should be involved at this point. Also, those who could block the activity should be identified and every effort made to intervene and contract with them.

Leadership development is another important process at this stage. Any health-education activity involving organizational or community leaders should have the specific objective of improving their knowledge about the nature of health education, as well as improving their communication, decision-making, and problem-solving skills. Moreover, as early as possible, the values of those who are involved—providers and consumers alike—should be clarified, for the likelihood of conflict will be far greater if there is basic value disagreement. This is not to suggest that there must be total agreement about values but only that unclarified values may result in counterproductive behavior.

Phase 2: Needs assessment

A vital phase of planning, needs assessment can range from merely asking a patient-education group why it has assembled to developing data-gathering instruments, sampling procedures, coding forms, and computer print-outs that categorize data according to a multitude of complex variables. In short, the technology for needs assessment can be simple and inexpensive or highly refined and very expensive depending upon the purpose for which the data are needed.

Generally speaking, if needs assessment is for helping a client deal with problems of learning and changing, and if the strategy is principally to involve the client in a process of discovery, the assessment can be made informally. But if the activity is a research and demonstration effort to be duplicated elsewhere, if it is a large-scale activity to be evaluated for cost-effectiveness, or if it is intended to change an agency's policies and priorities, thereby affecting other programs, the assessment should be made with strict care and accuracy.

The first step of phase 2 is to identify how the problem has been measured in the past. In terms of facilities, for example, measurements are often expressed on the basis of number of beds per 1,000 population or of basic facilities and services for a "catchment area" (a geographically based, population-oriented service area). For health behavior, however, establishing standards is difficult. While defining health as complete mental, physical, and social well-being may suggest goals, these characteristics are not functionally measurable.

The content of needs assessment consists of the standards and other criteria used as problem indicators; obviously, those used in relation to air pollution, for example, will differ from those used in relation to hospitals. On the process side, the individuals or organizations involved in an effort need to agree on the assessment's starting point, on its standards and criteria, and on the nature and extent of the problem.

The second step is to determine what data are to be collected, which, in terms of content, means knowing where they can be found and how collecting can best be accomplished. In terms of process, it means that the planning committee must agree on approaches and on why each is important. If standards for measuring the problem already exist, the committee can focus on the information to be collected and where it can be found—sometimes a simple matter of comparing existing resources with the desired standard and setting a goal of obtaining the additional resources needed to bring the client up to the standard. An absence of standards may mean collecting existing information about the problem, using these data to develop the health-education activity, and evaluating by re-collecting information later to see whether progress has been made.

The third step is data collection and analysis. The terminology of data collection, its range of procedures, its technical approaches and methods, its costs, practicality, and effectiveness—all compose the content aspect of planning, and both the health educator and the planning committee must be sufficiently familiar with this field to make sound decisions. In terms of process, several issues are important: knowing what the choices are; agreeing on approach; keeping open communications between the committee, the committee's client, and the educator; and being sensitive toward those asked to provide the data. If a household-interview survey is used, for example, interviewers should be sufficiently sensitive so that respondents are not disturbed by the experience.

In its 1976 *Social Needs Assessment Handbook,* the League of California Cities compared six basic methods of data collection with a number of different variables (see table 13).

Once collected, data must be tabulated and prepared for analysis. In highly complex situations, statisticians may be needed to determine which results are statistically significant. If data accuracy is less important than getting committee members to agree on the problems they want to solve, the problems may simply be listed on a chalkboard or sheet of newsprint and the committee helped to assign priorities among them.

The fourth step in needs assessment is to describe the nature and extent of the problem, and here accurate data are important for countering any unproved assumptions that people might harbor about a given situation. Whether data assessment has been formal or informal, the data must provide the assessors and health educator with an agreed-upon common base of facts, and participants in the planning should be involved in determining what the data mean to them.

Experts may provide the planning committee with their own conclusions, and the committee must either accept these conclusions or develop their own, for it is acceptance and assimilation of the data that make further steps possible. In some situations the committee may wish to conduct public meetings or hearings to present the problems for other peoples' reactions.

Phase 3: Goal setting

A *goal* is a future event toward which a committed endeavor is directed; *objectives* are the steps to be taken in pursuit of a goal. Establishing criteria for goals—the first step in phase 3—provides everyone concerned in a health-education effort with a consistent directional framework. The following criteria are those usually established or considered.

1. The goal should be a specific, stated, and measurable event so that the committee can later determine whether the event actually occurred.
2. Goal attainment should entail a reasonable time period. Goals that take more than five years to achieve are often perceived as too distant to be meaningful in the present. Also, any substantial change in interim conditions may cause an overdistant goal to become unrealistic or unimportant.

TABLE 13
Comparison of Data-Collection Methodologies

Method	Advantages	Disadvantages	Result Quality	Staff Requirements	Costs
Person-to-Person Interview	1. High response rate 2. Highly flexible 3. Visual aid opportunity 4. Community input and morale builder	1. High costs 2. Raises expectations 3. Travel expenses 4. Possible interviewer bias 5. Technical staff required 6. High agency effort 7. Possible computer needs 8. High call-back expenses	1. Yields detailed and high-quality results 2. Most representative results 3. Quantifiable results	1. Technical assistance for interview construction 2. Interviewer training 3. Technical assistance for data analyzation, processing, and interpretation 4. Several interviewers	High
Telephone Interview	1. Easy to administer 2. Low call-back expense 3. Community input and morale builder 4. High response rate 5. Relatively lower cost	1. Possible interviewer bias 2. Possible computer needs 3. Raises expectations 4. Representativeness and sampling problems	1. Quantifiable results 2. Relatively quality results 3. Unless corrected, some bias in results 4. Fairly detailed results	1. Interviewer training 2. Several interviewers 3. Possible technical assistance for data analyzation 4. Technical assistance for interview construction	Medium
Mail-Out Questionnaire	1. Low cost 2. Minimum staff time 3. Possible good response 4. Larger outreach 5. Community input	1. Generally low return rate 2. Possible bias and unrepresentativeness 3. Ineffective for illiterate people	1. Quantifiable results 2. Low to medium quality 3. Possible major biases 4. More candid results	1. Technical assistance for questionnaire construction 2. If hand-processed, one or two untrained staff	Low

	Advantages	Disadvantages	Results	Technical/Staff Requirements	Costs
Existing Records and Statistics	1. Relatively low cost 2. Minimum staff effort 3. Ongoing assessment and evaluation possible	1. No community input 2. Census data cost can be high 3. Possible agency uncooperativeness 4. Possible lack of question understanding 5. Possible computer needs	1. Relative quality results 2. Quantifiable results 3. Relative detail in results	1. Possible technical assistance for statistical interpretation 2. One or two staff 3. Technical assistance if computer-processed	Low to medium
Special Methodologies	1. Relative costs and staff effort 2. Possible community input	1. May require other methods for representativeness 2. Possible bias	1. Results can be quantified 2. Relative quality 3. Subjective	1. Relative—could be one staff	Low to medium, depending on scope and type
Meetings	1. Inexpensive 2. Community input and feedback 3. Flexibility 4. Opportunity for questionnaire distribution 5. Reflects aggregate community opinion	1. Hard to quantify 2. Possible result bias 3. Relatively low input for individual problems	1. Possible bias 2. Hard to quantify 3. Can be made quite representative	1. Minimal technical requirements 2. Sufficient staff to plan and organize meetings	Low monetary costs

SOURCE: League of California Cities, *Social Needs Assessment Handbook* (Sacramento, Calif., 1976), p. 115.

NOTE: Special methodologies include systematic field observations and investigations, the action-research approach to conducting the project activity, the anthropological technique of training those who regularly collect and report data, and others.

3. Goal attainment should be a realistic possibility. An unrealistic goal, such as the total eradication of disease, is meaningless and invites failure.

4. Goal setting should take into account probable costs, the availability and source of funds, and who will be responsible for managing expenditures.

5. Goal setting should take into account the population that will be affected by the goal and involved in its implementation.

6. Goal attainment should produce a behavioral result in terms of individual, organizational, or social change.

7. The goal must be relevant to the client system. If a goal statement does not match the problem situation, either the goal is unrelated to the problem or the problem has been ill-defined.

8. The goal must accord with the client system's existing policy (unless the goal is to change policy affecting the problem situation).

Ensuring that goal setting is linked to organizational or community policy development—the second step in phase 3—is important because policy is the key force behind the organization of systems. Particularly where large organizational or social systems are concerned, the health educator and planning committee must understand policy and its relation to the planned activity.

The third step in goal setting is to make a comprehensive statement of alternative goals and the consequences of carrying them out. If, for example, the people of a given neighborhood do not have access to an ambulatory-care clinic located elsewhere in the city, five alternative goals are possible: (1) helping residents to find ways of getting to the clinic, (2) developing a transportation system for getting them there and back, (3) obtaining a mobile ambulatory clinic that makes periodic scheduled trips to the neighborhood, (4) establishing in the neighborhood a storefront clinic that is managed within the organizational framework of the other clinic, or (5) creating a neighborhood health center to be operated by a neighborhood health association. All the previously listed criteria would be applied to each alternative to enable the committee to make the best possible decision.

In order for sound alternative goals to be established, the committee should be able to make projections over the next three to five years to anticipate any changes that are likely to affect the choice of alternatives. Testing the reality of a situation is part of this step; creative problem solving is important in developing potential alternatives; and force-field analysis is useful for diagnosing which forces need to be modified or changed and how this can be done. Again, the committee may wish to conduct open meetings or hearings to get citizens' reactions.

Deciding which goals are to be selected is the fourth step, which follows when all alternatives have been fully explored. A *decision* is a conscious choice between two or more courses of action, and its nature may well determine an effort's ultimate success or failure. Health educators may encounter four general methods of decision making.

1. Autocratic decision making requires a leader who controls important resources and a population that gives the leader its loyalty, a situation that is unlikely to occur in most health-education settings.
2. Minority decision making requires the impending issue to have a legal or power base (such as affirmative action) and a strongly cohesive minority in support of the issue. Health educators encounter this situation when they adopt an advocacy role for a minority group.
3. Majority decision making requires democratic discussions-decision processes, with options open for selection and opportunities for all opinions to be voiced. Majority decision making works best when the majority is committed to the decisions made. It is the basis of most decisions relating to health education.
4. Consensual decision making is the most effective method, but it requires total group support of the position to be taken. For this to occur, the committee must periodically ascertain who is still not in accord and why. By taking time to resolve minority concerns, the majority can move decision making from a majority to a consensual level.[9]

In all decision-making situations the health educator should first explore possibilities for using the consensual method. Next most desirable is the majority method. An important ground rule here is that silence does not necessarily mean assent; for if the dynamics of decision making are ineffective, some people—particularly those who are opposed to an idea or who are unskilled at seizing an opportunity to air their views—may not participate, allowing the decision to be made but later resisting its implementation. In effective decision making, all members volunteer or are asked to share their views before the decision is made.

The fifth and final step in phase 3 is the development of strategies for implementing the goals selected. If the committee's goal is to develop its own neighborhood health center within three years, for example, it may consider the following strategies: (1) persuading the local health-systems agency to include this as a priority in its area health plans; (2) persuading elected officials at city, county, or state levels to support the idea and to allocate resources from existing services; (3) seeking federal financial support by means of political contacts and by submitting a proposal through regular channels; or (4) seeking financial support from foundations and citizens.

Understanding general theories of change, as well as how changes are made in a given organizational or community setting, is important. To this end, it is sometimes helpful to ask someone with experience in getting things done to advise on strategies. For implementation purposes, consensual decision making should be the method used whenever practicable.

Phase 4: Planning/programming

Phase 4 converts the agreed-upon strategies into a rational implementation plan or program, designs systems and tools for managing the activity, and negotiates commitments among those to be involved. To complete the first step—developing a plan or written program—both the health educator and the committee may wish to learn something more about planning to discern which method best fits their situation.[10]

In a patient-education group, the plan could focus on the sequence of scheduled activities; in a school situation, on the educator's lesson plan; in a community system, on preparing a formal proposal for presentation to a decision-making body for approval and support. In any case, those to be involved in the plan must understand and be committed to it. In some cases it may be desirable or necessary to obtain letters of endorsement from key organizations and leaders.

The design of management systems and tools—the second step—is an important aspect of any health-education activity, though whether these are to be formal or informal aids will depend upon a situation's complexity. While management functions seem sometimes to be an intuitive part of the educator's style, they are being performed nonetheless, and their development requires some understanding of how organizations and systems work, how management should operate, and how individual roles can be made interdependent.

Basic management functions include the following related elements:

• *Assuring continuity of effort as an activity moves toward its goal.* In complex situations, use of a Management by Objectives (MBO)* system assures that all elements of a scheduled activity are purposeful and interrelated. On occasion, the educator and committee may want to design a Program Evaluation and Review Technique (PERT)* flow chart for a visual presentation of steps.

• *Monitoring the activity's implementation.* Exhibiting specific steps and relationships in MBO and PERT forms facilitates an ongoing monitoring of progress.

*See Glossary.

• *Keeping communications open between the plan's various elements and the people involved.* Keeping communications open has a "feedback loop" effect. People aware of what is happening as it is happening are better able to determine whether their remaining activities should be carried out as planned or modified to fit a changing situation.

• *Instituting a crisis prevention/intervention system (CPIS).* This enables the educator and committee to discern whether a problem is developing and to prevent it by dealing with the indicators as soon as they become evident.[11] Trustworthy indicators of a potential problem are the absence of key people from scheduled meetings and the failure of someone to honor a promise to cooperate. If such incidents are ignored or not dealt with openly, people make guesses about them, and a proliferation of untested assumptions eventually leads to conflict. Dealing with an event means finding out why it occurred and gaining assurance that the plan is still operational, or problem-solving the issue and revising the plan if need be.

The final step in phase 4 is that of negotiating commitments to participate in the activity through the use of the Memorandum of Agreement (MOA).[12] The *contract* (discussed under phase 1) enables the health educator to develop and maintain a healthy relationship with the client or committee. The *MOA* (about which more will be said in chapter 12) enables the committee to develop collaborative relationships with organizations that are to provide resources for the activity or to participate in some phase of the implementation. In negotiating involvement and commitments, the MOA somewhat resembles a political process. Health educators and committee members can learn effective negotiating skills through training.

Phase 5: Implementation

Implementation consists of initiating the activity, providing assistance to it and its participants, problem-solving issues that may arise, and reporting on progress. Assigning the initiation of activity to this phase is only a technicality insofar as the activity in its broadest sense was begun with the first entry or intervention by the health educator or planning committee. By other staff people, however, the activity may be perceived as commencing only on their first day of work; by participants, upon their first entry into the room in which it is to be conducted. To facilitate orientation and communication, these persons may have to undergo Lewin's "unfreezing" process before actually engaging in the health-education experience.

The second step—ongoing training, technical assistance, and consultation—heightens the learning value of the experience. Training and technical assistance (T & TA) includes:

1. Assisting in the design, development, and evaluation of the activities

2. Developing training courses in various areas
3. Developing technical manuals, brochures, or guidelines
4. Giving technical consultation to staff.

Subject matters may vary from stenographic to interviewing skills or how to use a new piece of office equipment. It is less essential for educators or committees to know a given subject matter themselves than to know when others need it and where they can acquire instruction in it. The test of T & TA is the extent to which people feel they have been helped to do a better job.

The third step is that of dealing with problems as they arise and attempting to resolve them constructively. Creative problem solving should be a part of the ongoing training of committee and staff alike. The final step is that of reporting, or documenting an activity's ongoing progress to keep everyone informed. Important here are skills in communicating information in ways that facilitate apprehension of what has been occurring.

Phase 6: Evaluation

Because chapter 13 is wholly devoted to the subject of evaluation, the description here will be brief. The steps are: (1) to clarify the evaluation measures, (2) to collect evaluation data and analyze them, (3) to provide appropriate feedback to the activity, and (4) to redefine the problem and standards.

If objectives were initially established with built-in measurement indicators, the evaluation can begin by identifying and reviewing those measures. If objectives were stated broadly and vaguely, however, experts may have to be brought in to help develop appropriate measures. Accounting for funds and equipment used is included in the evaluation, which is sometimes conducted by the committee and health educator, sometimes by outside evaluators and auditors. In either case, the measures themselves must be understood and agreed upon.

Data collection and analysis in this phase shares many of the elements discussed under phase 2. The difference is that needs-assessment data are essential for planning purposes, while evaluation data reveal results and the reasons for them.

Reporting the evaluation results has the same value as other feedback and assimilation processes, with the significant difference that evaluation tends to be threatening to those who were involved in the activity. Because errors and failures are not always accepted gracefully, evaluation is often treated lightly or left to the last when time and resources may be lacking to do an effective job. It cannot be overemphasized, however, that evaluation can be a powerful learning experience that increases participants' knowledge and skills, thereby enabling planning and programming to improve.

Finally, the learnings derived from the evaluation should result in a redefinition of the problem and a refinement of the measures and standards used to determine its nature and extent. The plan thus ends with a new look at the first step of needs assessment and can continue this process of self-renewal if so desired.

Health-education planning, then, is open, dynamic, and exciting hard work whose most important principle is to involve those who will be affected by the program. Donald N. Michael offers six rewarding precepts for all people, including health educators, who work in planning.

1. Acknowledge and live with great uncertainty.
2. Embrace error for learning purposes.
3. Accept the ethical responsibility and conflict-laden interpersonal circumstances that attend goal setting.
4. Evaluate the present in light of the anticipated future, and be committed to actions that respond to long-range anticipations.
5. Live with role stress and forego the satisfactions of stable, on-the-job social-group relationships.
6. Be open to changes in commitment and direction as suggested by changes in the conjectured future and by evaluations of ongoing activities. [13]

REFERENCES

1. The ten priorities are listed in the Health Planning and Resources Development Act of 1974 (P.L. 93–641), and in various materials describing the act, as approved and distributed by the U.S. Department of Health, Education and Welfare's Bureau of Health Resources Administration.
2. J. Simmons, ed., "Making Health Education Work," *American Journal of Public Health* 65 (supp.) (October 1975): 1–49.
3. H. L. Blum, *Planning for Health*, pp. 54–66.
4. H. L. Blum, *Expanding Health-Care Horizons*, p. 110.
5. L. Green et al., *Health Education Today and the PRECEDE Framework*, pp. 2–17.
6. D. Palmiere, "Types of Planning in the Health-Care System," *American Journal of Public Health* 62, no. 8 (August 1972); 1112–15.
7. D. Sullivan, "Model for Comprehensive, Systematic Program Development in Health Education," *Health Education Report* 1, no. 1 (November-December 1973): 4–5.

8. League of California Cities, *Social Needs Assessment Handbook*, Sacramento, p. 115.
9. P. R. Mico, *Program Budgeting for California Cities*, pp. 17–20.
10. See, for example, Blum, *Planning for Health*.
11. P. R. Mico, *First Tango in Boston*, pp. 10–11.
12. P. R. Mico, "Design for Macrosystem Change" and "Memorandum of Agreement (MOA)" (Papers produced in 1973 as part of the Developmental Approach to Community Change project, conducted by the NTL Institute for Applied Behavioral Science for the National Institute for Mental Health, 1971–74).
13. D. N. Michael, *On Learning to Plan and Planning to Learn*, p. 18.

12
Methods for health education

For the purposes of this book, *method* denotes the procedure of applying a set of directions or guidelines to a problem situation in order to resolve the problem. As the previous chapters have suggested, many existing methods are useful for health education, and many situations exist for which effective methods have yet to be developed. Resourceful health educators are adept at using the best methods at hand and continually seek more effective means of coping with problems that persist in delaying or obstructing the progress of learning and change. This chapter opens with a brief overview of the health educator's functions, then describes a number of methods in general use today.

FUNCTIONS OF A HEALTH EDUCATOR

So specific are most health-education methods that it is difficult to isolate a few and confidently term them "basic." It is perhaps more instructive to attempt an overview of a health educator's key functions and to relate appropriate methods to them. Though the list that follows is by no means complete, it does suggest ten functions expected of most health educators.

1. Intervening into various situations for educational problem solving requires conducting a diagnosis to determine where and how to

begin the problem-solving process, interviewing, developing initial contracts, and conducting third-party interventions in cases of conflict. *Methods include:* force-field analysis, contracting, interviewing, the Memorandum of Agreement, third-party intervention and arbitration.

2. Working with groups of people in a variety of situations requires an understanding of group processes and of the application of group dynamics methods. *Methods include:* group process, decision making, patient-education groups, team building, board training, conferences, meetings, group facilitation, nominal group process technique, role clarification, and role playing.

3. Problem solving requires knowing how to diagnose problems, how to give and receive help, and how to utilize creative energies in exploring alternative resolutions. *Methods include:* force-field analysis, planning, decision making, conflict management, case method, nominal group process technique, constructive confrontation, role playing, simulation, and consultation.

4. Collecting accurate information on which to base planning and problem solving requires knowing how to define a problem clearly, how to determine what information needs to be collected and where it can be obtained, how to use experts in data collection and analysis, and how to use information collected. *Methods include:* needs assessment, force-field analysis, nominal group process technique, and interviewing.

5. Planning and developing programs requires an understanding of planning as a structured technique and of program designing using a variety of methods. *Strategies include:* application of principles of planning, social change, and mass communications.

6. Communicating effectively, utilizing a variety of methods and media, requires an understanding of communication processes, the development of communication materials, and an awareness of various media and their uses. *Methods include:* diffusion and adoption techniques, mass communications, conference method, and lectures.

7. Developing and maintaining effective relationships with individuals requires respect for persons and their needs, communicating effectively, developing interdependent relationships, and resolving interpersonal conflicts. *Methods include:* application of principles and conditions of learning, contracting, group facilitation, life planning, constructive confrontation, coaching, consultation, role playing, personal and programmed instruction.

8. Working in and with organizations requires an understanding of organizational behavior and organizational development. *Methods include:* role theory, contracting, team building, group processes, group facilitation, decision making, conflict management, constructive confrontation, meetings, and role clarification.

9. Working in community and social situations requires an understanding of social behavior and of strategies for social change. *Methods include:* group facilitation, planning, contracting, board training, conferences, meetings, constructive confrontation, consultation, and mass communications.

10. Evaluating the effectiveness of educational efforts requires setting measurable goals and objectives, identifying expected outcomes, determining how to collect evaluation data, and utilizing these data for feedback and performance improvement. *Methods include:* evaluation and goal setting in planning and nominal group process technique.

Some of these methods have already been discussed. In the section that follows, the others will be described in their general usage, which means that they must be modified for specific usage and that appropriate conditions must either exist or be created for their use.

HEALTH-EDUCATION METHODS

Group facilitation

In health-care settings, groups are continually being formed to pursue some educational purpose or to enhance the availability, organization, and delivery of services. Helping such groups to improve their functioning is called *facilitation* and is an obligation of health educators. For overall effectiveness, the facilitator must be equally helpful to the group as its designated leader or as merely another group member, helping the group when it is on target and intervening when it becomes sidetracked or obstructed. Because each type of group has distinctive characteristics, however, the facilitator's role must be modified accordingly. Table 14 lists six types of groups together with their implications for the facilitator.

The ad hoc group is one that has been formed for a temporary assignment. Members are generally from different parts of the organization, ordinarily have little contact with one another, and tend to approach the assignment with low commitment and little desire to volunteer for additional work. The facilitator's role is to help the group to get organized and

TABLE 14
Group Facilitation

Type of Group	Characteristics	Role of Facilitator
Ad Hoc	Common task Outside responsibilities and loyalties Limited time for task	Help in forming Coordinating arrangements Help in communications Keep focus on task
Committee	Common purpose Outside responsibilities and loyalties Structure	Help in forming Help in setting agendas and conducting good meetings Help in communications Keep focus on task Test decision making and commitments
Social Group	Meets needs for identity High energy Low task No structure High flexibility	Help in maintenance needs regarding norms and processes
Training (Individual change)	Focus on individual needs (intra and interpersonal) Common educational objectives Structure	Formalized role, generally Help in forming Development of individual skills, life plans, support systems Help in interpersonal processes
Community Boards Interagency committees	Focus on social change Members represent constituents Turf protection Common goals Structure Problem solving Conflict	Formalized role, generally Help in forming and maintenance Help in confrontations and negotiations Test decision making and commitments
Organizational Teams	Focus on intrateam concerns Members work together in same unit Common task and objectives High energy Interdisciplinary	Help in formation and maintenance processes Role clarification Communications and problem solving Confrontation Test decision making and commitments

clear about its objectives, to help coordinate its meeting schedules and communication processes, and to keep the group balanced between task and process.

The committee is generally more structured around a common purpose relating to an ongoing organizational function. Though members are still from different parts of the organization and have differing responsibilities and loyalties, they meet more often and for longer periods of time. The facilitator's role is again to help the committee to get organized and to develop and maintain constructive meeting procedures, such as establishing agendas, focusing discussion on one item at a time, keeping communications clear, beginning and ending meetings on time, and, in general, maintaining an environment conducive to good meetings. The committee should be continually focused on its task; decision making and commitments should be understood and supported. The facilitator may wish to resolve any personal conflicts between members outside the committee's working time.

A legitimate informal phenomenon within the organizational setting, the social group may be confined to coffee-break or lunchtime grouping or extend to outside social and recreational pursuits. In either case, the group primarily enables its members to meet social and identity needs. Members enjoy being with one another, exhibit high energy and great operational flexibility, and voluntarily help the group to accomplish its purpose. Generally, there is no specific organizational task to be carried out, and, having no formal objectives, the group tends to have little or no formal structure.

The facilitator's role (often as a member) is to help the group to develop and maintain its normative structures and processes: to help members feel involved, to improve communications, to resolve problems of domination or manipulation, to enable members to confront one another on ideas and problem-solving approaches, and to engender respect for and sensitivity toward one another's feelings.

The training or educational group established to produce individual change generally focuses on individual needs, though the group will be well structured around common educational objectives, training designs, and schedules. Here the facilitator is likely to be formally designated as trainer or educational leader and will provide assistance in many areas: getting the group organized and oriented to the learning experience; conducting assessments of individual needs and group objectives; monitoring the training schedule and environment; maintaining norms for interpersonal processes and developing interactional skills; developing individual life or career plans and support systems for external implementation of personal learning objectives; and encouraging ongoing evaluation of the learning experience for purposes of feedback and improvement.

Groups organized for social change include such bodies as an elected group that is developing policies relating to health, a commission or board that has been appointed to advise city or county officials on health matters or to direct some established health-care function, a community board of directors for a neighborhood health association, an interagency committee composed of agency executives or representatives, or a coalition of organizations and groups organized for a special purpose, such as a consumer advocate coalition.

The members of such groups generally represent some constituency whose interests they protect, their decisions usually based on considerations of fairness and equity toward their constituents. The group is likely to have a well-established structure and purpose and the facilitator's role to be formalized in an organizing or training capacity.

These groups, too, need help in getting themselves organized, operating, and conducting meetings well: in establishing and following agendas, creating a climate conducive to constructive confrontation, clarifying whether a member's own or his constituency's interests are being represented, and testing whether decisions are sufficiently understood and supported, and commitments firm enough, for successful implementation.

Teams are groupings of people from the same organizational unit whose members, though of different professional background and experience, must work together in order to achieve a common objective. Since the team effort elicits their primary responsibility and loyalty, members' concerns are usually energetically centered on how to work together most effectively. The facilitator's role may be formally that of team builder or informally that of a team member who helps the team in its functioning while at the same time providing educational services. Whatever the group theory employed, the kind of help that teams need runs the full range of developmental procedures and processes, including how to develop and maintain effective working relationships with other organizational units and with groups and organizations in the community if it comes into contact with these outside resources.[1]

Interventions may be grouped into four broad categories, in each of which a comment or question is directed toward some aspect or element of the group. (1) *Content intervention* is directed toward the substance of a subject or film under discussion. (2) *Intrapersonal intervention* is directed at one person only. (3) *Interpersonal intervention* is also directed at only one person but in reaction to an action or comment by another member of the group. (4) *Group intervention* is directed toward the group as a whole or toward one segment of it.[2]

In the more definitive breakdown of techniques that follows, each item can be placed under one or more of the four general categories.

1. *Content focus* does not differ from the description of content intervention.
2. *Process focus* centers on what is happening in the group (e.g., "I wonder what is really going on in the group right now?" or "Are you aware that a decision has been made though only two persons voiced an opinion?"). How groups are made to focus on their own processes is determined by the facilitator's personal style or training strategy.
3. *Asking for feelings* centers on a voicing of personal feelings by group members, a technique which some facilitators and many participants find to be the most interesting part of the training process. For some participants, this provides the first opportunity to learn how others feel about their behavior, an important learning goal.
4. *Direction giving* sometimes takes the form of a suggestion; at other times the form of imposed actions, some facilitators feeling that group members should learn how to handle forced direction. A facilitator who recognizes that he has a high need to control may satisfy this need by direction giving or may overreact by failing to supply direction when to do so would be helpful. The facilitator must decide whether to let the group work through its own impasse at the possible cost of time wasted or to supply direction at the risk of reinforcing dependency. Relevant factors here include the length of the training program, the resources available, the group's level of dependency, and the facilitator's tolerance of ambiguity.
5. *Direct feedback*, whether to a member or to the group as a whole, may be given early, as a model to legitimate the giving of feedback, or later, after there has been some working through of authority problems. Here again the facilitator is faced with a dilemma, the more so since group members are often anxious to know how the facilitator sees them.
6. *Cognitive orientations* denote the provision of relevant theory or information. The facilitator must determine whether participants will learn more from a lecture or from their own experience, and whether the lecture merely satisfies a personal need for the facilitator to be seen as an expert.
7. *Performing group functions* means intervening in the task-maintenance dimension until group members are able to perform such functions for themselves. In relation to task functions, the facilitator may seek opinions or reactions from the group or offer a personal opinion; initiate a new goal, problem definition, or way of organizing for work; elaborate or summarize an idea or test the idea for consensus. To meet maintenance needs, the facilitator's intervention may take the form of

setting standards, keeping communications open, encouraging participation, harmonizing differences, and helping to release individual or group tensions.

8. *Diagnostic interventions* require the facilitator to diagnose group process—e.g., "There are several possible reasons for this group's apathy. First, our goals are unclear. Second, we're afraid that old conflicts may resurface if we start to work again." The group may then be queried for other possible reasons.

9. *Protective intervention* means that the facilitator may intervene to protect members from unnecessary trials: from sharing personal experiences or feelings that are inappropriate to the training goals, from creating situations that neither the facilitator nor the members can handle, from ill-timed or overly severe feedback, or by helping members to maintain their identity despite group pressure to conform. Some facilitators prefer to focus on process and to ask the group whether a given behavior seems appropriate to its goals.

Nominal group technique

The purpose of nominal group technique is to ensure equal participation in a problem-solving situation by means of a structured procedure for contributing ideas to the group. It is especially useful when group discussion tends to be dominated by a few members and when high agreement or consensus is required on problems and approaches to them.

Although the method can be used at any point in a group's work, it is most often used in the early stages of needs assessment and program planning. A group of eight to ten persons is an ideal size for this activity. Large groups can be divided into smaller groups of equal size to work concurrently on the activity, which takes about two and one-half hours to complete. The method presented here is a slight modification of the original designed by André L. Delbecq and Andrew H. Van de Ven[3] and has been found to work well in many different settings.

Activity begins with the facilitator introducing and clarifying the group's selected problem and describing the steps to be followed in the nominal group method. If the group is large, the means of forming smaller groups is discussed, and the participants move into these smaller groups. For ten to fifteen minutes each participant works alone and silently with paper and pencil, recording as many responses to the problem as he can recall. The facilitator should allow enough time for all participants to record whatever they can.

Next, the group selects an individual to record its collective ideas on newsprint before the group. In a round-robin procedure, each person in sequence orally relates his first idea, which the recorder records on the newsprint. A person whose first idea has already been given by someone else moves to the next idea on his list. When all persons have given their first idea, the sequence continues as established as long as anyone has ideas to contribute. A person who has run out of ideas passes a turn, and others continue to contribute until all ideas have been exhausted. The list is then open for discussion, the purpose being to clarify and understand the ideas. Debates, opposition, and promotion of ideas are not permitted.

When these ideas have been clarified and understood, each participant is asked to select a given number of the issues most important to him and to record them on a separate sheet of paper. These ideas are then called off to the recorder, who either lists them without duplications on a separate sheet (if time permits) or marks them off the original newsprint lists. If several groups are working at the same time, they come together with these "important listings." Each group should be given an opportunity to present its listings to the others and to clarify any ideas the others do not understand.

Each participant then selects the five most important problems on the lists, recording them on a separate sheet of paper and ranking them from 5 (the most important) to 1 (the least important). The rankings are read off to the recorder, and the ranking numbers for each idea are recorded alongside it. When all rankings have been recorded, the "scores" (the sum of the numbers alongside an idea) are added for each idea, and the idea having the highest score is regarded as the most important problem.

All the ranked ideas are then listed sequentially: those with the highest scores at the top, those with the lowest scores at the bottom. The facilitator leads a group discussion around the results. When the problem list has been accepted, the group is ready to move to the next step in problem solving.

Role clarification

Because role conflict is among the more persistent difficulties encountered in interdependent work situations, methods that help to clarify roles are a necessity for health educators. The method described here, developed by Ishwar Dayal and John M. Thomas,[4] is especially useful where teams and community boards are striving to achieve organizational or social change.

The method takes from two to three hours per role depending upon the number of people involved. It is helpful if instructions are distributed before the exercise begins. The facilitator introduces the exercise by orienting participants to its sequences, each of which centers on a focal role. Work should begin with the role regarded as most ambiguous or conflictive; the other participants should be those whose own roles are in some way affected by the focal role.

On newsprint sheets, the focal-role person (hereafter designated as A) describes his own *perception* of his role, how the role is carried out, and how it contributes to the team's objectives and the organization's goals. The other members likewise record their perceptions of the focal role. Discussions begin with A sharing his perception, following which the other participants contribute theirs. Agreements are noted and differences discussed and problem-solved, aiming at consensus if possible.

Next, A records his *expectations* of how others' roles should help him to function more effectively, while the other members record their expectations of the focal role as it affects their roles. Discussion focuses on agreements and on problem-solving any differences until general agreement is reached on mutual expectations. This concludes the initial work session.

From the results of this session A prepares a written role description, or modification of his previous statement, and distributes copies to the other team members. After reviewing the statement, the team caucuses with A either to affirm the statement or to negotiate refinements. The results of the caucus constitute A's clarified role, though most of the other team members become clearer about their own roles as well. If it is desirable to apply the procedure to other focal roles, the facilitator helps the team to arrange for as many more work sessions as needed.

Role playing

Role playing enables people to practice and experiment with a new behavior in a safe learning environment; it is also a helpful technique for restructuring a situation for the purpose of gaining greater insight into its problems.[5] The method has two approaches. *Structured* (or preplanned) role playing encourages learning by observing, doing, imitating, and sharing—in short, by conceptualization and analysis. *Spontaneous* role playing shares the advantages of structured role playing but minimizes analysis.

Role playing's components include, (1) enactment, or the actors' interactions, (2) the depiction of realistic behavior, (3) improvisation, (4) experimentation and practice until learnings have been attained, (5) formal or informal sharing of experience and observations, and (6) diagnosis of information for planning future training experiences.

Both structured and spontaneous role playing require some preplanning. The structured form requires identifying a problem, collecting information about it, setting objectives, describing the situation in writing, clarifying actors' roles, and providing guidelines for participants and observers alike. For the spontaneous form a warm-up discussion will suffice. Thereafter, both forms follow the same procedure: introduction to the exercise, discussion of its purpose and steps, enactment, and final discussion following the prepared guidelines.

Finally, five techniques have proved valuable. *Role reversal* enables one learner to discern another's view of a problem by playing that other person. *Soliloquy* stops the action at certain points to interview the actors on their feelings or attitudes at that time. In *doubling*, others sit beside or stand behind the actors, periodically interrupting them to express their view of what is occurring. In *multiple role playing*, several participants act a given role while several others act another role, all eventually engaging in simultaneous role playing around the same problem and then sharing their experiences. In *role rotation*, the same actor plays all the roles in a situation to broaden his personal learnings.

Third-party intervention and arbitration

Differences among the various parties to an interdependent effort often result in conflicts whose disruptiveness can cause the effort to fail. If there is reason to believe that the conflicting parties are willing to participate in problem solving, third-party intervention and arbitration is especially useful. The method described here, as it actually unfolded, was used by a colleague of the authors to resolve a conflict between a local, state, and federal agency over providing health-care services to a minority population and is appropriate only to the area of community or social change.[6]

In early 1972 a state migrant council and a local clinic identified the need for a health program for migrant workers in an agricultural area served by the clinic. The council was awarded a grant by the Department of Health, Education and Welfare (HEW), under the terms of whose contract the council was designated as the grantee and responsible for financial accountability; the clinic was to provide the health-care services. The council subcontracted the clinic to provide these services, and the program progressed well for a year.

Early in its second year, however, the council and clinic conflicted over the eligibility of those whom the clinic served. Learning that the clinic was using project resources to serve other than the seasonal and migrant workers for whom the resources were intended, the council advised the clinic to stop this practice, and the clinic refused to do so. Other differences caused mounting polarization between the two agencies, each of which appealed to HEW for support.

An HEW consultant, who had been providing the clinic with consultation on a related project, was asked by HEW to be the third-party facilitator, and at a conference all three parties to the arbitration agreed on its ground rules.

1. Each party was to have a four-member negotiation team with an additional person serving as the team's official negotiator. The council's

and clinic's chief administrators were allowed to participate as their teams' sixth member.

2. The consultant was designated as the convenor of arbitration.

3. The arbitration team was to consist of the three official negotiators and the convenor.

4. The plenary body was to include the official members of all three negotiating teams plus the convenor of arbitration.

The convenor called the plenary body to session by seating the three negotiating teams and reviewing the ground rules. Next, the consultant suggested that each team prepare its own history, to be shared with the others, of the events and processes that had led to the conflict, a history on whose details all agreed during the ensuing discussion. Asked to examine the process to this point and to decide the next step, the arbitration team decided that each team would present its mission statement and objectives to the planning body the next day, when they were discussed and accepted. The teams then prioritized their objectives and identified problems that would impede their achievement, following which they shared this information with one another.

Each team then agreed to prepare a proposal for presentation the next day: HEW, on the status of the contract; the council, on improving communications; the clinic, on how its services should be evaluated. On the last day the plenary body heard these proposals, the arbitration team discussed them, and detailed statements were agreed upon. Finally, the council requested, and all parties agreed to, an exchange of key program-services data with the clinic.

The consultant closed the arbitration by reviewing agreements made on mission, objectives, a communication system, a conflict-resolution mechanism, and a continuing negotiating process. Key decisions presented for final affirmation included: (1) a commitment by council and clinic boards to meet together with an arbiter whenever necessary, (2) a commitment to focus on resolving all issues necessary to develop a new contract that satisfies HEW, and (3) a commitment by all three parties to develop a management system in which all can collaborate effectively.

The arbitration was successful in four ways. It enabled all parties to engage in a face-to-face confrontation on all the problem issues. It demonstrated that agreement could be reached on mission statements, objectives, and problem lists. It resulted in important decisions being made, and it not only permitted the clinic's services to continue but provided a framework for agreement on their continuation. The ultimate mark of effectiveness was that, although the council and clinic continued to experience stress, the contract was successfully renegotiated and the health-care services continued.

Constructive confrontation

In human relationships, misunderstandings occur, mistakes are made, feelings are hurt, and communications break down. A response that further deteriorates a relationship is a *destructive confrontation*; one that resolves interpersonal conflicts that would otherwise inhibit a personal or working relationship is a *constructive confrontation*.[7] The degree of caring and collaboration exhibited by the confronter and the style of reaction exhibited by the confrontee together determine whether a confrontation will be constructive or destructive. Degree of caring and collaboration can range from high (win-win) to low (lose-lose), precipitating reactions ranging from highly explosive to suppressed or avoidance behaviors.

Described here is an eight-step method of constructive confrontation, followed by a review of the confronter's and confrontee's key roles and functions (see table 15).

(1) A precipitating incident is or is not mutually perceived by A and B. (2) If A exhibits a readiness to confront, B must be willing to collaborate. (3) A must ensure that setting, timing, staging, and climate are conducive to a good confrontation. (4) Both parties must clarify the precipitating incident, employing active listening and hearing. (5) Both parties give and receive feedback on their feelings to ascertain and apprehend the incident's relevance. (6) Attempts should be made to develop trust, to build on alternatives, and to test their feasibility. (7) Both agree on a creative resolution, seeking consensus and commitment and assuring built-in measures for test-

TABLE 15
A Constructive Confrontation

Confronter (A)	Confrontee (B)
1. Perceives incident	1. May or may not perceive
2. Initiates readiness to confront	2. Negotiates readiness
3. Initiates confrontation	3. Accommodates, responds
4. Describes incident	4. Clarifies
5. Feedback regarding feelings, seeks understanding*	5. Feedback acceptance and response
6. Suggests alternative courses of resolution, builds, tests	6. Suggests alternatives, explores, develops, tests
7. Resolve, pursues resolution*	7. Negotiates acceptable resolution
8. Process experience*	8. Process experience

*Key components.

ing and evaluating. (8) Both parties process the experience, seeking learnings that will reduce or prevent future incidents, a critical component of constructive confrontation.

Conflict is inevitable when people need one another because it is impossible in interdependent situations for everyone to meet everyone else's expectations all the time. But conflict is also essential, even in health situations where conditions are always in flux and needs keep changing. Instead of being viewed as fearful, then, conflict should be seen as a vital means of constructively improving interpersonal relationships. Constructive confrontation should become a way of life.

Consultation

The purpose of consultation is to provide help to a client. This may mean focusing on human relationships, helping clients to perceive, understand, and act on events in their environment. It may mean offering technical assistance in carrying out an organizational task or function, such as constructing a better records system, reorganizing the delivery of services to consumers, or developing a detailed implementation plan for a community project. It may mean providing the client with expert information: clarifying a federal or state program's participation guidelines, a new certification procedure, or the meaning and implications of a new law.

In brief, consultation applies alike to individual, organizational, and social forms of learning and change. Though generally associated with the last two forms, it is occasionally used effectively by managers who want personal help in dealing with problems. Insofar as every person is ideally capable of being helpful to another, every person can be a client seeking help from someone else.

Process consultation, the method most likely to be employed by health educators, usually involves three sets of relationships: (1) two-way, a direct engagement between consultant and client; (2) three-way, in which the consultant helps to resolve a problem between the client and the client's client, such as helping a manager to resolve a staff problem; and (3) third-party, in which the consultant helps two parties in the client system to resolve a problem between themselves.[8]

The effective consultation relationship is a shared one requiring of both parties a body of knowledge and skills as well as an understanding of the problem and of the actions to be taken toward resolving it. The relationship must be voluntary and trusting, both parties understanding that it exists solely for the purpose of focusing on a given problem and will terminate when the problem has been eliminated. Finally, it must be mutually supportive and disciplined, both parties acknowledging the necessity of clear agreements on work and on mutual responsibilities. The basic elements of this relationship should be spelled out in the psychosocial contract described in chapter 11.

Determining work procedures and setting will be greatly facilitated if the client is directly involved in the determination. A time schedule should likewise be developed with the client's cooperation, and the problem should be clearly defined to minimize any untested assumptions or unrealistic expectations. If the work requires hierarchical decision making, people at each hierarchical level should be involved in the problem-solving process.

Needs assessment is essential to process consultation, whose procedures must be congruent with the client's situational requirements. The collected data can be used for three purposes: (1) diagnosis, in which the consultant helps to analyze their implications for a reassessment of the problem; (2) reflection, in which the client is helped to apprehend the larger problem-situation and to identify feelings about it; and (3) response, in which the client is helped to develop an appropriate plan of action.

Several types of intervention are useful in meeting a consultation's purposes. Agenda setting sensitizes clients to their own procedures and processes, stimulating a desire for analysis and improvement. Data feedback reveals clients' processes in such a way as to aid problem solving. Coaching, a third method, is described elsewhere in this chapter. Making structural suggestions helps to clarify membership and role issues, communication and decision-making patterns, work and resource allocation, authority alignments, and assignment of responsibility.

Certain stresses are inherent in a consultation situation, and, while these cannot be totally eliminated, they can be minimized through awareness and understanding. Perceiving the consultant as an authority or power figure, for example, can arouse resentment, suspicion, and distrust among clients, especially if this outsider's apprehension of their situation does not inspire credibility, if he errs through overeagerness to demonstrate his worth, or if he seems more devoted to fulfilling his own rather than clients' needs.

Out of fear of the unknown or of failure, clients are, for their part, sometimes visibly insecure. Manifestations of insecurity may range from an overdependence on the consultant to a difficulty in asking for help and, in some instances, to outright rejection of the consultant's authority. Clients with exploitative motivations may wish to use the consultant to pursue some hidden agenda. Finally, because of insecurity on the part of the client or an exploitative motivation on the part of the consultant, either or both parties may resist terminating the relationship when the assignment has been completed.

It is not surprising, then, that the consultant must bring special abilities and traits to the consultation process. These include:

1. an ability to empathize with clients' problems and adjust to their environment.
2. a confidence in clients' ability not only to resolve their problems but to learn and grow
3. a willingness to share approaches and experiences, to explore and experiment in the interests of creative solving, and an ability to enable clients to adapt new learnings to new situations
4. a sensitivity to timing so that interventions are suited to clients' readiness to move ahead
5. an ability to listen to, and actually hear, clients' accounts of their processes
6. an objective self-awareness that prevents sacrificing clients' needs to one's own needs.

Terminating the relationship is jointly resolved when the assignment has been completed (or earlier, if either party so prefers). Whenever it occurs, a termination interview should be conducted so that both parties can review the experience in the interests of future improvement. At the end of a consultation, clients should feel that they have been helped on the evidence of a solved problem; improved skills or performance; changes in basic values, motivations, or attitudes; or a greater understanding of, and concern for, the processes of learning and change.

Memorandum of Agreement

A written agreement, though not a legal contract, the Memorandum of Agreement (MOA) enables two or more organizations to form and sustain a collaborative relationship to bring about community or other social change.[9] Clearly, the better prepared the organizations are to engage in MOA transactions, the more binding will be their agreements. Preparedness means:

1. Having enough internal security to devote energy to a collaborative effort
2. Understanding the social problem to be resolved
3. Accepting the collaboration's larger common goal
4. Participating in a determination and clarification of purposes
5. Identifying MOA approval procedures
6. Designating and training teams that will represent their organization in the negotiation.

For a macrosystemic effort to be effective, three conditions must exist. First, the effort must be fantasy-free: assumptions must be tested and expectations met. The MOA helps in this regard by identifying and clarifying any such obstacles. Second, the effort must have full organizational commitment. The MOA brings this about by enlisting the support of each organization's top policy-making and decision-making structures.

Third, conditions must exist for continuing problem solving, confrontation, and negotiation. A trusted third-party resource is essential in creating these conditions, as well as in instituting evaluation and feedback procedures that will help the organizations to improve their internal functioning to participate better in future efforts. The third-party resource may consist of outside consultants or of a policy-level committee composed of representatives of the participating organizations.

As noted, the MOA should be a written document, and all participating organizations, as well as the third party, should have a copy of it. The agreement should include:

1. An identification of the participating organizations
2. A statement of the problem, goal, and objectives
3. A description of the interagency management structure
4. Descriptions of how each organization will participate in, and contribute to, the joint effort
5. A description of procedures and ground rules for meeting and working together
6. A delineation of the third party's role
7. A statement of conditions for renegotiating the MOA.

Any participating organization can request a renegotiation of the MOA if it feels that a changing situation warrants a reconsideration. If a fixed period of time passes without one, the third party should undertake a general reconsideration among all parties, in this way assuring ongoing discussion and negotiation of interagency working conditions and relationships.

Mass communications

Radio, television, films, newspapers and newsletters, magazines and journals, books, pamphlets, and posters—all are communications media of great utility in conveying information to vast numbers of people. Mass media are often used when a serious threat to health requires reaching as many people as possible as quickly as possible; when it is desirable to change health perceptions, attitudes, and behaviors over an extensive period of time; and when it is useful to coordinate a variety of forms of education.

According to Jack Smolensky and Franklin B. Haar, seven factors are highly important to mass media effectiveness.

1. Credibility: The source must be competent and reliable so that the receiver can trust the message.
2. Context: The message must be relevant to the receiver and provide a link with participation.
3. Content: The message must have genuine meaning.
4. Clarity: The receiver must be able to understand the message.
5. Continuity: Though repeated with variations, the basic message must be consistent enough not to confuse the receiver.
6. Channels: The message must use such established communication channels as the receiver is likely to use.
7. Capability: The receiver must be capable of doing what is asked and with the least amount of effort.[10]

To this list the authors would add an eighth factor: collaboration with media professionals to determine how media can best be used for an educational effort.

Smolensky and Haar offer the following suggestions for using communication tools.[11] Newspaper articles, which should first be discussed with the appropriate editor, must be written briefly, simply, and clearly, answering the questions Who, What, When, Where, and Why. Copy should be typed double space and given to the editor at least twenty-four hours before release time. The same writing guidelines apply to pamphlets, which should, of course, be well designed and attractive. In this case, however, special attention should be given to reaching speakers of languages other than English, and the pamphlet should be tested for reader comprehension before it is reproduced.

All aspects of a proposed radio or television program should be discussed in advance with the program manager or public service director. For both media, possibilities include spot announcements, news items, and talk show interviews. Public broadcasting is often receptive to developing health-education programs, and closed-circuit TV should not be overlooked. Educational films should be appropriate to the occasion and introduced before presentation to facilitate later discussion. New films should be previewed before presentation to an audience.

Finally, health fairs and well-designed exhibits located in high-circulation areas can be especially effective when someone is present to discuss the subject and distribute related information. All mass communication methods are useful when people are already motivated to improve their health, but they have limited effectiveness where such motivation is absent.

Conference method

In the conference method, a group of people (such as an association) learns by sharing information, ideas, and experiences, during the course of which attitudes and opinions are periodically checked for evidence of progress.[12] Periodic checks may be routinely performed once a year or at the beginning, middle, and end of a program. They may take two to three days or more depending upon the number of people involved and the issue that has brought them together.

An effective conference requires setting up a planning committee composed of participants for the following purposes: determining costs and budget, setting goals, designing the conference agenda, locating a suitable facility, inviting resource personnel, preparing and distributing information to participants, arranging for registrations and other maintenance or comfort considerations, agreeing on management and monitoring processes, continuing the planning committee's function during the conference in case the design should need to be changed, and developing procedures for evaluation and for any follow-up that may be indicated.

The conference itself consists of three parts: opening, program presentation, and closure. For each part, the leader's tasks are as follows.

Opening: Providing orientation and introductions, explaining objectives, presenting an overview of the conference, and explaining procedures.

Program: Introducing each topic and its presenters, reviewing procedures and what is expected of participants, using audiovisual resources where appropriate, and involving participants in conducting the program.

Closure: Summarizing conclusions and results and evaluating the conference.

Meetings

As the need for participatory processes grows, the need for better meetings grows perforce. Meetings bring small groups together for information sharing, planning, problem solving, and decision making.[13] The following guidelines should help to clarify procedures.

Several planning steps should precede the meeting. Answer the questions Who, What, When, Where, Why, and How Many. Prepare and distribute an agenda, and set up a meeting room. Begin the meeting on time, and clarify time limits. Ask participants to introduce themselves and to state their expectations of the meeting. Define planners' and participants' responsibilities. Participants may be asked to review and revise the agenda. Review action-items from previous meetings. During the meeting, focus on only one problem at a time to reduce confusion and straying.

At the meeting's close, establish action-items, who should be responsible for carrying them out, what should be done, and when. Review recorded notes. Establish the date, time, and place of the next meeting, set a preliminary agenda, and evaluate the meeting. Closing the meeting on a positive note helps to bridge the business of one meeting to that of the next. After the meeting, distribute minutes to participants, and follow-through on action-items in preparation for the next meeting. While health educators may not be required to perform all these tasks themselves, they should see to it that someone is charged with so doing.

Simulation

Experience is the best teacher; simulation is the next best thing to direct experience; therefore simulation is the next best teacher. Frequently used in training programs and in the classroom, simulation helps to demonstrate problem solving, decision making, values clarification, and other basic learning processes and can be employed in connection with individual, organizational, or social change.[14]

Simulation can take the form of one person's flexibly performing the role of another person; it can take the form of a structured game having established procedures and rules, constraints of time, resources, or resource allocation, and a specific objective and end; or it can be a combination of the two, both structured and flexible. It can occur spontaneously, taking advantage of an on-the-spot learning opportunity, or it can make use of an expensive kit with printed instructions and manufactured materials.

If the health educator decides that a simulation can be useful, instructions and materials should be at hand and ample time allowed for explaining, using, and learning from the method. Because confusion diminishes its effectiveness, rules and procedures must be well understood before enactment, and the event should be monitored thereafter to assure that implementation is carried out correctly. After the simulation, learnings are summarized by means of four steps: (1) reviewing the experience's sequence, (2) identifying events that held the greatest meaning for participants, (3) analyzing that meaning, and (4) drawing generalizations for future situations.

Simulation is especially useful for health education. It images the physical, social, and emotional factors that help to shape health behavior. It offers serious, challenging, and exciting objectives and stratagems. From it participants may gain greater sensitivity toward health status, new insights into health-behavior motivations, practice in critical thinking and decision making about health practices, and a better understanding of alternative behaviors available in their own lives.[15]

Case method

Popularized by Harvard University's schools of law and business, the case method focuses on developing independent thinking, analytical concepts, and skills for putting knowledge to use in organizational and social problem solving.[16] The method is composed of three elements: case report, case analysis, and case discussion.

The case report offers a detailed picture of an actual problem-situation. Though usually written, it can be presented on videotape or film, on cassette recordings, or as a role-playing simulation. In all cases, names are changed to protect confidentiality. The case should be based on firsthand observation and show more than it tells about interpersonal relationships, progress, and effects of change. After learners have studied the incident by themselves for a few minutes, the instructor spends twenty to thirty minutes interviewing the group to gather as much information about the case as possible (no presentation can provide all the needed information or totally avoid bias).

The case analysis should be rational, systematic, and comprehensive enough for learners to take a broad view of the situation's difficulties and to reflect on issues for both short- and long-term actions and on valid principles for achieving organizational or social goals. For five to ten minutes the group considers two questions: What is at stake in this situation? and How shall we state the critical question for action now?

The next step takes from twenty to thirty minutes and consists of four parts.

1. Working individually, participants write responses to, How would I handle the incident? Why?, and give their papers to the instructor.
2. Based on these responses, small opinion-groups are formed, each to present the strongest case for its position.
3. Groups engage in brief debates about their positions.
4. With the instructor's assistance, the problem is resolved.

Build-in biases and the failure of some learners to make a maximum effort are common limitations in case analysis.

The case discussion, which may take as long as an hour, focuses on the case as a whole, reflecting upon, discussing, and summarizing the general ideas raised by the case and the learnings derived from it. Discussion should take place in an informal and freely experimental atmosphere and provide experience in accommodating disagreement.

Coaching

Insofar as it provides step-by-step guidance in learning a new behavior or acquiring a new skill, coaching is essentially a strategy for individual learning and change, though by improving individual role performance and coordination with the roles of others it clearly has team application as well.[17] It is a vital method for health educators who are helping health professionals to impart a specific skill, such as self-medication, to patients or clients. The basic dynamics of the coaching relationship are the learner's need for close guidance in progressive mastery of the learning matter and the coach's techniques for keeping the learner in a developmental sequence.

Coaching is not a passive process of merely enabling a learner to experience something new and then commenting on it. At the initial stage, the effective coach adopts a strongly active role: setting the stage for the learning experience, becoming an active partner to the learner's role, getting others to play supportive roles, demonstrating how the skill should be performed, and showing which steps are being performed incorrectly. Coaching is also a structured experience consisting of an overall plan or schedule, of the step-by-step lessons or exercises themselves, and of measures that enable the learner to know how well the skill is being apprehended.

If coaching is to be effective, a strong psychological relationship must develop between coach and learner demonstrating great sensitivity on the part of the former and trust on the part of the latter. The coach must be acutely sensitive to personal forces acting within the learner, for example, in order to heighten those that motivate learning and change and also to control the delicate balance of pressure and relaxation that guides the timing of the learning experience. If the coach moves too fast, the learner may feel distressed, confused, or lost; if movement is too slow, the learner may become bored and disinterested or impatient and angry. The coach must know precisely when to encourage risk taking and when to confront an avoidance of new learning or a reversion to old behavior.

Because learning new practices often involves relinquishing old perceptions, the learner's perception of self is likely to undergo change as well, with the result that the coach-learner relationship will eventually become more collaborative than it was at the beginning. Instead of merely adopting a new skill modeled by the coach, the learner will increasingly perceive alternatives for refining its expression. At this final stage the coach's role is to collaborate with the learner in cultivating a personally unique style of performance.

Interviewing

Gathering information for purposes of planned change requires an appropriate fusion of three methods: interviewing, observation, and the judicious use of documents. Whether in the form of a highly structured experience involving trained personnel and precoded instruments or that of an informal contact with respondents, interviewing is the primary method of collecting information. It can be used wherever the planning and action processes of a change effort require information to be collected from individuals, and it is a highly complex social interaction involving interviewer and respondent in an exchange of perceptions, feelings, values, interpersonal communications and relationships.

Closely related to and supplementing interviewing is observation, by which is meant selective, purposeful watching, listening, or counting. On some occasions, observation may be necessary before interviewing can be conducted; on others, it may be necessary for checking the accuracy of interview responses. Observation is essential when interviews alone fail to provide all the needed information or when documents needed for further study do not exist. Sometimes, as when a health educator is unable to speak a client's language, observation is the only method that avails for gathering information.

To the extent that they are comprehensive, accurate, pertinent, and well prepared, documents, too, constitute a rich source of information. Documents are recorded evidence of past experience and exist in three forms: written media (newspapers, magazines, reports, files, medical histories, memoranda, vital statistics, etc.); audio media (tape recordings); or visual media (television, films, photographs). With these distinctions in mind, the following guidelines should help to illuminate the most important features of the interview method for the health educator.[18]

1. *Interview approach.* Factors to be considered in selecting the interview approach include accessibility of information, the method's costs, and the importance of the information's relevance and validity. First, it must be determined whether the desired information is even obtainable through interviewing, observation, and documents, and, if so, whether respondents will be willing to yield it to the interviewer. Second, costs must be determined for the time required to arrange for and conduct the interview (preparing forms, training interviewers, coding and tabulating data for analysis, etc.).

Third, the importance of the information to the interviewer must be established. In general, only that which is strictly relevant to the health-education program should be collected. Fourth, the interviewer must decide how important will be the information's reliability. Because distortion and error can occur in any method, expert consultation should be sought where accuracy is important.

Setting the stage for an interview may be done in either of two ways. (1) The interviewer may call the respondent to explain the interview's purpose and to schedule a convenient time and place for it. (2) Letters may be sent out in advance, or publicity transmitted to a neighborhood via mass communications, then followed-up with telephone calls or direct contacts.

2. *Interview styles and types.* Interview styles range from engaging the respondent in informal open-ended discussion to directing formally structured questioning to each respondent in the same way. The nondirective interview, developed by Carl Rogers and used extensively in psychotherapy and counseling, requires a passive interviewer who allows the respondent to decide what and how much is said. In the highly directive Kinsey method, respondents are asked questions rapidly for the purpose of maintaining spontaneity of response. [19]

More particularly, three types of standardized interviews are currently in use: (1) limited response (respondent has limited role in selecting topics or responses); (2) free response (respondent is free to discuss any area of inquiry); and (3) defensive response (interviewer attempts to force respondent into a particular position on a given topic). A *closed question* is one that can be answered by a yes or no; an *open question* allows as full a response as the respondent wants to give. Researchers generally agree that *leading questions*—those suggesting a desired answer—should be avoided. The interviewer's role may range from one of initially active questioning and recording to one of listening and recording once the respondent has begun to provide information freely.

3. *Factors influencing participation.* Numerous factors influence the respondent's degree of participation in the interview process, and the interviewer must be aware of these in order to make appropriate choices. Matching the interviewer to the respondent, for example, is important insofar as a female respondent may be reluctant to confide intimate aspects of family planning to a male interviewer. Demonstrating a shared interest can increase the respondent's participation by enhancing the interviewer's credibility.

Further, the interviewer should be willing to conform to respondents' customs. Wearing ranch attire to interview respondents in the business world would be as inappropriate as wearing business attire to interview ranch hands or migrant workers. Clearly, too, the interviewer's verbal and nonverbal behavior, apart from direct questioning, can give subtle cues that encourage or discourage the respondent's participation.

Choice of language, making comfortable transitions between topics, the pace of the interview, the respondent's previous experience in being interviewed—all affect respondent participation to some degree. Other factors may include the respondent's desire to be of help to others and the emotional satisfaction of expressing one's own opinions or of feeling that someone else is interested in what one has to say.

4. *Interview quality.* Asking respondents for feedback on their perception of the interview's purpose is a useful means of clarifying purpose and approach and of gauging the interview's effectiveness as well. Other criteria for judging effectiveness include covering the full scope of the interview,

obtaining and maintaining a high degree of participation, eliciting responses that are neither too long and rambling nor too short and uninformative, getting in-depth information about a particular issue, and having evidence that the information is accurate.

Health educators involved in patient-education programs may be asked merely to train other health professionals in interviewing techniques. Where community health problems are being assessed, however, they may themselves be directly involved in the interviewing process. Whatever the case, interviewers must uphold professional ethics in the following ways: by taking seriously the interview's purpose and being committed to the scientific approach, and by exhibiting respect for the respondent's values, avoiding a judgmental attitude toward their behaviors or social systems, protecting the confidentiality of their responses, and refraining from criticism and gossip.

Lectures

Because the lecture (or speech) is used to inform, motivate, or influence the thinking of a group on a particular subject, a good lecture must be well organized, well developed, clearly presented, and stimulate group interest.[20] The method is appropriate when:

1. the lecturer knows more than the group about the subject
2. all participants need to hear the same information in the same way
3. the group is too large for small-group activity
4. time is scarce
5. there is take-home reading and discussion material for follow-up purposes.

Involving learners in the learning process has been emphasized throughout this book on the principle that this enhances learner motivation. Because the lecture method offers little opportunity for such involvement, health educators prefer to adopt other methods for informing people.

Personal instruction

Face-to-face instruction is one of the most effective strategies for individual change when the instruction is especially tailored to the individual's needs and interests. It is used whenever a doctor, nurse, or health-education specialist decides that a particular individual needs a health-education experience. Many aspects of the interviewing method are germane here, especially those dealing with the complex interrelationship between interviewer and respondent. Other considerations include the following.

1. When personal instruction is to be given, the instructor and assisting specialist (if other than the instructor) should plan objectives and pro-

cedures, and a lesson plan should be developed that obviates repeated replanning in the future. The patient should be involved in scheduling the activity in order to feel himself to be a part of the planning and implementation processes.

2. In a large health-care organization, scheduling and conducting the personal instruction must be organized, for these involve personnel time, patient treatment schedules, and, if the instruction cannot be given at the patient's bedside, the use of special facilities, such as a private room set aside for such purposes.

3. When the instruction has been completed, records should be made for documentation purposes—in the case of a patient, the education notes that go into the medical record. Such records should include the patient's evaluation of the activity for use in improving future lesson plans and teaching procedures.

Programmed instruction

Most commonly encountered in the form of programmed books and teaching machines, programmed instruction is useful for imparting a body of information to a large number of people on an individual basis when they are ready to receive it. Generally speaking, programmed instruction is used for individualized education and change efforts, particularly in patient education and in some instances in career development programs as well. Ideally, it permits learning at the individual's own pace, allowing frequent self-testing for comprehension.

Programmed instruction works best when the health-care organization has the resources to produce its own educational modules and has the audiovisual equipment for patients to use the modules as prescribed. The modules must be developed with overall staff agreement so that all will know what they contain and when they should be prescribed. The material within the module must be attractive, well written, accurate, and geared to the learner's needs and interests. Audio or visual aids used with the material should complement its content. Ordinarily, a scheduling system must be developed for programmed instruction, as well as a system for recording its usage.

This discussion focuses on the use rather than on the preparation of modules because their preparation is a highly developed technology in its own right and because preparation is seldom a health educator's responsibility. Ideally, then, the health educator, working with a health-education policy or advisory group, decides that a body of patient or individual education is used frequently enough to warrant its development into a programmed module and works with audiovisual personnel to prepare and pretest one.

The new module is then incorporated into the organization's resource library, and the health educator helps to develop guidelines to illuminate its purposes and content for physicians and other treatment personnel. The health educator then works again with audiovisual personnel to develop instruments and procedures for the module's use by patients and to evaluate the effectiveness of such use.

It is very difficult in reviewing so many methods to describe their detailed application within the broad field of health education or to provide enough in-depth discussion to satisfy those whose interests center strongly on any one or another method. Many books have been written on each of these methods, and references to them have been cited throughout the chapter. What should be understood here is that health education draws upon many methods, that the methods themselves have multiple uses, and that resourceful health educators should assess their mastery of these to determine which new methods can be learned to enrich their key functions.

REFERENCES

1. I. M. Rubin, M. S. Plovnick, and R. E. Fry, *Improving the Coordination of Care*, p. 88.
2. NTL Institute for Applied Behavioral Science, "An Inventory of Facilitator Interventions" (Alexandria, Va., 1973).
3. A. L. Delbecq, A. H. Van de Ven, and D. H. Gustafson, *Group Techniques for Program Planning*.
4. I. Dayal and J. M. Thomas, "Operation KPE: Developing a New Organization," *Journal of Applied Behavioral Science* 4, no. 4 (1968): 473–506.
5. M. E. Shaw, "Role Playing," in *Training and Development Handbook*, ed. R. L. Craig and L. R. Bittel, pp. 206–24.
6. P. R. Mico and H. S. Ross, *Health Education and Behavioral Science*, p. 159.
7. P. R. Mico, *Win-Win–Person-to-Person: The Art of Constructive Confrontation* (Oakland, Calif.: Third Party Associates, forthcoming).
8. E. H. Schein, *Process Consultation*, pp. 1–30.
9. Mico and Ross, *Health Education and Behavioral Science*, pp. 130–134.
10. J. Smolensky and F. B. Haar, *Principles of Community Health*, p. 105.
11. Ibid., pp. 120–31.
12. L. W. Lerda, "Conference Methods," in Craig and Bittel, *Training and Development Handbook*, pp. 154–73.
13. M. Doyle and D. Straus, *How to Make Meetings Work*.
14. D. A. Sleet, "The Use of Games and Simulations in Health Instruction," *California School Health* 9 (January 1975): 11–14.
15. Society for Public Health Education, "Gaming-Simulation and Health Education," *Health Education Monographs* 5 (supp. 1) (1977): 4–90.

16. P. Pigors, "Case Method," in Craig and Bittel, *Training and Development Handbook*, pp. 174–205.

17. A. Straus, "Coaching," in *Role Theory*, ed. B. J. Biddle and E. J. Thomas, pp. 350–53.

18. For technical details, see S. A. Richardson, B. S. Dohrnewend, and D. Klein, *Interviewing: Its Forms and Functions* (New York: Basic Books, 1965).

19. Ibid., pp. 138–70.

20. H. P. Zelco, "The Lecture," in Craig and Bittel, *Training and Development Handbook*, pp. 141–53.

13
Evaluation of health education

Evaluation is a continuous, systematic process of directly or indirectly observing, keeping a pertinent record of, and objectively judging the extent to which a target behavior has changed so that the new behavior can be supported and reinforced and its future trend predicted. Not an end in itself but rather a means to an end, it should be an integral part of any health-education activity from its initial planning stages through the activity's close.

Although all too often neglected in the past, the necessity for measuring effectiveness has grown more pressing as health education has ascended the list of national priorities, especially as a strategy for reducing the costs of health care. In the long run, this pressure on health education to prove its worth will benefit professionals and clients alike as enhanced effectiveness and greater resources stimulate and complement each other. To illuminate this important activity, then, chapter 13 presents an anatomy of the evaluation process, offers two examples of evaluation programs, and concludes with a discussion of some of the problems that impede effective evaluation.

ANATOMY OF EVALUATION
Before undertaking a step-by-step examination of the evaluation process, a few preliminary observations should be made. First, it is assumed that people who are taught the seven basic health practices, for example, will

succeed in learning them, having learned them will practice them, and by practicing them will become healthier. It is assumed further that this chain of events can be tested: hence, the clearer the assumptions, the clearer the evidence for evaluation of success or failure. Evaluation should occur, however, only if a problem or behavior is susceptible to change; it is pointless to evaluate an activity in which no change is possible.

Second, health professionals, particularly those specializing in medical care, are trained in the scientific method and are more responsive to evaluations based on objective evidence than on subjective observation. For this reason, clear touchstones should be established against which change or lack of change can be measured. For example, behavioral objectives, which in turn become criteria for judging achievement, should specify who will benefit from the activity (e.g., weight-reduction patients), precisely how they will benefit (by losing an average of twenty pounds), and when the benefits are expected to materialize (within six months).

Further, demographic data pertaining to the health problem, and to the patients as well, can help not only to isolate the central problem but to forecast the potential for making a significant impact upon it. Such data are available from many sources, including hospitals (medical, admission and discharge, and billing records) and community resources, such as the local health-planning agency (census data, disease and death records, community problems and priorities). Other information sources are community surveys, interviews, and observation; for subjective observation can be useful if the criteria for measurement are clearly stated, if the activity is carefully documented in writing, and if the writing makes extensive use of numbers.

Third, the quality of an evaluation effort can be improved by attention to several basic principles. (1) Because human behavior is complex, more than one intervention is usually required to bring about change. Interventions should therefore be planned, consistent, and mutually reinforcing. (2) Because not all messages and formats appeal equally to everyone, varying the messages and formats enhances the potential for impact. (3) Careful diagnosis of the factors that predispose a person toward, activate, and reinforce a desired behavior increases the likelihood of success. (4) Group methods not only provide peer support and reinforcement but are cost-effective in terms of staff time.

Finally, when it is said that evaluation serves to measure changes in the condition of the target population, it must be remembered that the target population can be an organization as well as a group of patients. In this case, an evaluation identifies and analyzes organizational problems, examines the process of delivering services or of meeting project objectives, and keeps track of outputs to measure progress in the achievement of service objectives. It collects and communicates feedback about clients' satisfaction with the organization and its activities, assists management in modifying goals and objectives and improving work methods, and even questions the necessity and appropriateness of the entire service effort. All these introductory thoughts should be borne in mind as the evaluation process is here broken down into its component parts.

Approaches and types   There are two primary approaches to program evaluation. *Formative evaluation* aids the development of a program that is still in its planning stages in order to lay the foundation on which the program will be built. *Summative evaluation* measures the program's worth after it has been put into action.[1] In addition, five types of program evaluation have been identified.

1. *Surveys of need* are undertaken to determine whether a program is required at all and should precede any decision making about choice of program.
2. *Operations analysis* focuses on the program's process to discover whether guidelines are being complied with, basic standards are being met, and basic criteria are being applied.
3. *Effect studies* focus on the program's end results, ascertaining to what extent the program is or is not accomplishing its goals.
4. *Effective status monitoring* attempts to identify program-related changes, even if these changes cannot be proved to be program related. If, for example, a decline in county death rates follows a year of county education in basic health practices, a relation between the two may be assumed even though the relation is not strictly demonstrable.
5. *Event investigation,* sometimes making use of outside evaluators or auditors, attempts to ascertain whether a program should be kept or abolished.[2]

Ten steps   Health-education personnel work in highly ambiguous, flexible situations and tend to describe the sequence of their evaluation steps accordingly. Evaluators, however, want the kind of simplicity and precision that is reflected in the model shown in figure 15. These ten steps are especially useful to health educators who are new at conducting evaluations. More experienced personnel can reduce them to five: defining goals, transforming goals into measurable indicators of achievement, collecting data from the study group, collecting data from the control group, and comparing the data.[3]

Steps 1 and 2 are largely self-evident. Describe the problem and the obstructive attitudes and behaviors of those who are experiencing the problem. Describe the program's general approach and whether it will be a

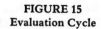

FIGURE 15
Evaluation Cycle

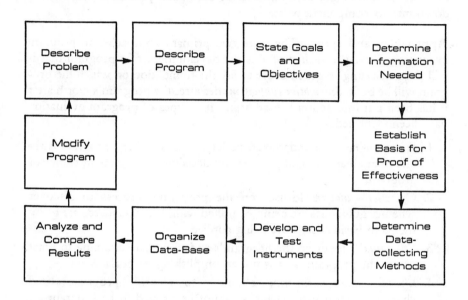

patient-education activity conducted in a hospital setting, for example, or an attempt to gain a particular group's participation in an immunization program.

Step 3—making a precise statement of goals and objectives—is essential for determining what the activity should accomplish and whether it is ultimately successful in this regard. A *goal* provides general direction for a long-term program (three to five years); an *objective* provides precise direction for a short-term activity (usually less than one year). In either case, the statements should contain specific quantifiable terms (numbers, percentages, frequencies) against which success or failure can later be measured, and it should be ensured further that the stated goals and objectives address the heart of the activity to be conducted so that educators are judged on the basis of what they set out to do.

If goals and objectives have been properly stated, step 4—deciding the type and source of data to be collected—is easy. Data should be looked upon as units of measure: the *number* of people who quit smoking, the *percentage* of the population that obtained immunization, the *frequency* with which a patient missed appointments. It should then be decided whether additional information is necessary, would be useful, or would be merely interesting.

Evaluators tend to collect more information than is generally necessary or manageable.

Step 5—establishing a basis for proof of effectiveness—generally requires the use of a *study group* that participates in the activity and a *control group* that does not participate, the two groups otherwise identical in all significant features. If the evaluation shows that the former has changed and the latter has not, the change can be attributed to the activity and cited as proof of its effectiveness. For evaluation purposes, data are collected from both groups both before and after the activity, and it is wise to obtain consultation on this from an evaluator during the planning phase. Unfortunately, however, all this takes time and money, and most health educators do not bother with it unless they are required to do so in order to obtain funds for special demonstrations.

Step 6 involves deciding how best to collect the evidence needed for evaluation purposes. Depending upon the activity, one or several methods may be used: studying patients' records or other relevant documents, interviewing, using questionnaires, counting the number of events that occur, or merely watching to see what happens. Whatever collecting method is employed, however, some instrument for collection will be needed, such as a questionnaire or an item checklist. Developing and testing such instruments to ensure that the data collected is valid and reliable constitutes step 7 of the evaluation cycle.

If trustworthy instruments already exist for step 7, they should be used; if not, new instruments should be designed. The items on the instrument should be arranged or worded in such a way as to prevent misunderstanding or confusion on the part of collector and respondent alike. The instrument should then be pretested on a group of people who fundamentally resemble, but are not members of, the study and control groups, the purpose being to see to it that the instrument collects what it is supposed to collect in the least troublesome, least expensive way. If enough money has been allocated to make use of computers, the instrument will have to be coded so that information can be fed into the computer system.

Step 8 is to organize the data-base for tabulation and presentation. By *data-base* is meant the sum of information on which the program has been built: information about the health problem or disease entity, or about such patient characteristics as sex, age, race, and educational level. Of great statistical importance here are the units of measure from steps 3 and 4 and the size of the study population.

Once the evaluation data have been tabulated, they are ready for step 9, analysis and comparison of results. Comparing the pre- and postactivity condition of the study and control groups, ask: Did the activity make any difference at all? If so, how much difference? How significant is the difference? Measures of difference and significance vary according to what is being measured and why, but an evaluation consultant or statistician can be helpful in answering these questions.

Results can also be measured against a fixed standard, of which Sigrid G. Deeds has listed five:

1. historical: before-after measurements, such as fewer deaths this year than last year
2. normative: comparing local with state and national death rates
3. theoretical: accepting the theory that a certain percentage of people will respond to a nationwide immunization program, checking the local response, and comparing the figures
4. negotiated: a combination of historical, normative, and theoretical standards designed for a specific program
5. absolute: requiring total compliance.[4]

In addition to developing new knowledge for future problem solving, evaluation is intended to improve the performance of activities already under way. Hence, step 10 calls for modification of the health-education program. Those activities that are already successful should be enhanced; those that are not successful should either be improved or eliminated.

Method of reporting, an infrequently discussed aspect of evaluation, can be decided only after weighing three factors:

1. Setting: Formal or informal, internal or external.
2. Content: Early decisions about what will constitute the report's content help in organizing the material, making transitions, and focusing on audience compatibility.
3. Media: The reporting media must communicate the complexities of the information to the audience's diverse needs. Techniques and media are limited only by the imagination (see table 16).

CIPP evaluation model Dale G. Lake developed a model in which evaluation is viewed as a process of using information to make planning, programming, implementing, and recycling decisions based on evaluations of content, input, process, and product (the first letter of each of these words forming the acronym *CIPP*)[5] (see table 17).

1. Planning decisions focus on needed improvements by specifying the domain, major goals, and objectives to be served. Hence, *content evaluation* identifies the environment in which change is to occur, the environment's unmet needs, and the problems underlying those needs.
2. Programming decisions specify procedures, personnel, facilities,

TABLE 16
Methods of Reporting Evaluation

	Internal	*External*
Oral	Reports to committees One-to-one feedback Professional staff meetings • Television • Radio	Television reports Radio reports Newspaper interviews Speeches Reports to the public via board of education meetings
Written	Required evaluation reports Ad hoc project evaluation reports: interim and final Office bulletins Office memoranda Position papers Required system reports	Mandated federal-state reports Public reports Pupil and school profile School newsletters, bulletins Reprints Press releases Occasional papers Periodicals, magazines
Graphic	Flip charts Overhead projector Slides Films	Flip charts Overhead projector Slides Films

SOURCE: D. G. Lake, "Formulating a General Evaluation Approach" (Prepared for the Organization Development Network Meeting, Spring Conference, Philadelphia, Pennsylvania, 1976).

budgetary and time requirements for implementing planned activities. *Input evaluation* therefore determines how to utilize resources to meet program goals and objectives. Its end result is an analysis of alternative procedural designs for cost-effectiveness.

3. Implementing decisions direct programmed activities. To this end, *process evaluation* can be used during implementation to provide periodic feedback to those responsible for the continuing control and refinement of plans and procedures.

4. Recycling decisions pertain to the continuation, development, drastic modification, or termination of activities. *Product evaluation*, which usually occurs after a project's complete cycle or termination, relates outcomes to content, input, and process information.

TABLE 17
CIPP Evaluation Model

	Context Evaluation	Input Evaluation	Process Evaluation	Product Evaluation
Objective	To define the operation context, to identify and assess needs in the context, and to identify and delineate problems underlying the needs.	To identify and assess system capabilities, available input strategies, and designs for implementing the strategies.	To identify or predict, in process, defects in the procedural design or its implementation, and to maintain a record of procedural events and activities.	To relate outcome information to objectives and to context, input, and process information
Method	By describing individually and in relevant perspectives the major subsystems of the context, by comparing actual and intended inputs and outputs of the subsystems, and by analyzing possible causes of discrepancies between actualities and intentions.	By describing and analyzing available human and material resources, solution strategies, and procedural designs for relevance, feasibility, and economy in the course of action to be taken.	By monitoring the activity's potential procedural barriers and remaining alert to unanticipated ones.	By defining operationally and measuring criteria associated with the objectives, by comparing these measurements with pre-determined standards or comparative bases, and by interpreting the outcome in terms of recorded input and process information.
Relation to Decision-Making in the Change Process	For deciding upon the setting to be served, the goals associated with meeting needs, and the objectives associated with solving problems, i.e., for planning needed changes.	For selecting sources of support, solution strategies, and procedural designs, i.e., for programming change activities.	For implementing and refining the program design and procedure, i.e., for effecting process control.	For deciding to continue, terminate, modify, or refocus a change activity, and for linking the activity to other major phases of the change process, i.e., for evolving change activities.

SOURCE: Developed by Daniel L. Stuttlebeam, from "Formulating a General Evaluation Approach" (Prepared for the Organization Development Network Meeting, Spring Conference, Philadelphia, Pennsylvania, 1976).

Experimental designs As health-education evaluation grows in sophistication, increasingly greater use will be made of experimental designs, which, in Lake's view, are highly useful for purposes of comparison. In true experimental designs, subjects are randomly assigned to alternative treatment groups for the purpose of yielding information on the program's own relative impact. If random assignment is too costly or difficult, however, a quasi-experimental design may be used in which comparison groups are formed for the purpose of yielding information on this program's performance in comparison with the performance of other currently existing programs.

If comparative results are to be valid, close attention must be given to three factors. First, to the greatest extent possible, bias must be eradicated from preexperiment comparisons in order to permit meaningful postexperiment comparisons of program impact. Second, the selected treatment alternatives must be feasible, for it is pointless to make comparative performance evaluations of experimental programs that have little practical likelihood of being adopted in the future.

Third, it should be realized that judgments of comparative program impact will depend upon whether a program was implemented as intended, for innovative programs often experience great difficulties during their initial implementation. Maintaining a clearly defined target population and a constant treatment condition is important to any controlled experiment. More important, however, is the necessity of constantly improving a program's functioning toward meeting its objectives. In this regard, especially, formative evaluation may transform an apparent loser into a winner.

TWO EXAMPLES OF EVALUATION

Described here are two examples of evaluation, both conducted in hospital settings: the first, a New Jersey program to reduce preoperative psychological stress; the second, a patient-education project in Minnesota. The first case is narrated briefly to provide an overview of a somewhat limited but nevertheless relatively effective process. The second case offers a more detailed view of the program evaluation cycle.

Reducing preoperative stress

In January 1974 Our Lady of Lourdes Hospital, a 400-bed community hospital in Camden, New Jersey, initiated a program of evening classes for surgical patients for the purpose of reducing preoperative psychological stress, lessening postoperative discomfort, and hastening recovery.[7] When it was found after a three-month trial period that only 50 percent of the target population had attended these classes, the program was changed. Thereafter, nurse instructors taught surgical patients on a one-to-one basis, discussing pre- and postoperative details, demonstrating simple breathing and leg exercises, and encouraging patients and family members to ask questions.

At the end of the program's first year, evaluation questionnaires were distributed, several days postoperatively but before discharge, to all except pediatric, local-anesthesia, and cardiac patients. Six patients per day were then surveyed at random until 100 questionnaires had been completed. The purpose of the questionnaire was to determine whether the program was being carried out properly and meeting its objectives—important information for hospital administrators because the program constituted an additional, though not a large, per-diem item on the budget.

The findings indicated that patients regarded the program as helpful and wanted it continued, though with more instruction in postoperative exercises. A majority of patients responded that preoperative instruction had caused them to feel more relaxed, and more than one-third indicated that it had reduced their anxiety, although in some cases this may have been owing more to the presence and attitude of the instructor than to the instruction itself.

For one of the inherent limitations of subjective evaluation is that respondents tend to give answers that they believe the investigators want, especially when they have undergone a recent ordeal and want to appear grateful for the help they have received. In an effort to overcome this tendency, the survey was conducted, not by the nurse instructor, but by the patient-education coordinator, who had had no prior contact with the respondents and whom they had therefore no desire to please. To what extent this strategy succeeded is unknown, however.

Another limitation in this case was the absence of a control group, but it had been decided that it would be wrong to deny such a group a health service as essential as preoperative teaching just to refine the results of the survey. Finally, although no statistical analysis was forthcoming from this evaluation, the hospital and its teaching personnel concluded that the program was reaching its goals.[6]

Evaluating patient education

United Hospital in St. Paul, Minnesota, regards patient education as an integral part of total health care and believes that it can be approached as a specific treatment modality to meet the patient's individual needs, interests, and capabilities. At this hospital, education programs are designed collaboratively by the patient and family members, the attending physician, and professional health workers (nurses, pharmacists, dietitians, etc.) who are already caring in their respective ways for the patient s various health needs.

Programs are multidisciplinary and employ team teaching, using professional health workers as teachers. Standard methods are used to initiate a program, determine the services needed, set reasonable behavioral objectives, deliver activities, and make available further guidance in self-care after the patient is discharged from the hospital.

In 1974–75 United Hospital was one of six agencies selected by a local consultant firm to participate in a project whose object was to develop a system for measuring the efficiency and effectiveness of patient-education programs. To this end, United adopted a formative evaluation system, based on the assumptions that a causal relationship exists between services provided and results obtained and that a knowledge of results improves program productivity.

Evaluation was thus seen as a systematic service-oriented procedure both for ascertaining a program's results and the efficiency with which the results were obtained. The system included evaluation measures for what occurred within the facility, evaluation measures for what occurred outside the facility, and interval reports (quarterly, monthly, etc.) on results. The eight basic elements established for United's program evaluation system were as follows.

1. *Statement of organizational purpose.* The statement of purpose or mission describes in general terms what the organization hopes to accomplish, by means of what services, and for whom. The statement should be broad enough to cover all the organization's programs but specific enough to distinguish this organization from all others in the community. For United Hospital's educational program, the stated mission was to provide educational services, under medical supervision, to the chronically disabled in order to reduce premature mortality and to enable patients to maximize their capacity for independent living.

2. *Statement of program goals.* Goal statements specifically identify the clientele to be served, the services to be provided, and the results to be achieved by each program; hence, an organization with three programs must have goal statements for each. The stated goals must be specific enough to allow formulation of program objectives, and the goals must be achievable by means of the services provided. For United Hospital's cardiac program, the stated goal was to provide cardiac patients with a program of individualized education, skill development, and counseling to minimize premature mortality, reduce unnecessary hospitalization, and facilitate the ability to live independently.

3. *Statement of program objectives.* Stated objectives are the touchstones

against which achievement is measured. Hence, objectives must be measurable, must include efficiency and effectiveness among their number, and their sum must equal achievement of the goal. For United's cardiac program, the stated objectives were: to maximize use of the educational program; to minimize the number of patients requiring institutional care and unnecessary rehospitalization; to maximize the number of patients who could profit by, and follow recommendations for, home treatment; and to minimize social isolation, maximize personal independence, and, if possible, secure employment.

4. *Development of measures.* Quantifiable data developed for measuring the achievement of objectives should be accurate and reliable, specify precisely to whom they are being applied, and be applied after services have been delivered. The measures used in United's cardiac program included the percentage of:

- primary and secondary patients who had been ordered to receive cardiac education
- cardiac patients no longer institutionalized
- patients who had followed critical recommendations in the home-treatment plan
- patients who now independently performed living skills learned in, or encouraged by, the program
- patients who had left their place of residence for social or recreational purposes during the month immediately preceding follow-up
- patients who had not required in-home service during the two weeks immediately preceding follow-up
- patients who had not been rehospitalized for the same cardiac condition
- patients who had either returned to work or secured new employment.

5. *Setting performance expectancies.* Expectancies are relative criteria against which the performance of objectives can be compared. In developing them, several factors should be considered: past performance, who is to be served, the control environment, and the quantity and quality of service to be provided. Expectancies make the system explicit so that everyone is observing the same rules. They should be negotiated with the staff that will actually do the work, and they should at all times be reasonable for the program's clients. Finally, expectancies are set at three levels: optimal level (not necessarily the maximum possible but what can be achieved if all goes well), goal level (satisfactory performance), and minimal level (if no improvement is possible, the program should be eliminated). For United's cardiac program, a sample expectancy was as follows:

	MINIMAL	GOAL	OPTIMAL
Percentage of patients not requiring in-home service during the two weeks preceding follow-up	70%	80%	90%

6. *Assignment of weights.* If a program's objectives are not of equal importance, they should either be rank-ordered or assigned relative weights in terms of percentages, the total equaling 100 percent. The objective with the heaviest weight is the highest priority. Weights can help to change both staff and patient behavior. In patient education, the balance between acquiring and actually practicing behavior should be assessed.

7. *Description of clients.* To facilitate interpretation of results, the persons being served should be described along with the problems to be resolved and the major barriers to their resolution. Examples from the cardiac program include the percentage of patients over sixty-five years of age and the percentage with diminished mental capacity.

8. *Management reports.* Finally, reports must be distributed regularly to persons both inside and outside the organization indicating actual performance on all objectives, expected levels of achievement, and including a summary description of the clients. Index scores indicate the degree to which each objective has been achieved; e.g., 50 = minimal performance, 100 = goal performance, 150 = operational performance.

Combining this evaluation system with other current methods (chart-audit case studies, pre- and posteducation assessments, verbal feedback) and incorporating the three major variables that affect the attainment of goals (the medical management plan, the patient's physiological and psychological state, and the patient's behavior) should provide a clear picture of the efficiency and effectiveness of patient-education efforts.[7]

EVALUATION PROBLEMS

A number of problems impede the proper measurement and evaluation of health-education efforts, and among them are the following common forms of error.[8]

1. Halo effect: the tendency of a factor other than that being studied to influence the factor that is being studied, as an unfavorable first impression might bias a rater's perception in a subsequent situation.

2. Rating error: the disposition of a rater to assign positions to others at the top, middle, or bottom of a scale.

3. Hawthorne effect: the effect on behavior or performance of singling out individuals for special treatment.

4. Self-fulfilling prophecy: forcing a situation to affirm a preconceived notion, as when a teacher expects students from disadvantaged background to perform poorly and the expectation produces a poor performance among them.

5. Post hoc error: confusing a time sequence with a causal relationship; e.g., A caused B because it preceded B.

6. Initial differences: observing and ignoring great differences between experimental and control groups at the beginning of an educational treatment. It would be unfair, for example, to compare the gain scores of gifted readers with those of persons with severe reading problems in a special reading program.

Further, Lawrence W. Green has identified seven dilemmas of evaluation posed by the very nature of health education.[9] First among these is the dilemma produced by the rigors of experimental design versus the significance of program adaptability. That is, the scientific rigor required of evaluation research forces strict compliance with procedural details that may constrain educational efforts. The result is either a rigorously defined but trivial intervention or a significant intervention that is too vaguely defined to be duplicated. The exits from this dilemma are to be found in more complex experimental designs, more detailed documentation and reporting of procedures, and more attention to the cumulative building of theoretical and research literature in health education.

Second is the dilemma of internal versus external validity. *Internal validity* denotes the degree of certainty with which program results can be directly attributed to the educational activity; *external validity,* to what extent such results can be expected to recur elsewhere and at other times. The dilemma is that the greater the striving for the one, the more the other is sacrificed. This dilemma can be eluded by developing decision rules for striking a balance between internal and external validity on the one hand and between resources and circumstances on the other.

Third is the dilemma of experimental versus placebo effects, which means that whereas medical researchers strive to eradicate patient involvement from their studies, health education strives to increase and enrich it. Fourth is the dilemma of effectiveness versus economy of scale—the need to respond to measures of quality and of cost-effectiveness at the same time. Sacrificing effectiveness to economy can be avoided by working with groups rather than with individuals, by using other technologies, such as teaching machines, and by employing a variety of approaches since one approach cannot work for all.

The fifth dilemma, of risk versus payoff, pertains to the expense of working successfully with fewer patients versus the economy of working less successfully with more patients. The sixth dilemma, of long- versus short-term evaluation, means that the effects of some health-education activities are immediate but temporary, while others may be slower in developing but longer lasting. Finally, the dilemma of how much to spend on health education may be resolved by means of evaluation, which should produce a knowledge of how much to budget. In the absence of good evaluation, health-education budgets have lower priorities.

In conclusion, the evaluation of health-education programs can be greatly improved if the following points are understood and acknowledged.[10]

1. Evaluation requires investments of time and money if it is to be planned carefully and productively.
2. The purpose of evaluation must be clear at all times to ascertain whether money was well spent, whether desired actions actually occurred, whether the selected approach was better than a previous one, and whether it contributed to solving the problem.
3. Good judgment should dictate what is measured and how. Some efforts cannot be measured for immediate results because they focus on such intangibles as enhancing self-esteem. Further, because health education adopts a collaborative approach toward problem solving, it is not always possible to establish at the beginning a measurable goal for some later action.
4. If an activity undergoes constant change, the bases for periodic and final evaluations must change as well.
5. Feedback of evaluation data should be constantly improved.
6. Those who helped to plan, and who participated in, an activity should likewise participate in its evaluation.

REFERENCES

1. R. A. Gabriel, *Program Evaluation*, pp. 12–15.
2. Ibid.
3. Ibid.
4. S. G. Deeds, "Overview of Evaluation" (Paper presented at National Conference on Hospital-based Patient Education, Chicago, 9–10 August 1976).
5. D. G. Lake, "Formulating a General Evaluation Approach" (Prepared for the Organization Development Network Spring Conference, Philadelphia, 1976). The experimental-design portion of the model was excerpted from AIR Educa-

tion Evaluation Module. For the entire module, write to Dr. Marshall Frinks, Florida State Education Department, Tallahassee, Fla. 32304.

6. N. H. Bryant, "Practical Considerations in Evaluating Patient/Consumer Health-Education Programs" (Paper presented at National Conference on Hospital-based Patient Education, Chicago, 9–10 August 1976). The case study reported in Bryant's report was from J. Hannabery, "Process Evaluation of Preoperative Teaching" (Paper presented at First International Congress in Patient Counseling, Amsterdam, April 1976).

7. M. Ulrich, "How Hospitals Evaluate Patient-Education Programs" (Paper presented at National Conference on Hospital-based Patient Education, Chicago, 9–10 August 1976). Ulrich credits Bob Walker and Associates, 23 East Grant St., Minneapolis, Minn. 55403, for the evaluation methodology employed.

8. Lake, "Formulating a General Evaluation Approach."

9. L. W. Green, "Evaluation and Measurement: Some Dilemmas for Health Education," *American Journal of Public Health* 67, no. 2 (February 1977): 155–61.

10. J. Simmons, ed., "Making Health Education Work," *American Journal of Public Health* 65 (supp.) (October 1975): 28.

14

o Call home:
+ Get-together 1st Sun.   - Dad scout salmon
- Kaplan $500   @ St Olaf

<u>Journals for Lit Review:</u>

Nursing Clinics of N Am
RC 356.5 N485

American Journal of N
PERIODICALS v.49

Am J of Pub Health
Nov 2008

RC440.R39
RC2066
001/24
22/25
24

Bell, William J., 1902-

Arban, J.-B. (Jean-Baptiste), 1825-
1889.
[Méthode complète de cornet à pistons
et de saxhorn. Selections; arr.]
Arban-Bell interpretations : for all
tubas, trombones and baritones : from
the William J. Bell Complete tuba
method. -- New York : C. Colin, c1975.
p. 82-206 of music ; 31 cm.
Arban studies and exercises,
transposed and with commentaries by
William J. Bell.
1. Tuba--Studies and exercises.
2. Trombone--Studies and exercises.
3. Baritone (Musical instrument)--
Studies and exercises. I. Bell,
William J., 1 902-   II. Title
III. Title: T   he William J. Bell
complete tuba   method.

Guidelines
for professionals

Professions are not born fully grown; they evolve from previously established bodies of knowledge, and when conditions are right new professions will evolve from them. If they are to survive and grow, then, professions must contain within themselves the means for their own advancement. Health education has such means—in numerous professional associations that are committed to the field's development, in having well-defined guidelines for preparation and practice, in holding continuing education in high regard, and in being guided by moral principles. This concluding chapter will discuss aspects of all these matters. For an expanded view of professional guidelines, the reader should consult appendixes A and B.

PREPARATION AND PRACTICE
Generally speaking, regulations governing the certification and licensure of health professionals exist to minimize or prevent malpractice and quackery within the conduct of the field. Although most such regulations are established by individual states, definitions vary greatly concerning the human-services areas to be protected, the professions that should be regulated, and the practices that are considered to be potentially dangerous.

Further, some health-education practices are governed by regulations for other professions. Because fine lines differentiate educational from therapy groups, for example, several states are now regulating encounter and personal-growth groups, which are usually defined as educational, because the regulators perceive them as being essentially devoted to therapy. Certification and licensure, then, may not always be matters of choice for health education. Merely by expanding a definition here or there, a state legislature can unintentionally and unexpectedly impose state licensure on the field; and once the procedure has been established in one state, other states may wish to follow suit.

Health-education professionals employed in elementary and secondary school systems are required to meet certification standards in their states. Otherwise, no state requires either certification or licensure of specialists; it suffices that the schools from which they graduated are accredited. For the master's degree in public health education (MPH), the accrediting body is the Council on Education for Public Health (for the Council on Postsecondary Accreditation). At present there is no accreditation body for the baccalaureate degree in community health education.

But accreditation of training institutions does not alone satisfy regulators' concerns about quality practice. Many health-education specialists who have been in practice for years need updated education, and there is no way at present of guaranteeing that they will pursue it. Moreover, federal involvement in health-care programs is increasingly being tied to demands for quality controls governing the providers of services.

If the costs of educational services are to be reimbursed under a (possible) national health-insurance program, the educators who provide those services may have to be certified or licensed. Working with various health-education associations, the federal government awarded a contract to the National Center for Health Education to study the roles of health-care, school, and community health educators. It is hoped that developing standards for their certification will be the next step. Meanwhile, the profession must oversee quality control itself.

Setting standards

SOPHE guidelines In 1977 the Society for Public Health Education (SOPHE) updated its "Guidelines for the Preparation and Practice of Professional Health Educators" to refine the functions of practice as a prerequisite to developing standards for distinguishing between levels of performance.[1] Written for academician and practitioner alike, this document covers six areas of preparation and practice: foundations for health education, administration, program development and management, research and evaluation, professional ethics, and special applications. It outlines the minimal level of needed preparation for baccalaureate and master's graduates, as well as the functions to be performed at each level.

Another SOPHE document, "Guidelines and Standards for Baccalaureate Preparation in Community Health Education," covers program objectives and goals, stature and number of faculty, and interrelationships between universities and community agencies.[2] Further, SOPHE is at present developing an approval mechanism for encouraging bachelor-level preparation programs to engage in self-study procedures.

In the preparation of professional health educators, these two documents cover the areas of community health education and of health education in health-care, industrial, and labor settings. Organizations interested in the preparation of educators for community and school health include the Society for Public Health Education, Public Health Education and School Health Education sections of the American Public Health Association, the American Association for the Advancement of Health Education, the American School Health Association, the Health Education section of the American College Health Association, and the American Alliance for Health, Physical Education, and Recreation.

Standards for health-services agencies In 1975 the federal Bureau of Health Education convened a three-day conference of health educators and health-planning leaders to develop standards for use by health-services agencies and for help also in developing national health-planning guidelines.[3] These standards, adopted by SOPHE in 1977, fall into three categories: standards for education of the individual in healthful behavior, standards for education within the health-care system, and standards of education for citizen participation.

For education of the individual, the following eight standards were established.

1. An organizational mechanism shall exist within the health-services area to determine the need for educational and promotional services, to inventory available services and resources, and to design a plan for developing, maintaining, and evaluating such programs in accordance with consumers' needs and interests.

2. A comprehensive, coordinated, and identifiable program component shall be included in the health or education plans of all appropriate departments, districts, and agencies at federal, state, and local levels. So that users and providers have a common understanding of program goals, priorities, scope, and costs, such matters should be set forth in writing and incorporated into these entities' overall plans.

3. Services shall be equitably distributed throughout the health-services area and be accessible to all communities within the area, including rural or economically depressed populations.

4. For help in planning, implementing, and evaluating programs, technical assistance and consultation services shall be provided by the health-systems agency, the state health-planning and resources-development agency, state health and education departments, centers for health planning, agencies of the Department of Health, Education and Welfare (HEW), and other consultative resources.

5. Programs under full-time professional direction, and having adequate funds, facilities, personnel, and materials, shall be located in health departments and federally funded health agencies serving 10,000 or more people, as well as in federal agencies that have identifiable employee-health programs. Program directors should have a master's degree in public health education or a related field, training in health and educational methodologies, and experience in providing health-education services. In the absence of such persons, individuals with baccalaureate degrees are acceptable if they are experienced and have consultative arrangements with a master's-level educator who meets the above qualifications.

6. To the maximum extent feasible, staff shall be made up of qualified persons who reflect the area's racial and ethnic background. Staff employers shall follow affirmative action procedures in recruitment, training, and promotion.

7. Educational institutions and funding sources shall be encouraged to develop a preparational hierarchy for health educators, the steps ascending from outreach workers and associates to personnel at the bachelor's, master's, and doctoral levels.

8. Educational institutions preparing students for careers in health education and allied health professions shall be asked to require at least one course in educational concepts and methodologies and to encourage continuing courses in these subjects.

For education within the health-care system, nine standards were set. Continuing to number consecutively, these were as follows.

9. Identifiable patient and family programs shall be available in hospitals having 150 or more beds, in health-maintenance organizations having 25,000 or more enrollees, and in federally funded health-care programs serving more than 5,000 persons.

10. Patient and family programs in such facilities shall be under full-time professional direction and have adequate resources.

11. Facilities serving fewer persons shall be encouraged to obtain part-time professional health-education specialists or other qualified personnel and to share their services whenever feasible.

12. Resources shall be distributed within the health-services area so that they are available to those receiving services at any of the facilities described above.

13. For help in planning, implementing, and evaluating such programs, technical assistance and consultation services shall be provided by the health-systems agency, the state health-planning and resources-development agency, state health departments, centers for health planning, HEW, and other consultative resources.

14. Identifiable patient and family services shall be reimbursable by third-party payers.

15. Agencies and organizations that administer federally funded health-care programs shall inform those eligible for services of their eligibility and shall inform providers eligible for reimbursement of that fact. These efforts shall be evaluated periodically.

16. An organized patient-advocacy system shall be established in the health-services area to interpret the nature and scope of available services to potential users, to hear their grievances about the quality of services, and to represent them in suggesting improvements.

17. Educational institutions preparing students for careers in health and allied professions shall be encouraged to provide preservice and continuing education and training for all direct providers of personal health care.

Finally, five standards were set for education for citizen participation.

18. An organizational mechanism within the health-services area shall ascertain the interests, skills, and availability of concerned citizens, find ways of including them in the agency's work, make their availability known to other agencies seeking citizen participation, and systematically encourage other citizens to become involved in resolving local, state, and national health problems.

19. Agencies involved in health-education and promotional planning, resources development, and services operation shall use both direct and indirect means of obtaining significant citizen input and participation: e.g., conducting opinion surveys on policies and programs, employing indigenous outreach workers to serve as patient advocates, and recruiting personnel who reflect a population's major racial and ethnic groups.

20. Technical assistance and consultation services shall help in the planning, implementation, and evaluation of citizen-participation activities with the help of the health-systems agency, the state health-planning and resources-development agency, HEW, and other consultative resources.

21. The health-systems agency and its state and national counterparts shall provide, or arrange for, ongoing orientation and training of the agency's governing body, development committees, task forces, and other appropriate citizens' groups. Such training shall include models of health

programs, decision making, and policy development, as well as illumination of citizens' opportunities, roles, and responsibilities in the formulation and assessment of health policies and programs. Other health agencies shall be encouraged to do likewise.

22. Educational institutions shall be encouraged to provide continuing education and training for health professionals on increasing informed citizen participation in the formulation and assessment of health policies and programs.

Standards for community preventive health services In 1978 the Health Services Extension Act mandated the development of standards for community preventive health services. To discuss the feasibility of establishing a collaborative work group to postulate model standards for such services, HEW's Center for Disease Control conducted discussions with the Association of State and Territorial Health Officials, the National Association of County Health Officials, the U.S. Conference of City Health Officers, and the American Public Health Association.

The model's purpose was twofold: (1) to establish minimum tolerable levels of preventable disease and of public-health conditions in a community, and (2) to describe the basic disease-prevention and health-promotion capacity that should be available to all communities. To this end, standards were drafted for twenty-eight areas of public health.

For health education specifically, the following goal was established: "Residents of the community will be provided information to help them assume a greater responsibility for disease prevention and health promotion; utilize health services and resources appropriately; understand, participate in, and comply with recommendations of health staff; participate in community-health decision making."[4] In addition, several focal points were established along with specific objectives and indicators of attainment (see table 18).

Continuing education Professional education should not be a one-shot endeavor; for as long as the profession faces problematic accreditation and credentialing issues, so long will an urgent need for continuing education persist.[5] To meet this need, the Western Consortium for Continuing Education for the Health Professions, for example, has conducted programs in conjunction with the Schools of Public Health at the University of Hawaii, the University of California at Berkeley and Los Angeles, and the Seventh-Day Adventist University at Loma Linda, California, as well.

Two federal trends suggest a further reason for continuing professional education. First, the federal government is increasingly consolidating categorical programs into more comprehensive integrated programs both

TABLE 18
Model Standards for Health Education in Community
Preventive Health Services

Focus	Objectives	Indicators	Population in Need
Integration of Health Education Services	By 19–, health-education services will be an identifiable and integral component of all appropriate preventive health services programs which serve the community.	Identifiable health-education services in programs	The community
	By 19–, individuals will receive health-education services as an element of their personal preventive health care.	Proportion of individuals receiving health-education services as part of personal preventive health care	
Promotion of Individual Health Maintenance	By 19–, health-education programs will be designed to increase the knowledge, skills, and motivation necessary for each individual to assume a greater responsibility for his health status. The public media will be an important source of such information.	Documentation of emphasis on individual responsibility for health Level of public media involvement	
Appropriate Use of Health Services and Resources	By 19–, the community will participate in a program which promotes appropriate use of health services and resources.	Existence	
	By 19–, the community will have access to a current inventory of available health resources and services.	Access to inventory	
	By 19–, the community will be covered by a health-resource information referral service.	Presence of formal and informal means of obtaining such input Information and referral service use	

TABLE 18 (continued)

Focus	Objectives	Indicators	Population in Need
Compliance with Medical Recommendations	By 19–, each patient receiving a personal preventive service will: • Be informed of the relative benefits and risks of receiving that service.	Documentation in patient record	Patients receiving preventive care
	• Be involved in the development of his health-care plan if he chooses to do so.	Documentation in patient record	
Staff Training	By 19–, staff providing health-education services will have necessary skills and knowledge.	Proportion of staff with health-education training	Staff providing health education
Citizen Involvement in Community Health Decisions	By 19–, a mechanism will exist in the community to ensure that: • Health-related boards and committees obtain advice and guidance from consumers.	Presence of formal and informal means of obtaining such input	Citizens involved in health decision-making groups
	• Orientation and training is provided for members of boards, committees, task forces, etc.	Documentation of action taken as a result of such input Documentation of programs presented	
	• Citizen participation in health-related decision making is assured.	Documentation of outreach activities and responses	

SOURCE: U.S., Department of Health, Education and Welfare, "Model Standards for Community Preventive Health Services," August 1978.

within and between major service areas, such as health and community development programs funded by the Department of Housing and Urban Development. Second, the federal government is increasingly shifting planning and implementation responsibilities for these integrated programs from national and state levels to local levels of government.

Thus, health educators, particularly those working in community and social change, must increasingly relate to public administrators, urban planners, economists, elected officials, and city-county-regional managers—in short, to social-change agents from a variety of other professional backgrounds. If they are to function effectively in these settings, they must expand their cognitive maps in order to interrelate health care with the broader functions of social systems.

To bring about a more effective attainment of objectives, managers of multipersonnel health-education units should be responsible for planning, organizing, and implementing in-service training programs. These can be carried out on an in-house basis with all staff members participating simultaneously, or they can be conducted elsewhere with only a few staff members at a time in attendance. In either case, the experience should be congruent with a planned program of staff development. An allotment of 5 percent of the budget and of one half-day per week for each staff person is a useful guideline here.[6]

Those who wish to proceed in a solo direction may pursue a separate, individualized course of study, ideally based on a lifetime career plan.[7] Having developed such a plan, individuals are better able to select developmental workshops or seminars that relate to their job requirements and that do not exceed what they can afford to pay. For such individuals, continued learning and development can be challenging, exciting, and self-actualizing, though it means regarding enhanced knowledge as its own reward.

The training of a health-education specialist should not be left to chance. While members of many other professions can perform health-education functions as a sideline, the shaping of a specialist is a highly complex endeavor. The knowledge base is there for the asking. What impart special dignity to the profession, however, are the moral principles by which it is guided.

VALUES AND ETHICS

By teaching people about the forces that affect their health, health educators hope to bring about changes that will conduce to healthier living; and because learning and change are deeply personal experiences, those who influence them must be guided by the highest ideals. *Values* are beliefs that are held in high esteem, *ethics* are often the behavioral expressions of values, and both are vitally important to institutions and professions that exercise any control over individuals.

To what extent may government exercise control over individual behavior? In response to this question, Raymond P. Shafer cites two principles: "*First*, that for a government to be of the highest character it must be shaped by individuals, initially and constantly, who understand that to be truly free and independent, they must be first interdependent. *Second*, that to be interdependent, a government with the highest character must permit the individual the most far-reaching exercise of freedom."[8]

This view suggests that government should intervene in the conduct of human behavior only when any individual, group, or thing becomes a serious threat to the safety or life of others and when traditional means of control have become ineffective. Government's proper role is to encourage the development of institutions and agencies that help individuals to help themselves.

It is the task of society to refine the principles that enable individuals to live satisfying and enjoyable lives. Hence, the development and transmission of sound values should be society's highest priority, and the societal institutions that are basic to this process should be continually revitalized. Whether governmental or societal, all the forces that help to shape national values will eventually affect the functioning of health educators, but this is especially so now when the profession's overall contours are rapidly taking shape.

Issues for health education

To what extent can health-education professionals impose their own values on patients? According to Pearl S. German and A. Judith Chwalow, " . . . this question, raised by sensitive and concerned health educators, resulted in ambivalence in the presentation of specific interventions, defensive postures with resistant patients, and possible vitiation of the effectiveness of the health-education strategy."[9]

German and Chwalow concluded that the greater the certainty of health educators of the soundness and defensibility of their interventions, the less they are troubled about imposing their values. In addition to attitude, however, two techniques are useful in handling such questions. (1) The "educational contract," which shapes the educator-patient relationship, enables patients themselves to decide what they wish to learn or change. (2) Clarifying both roles in their relationship bespeaks the educator's view that the patient is a responsible working member of the team.

Manipulation *Manipulation* denotes deliberately withholding a behavioral choice from a client, either because the withheld option is believed not to be good for the client or because the educator has a personal investment in a particular option. In both cases, the educator's values and ethics are brought into question.

Manipulation may also occur in relation to behavioral modification and the use of fear-arousal techniques. Behavioral modification consists of altering environmental conditions on the theory that as these conditions change, responsive behaviors will change as well.[10] The issue of concern here is the extent to which those who are to undergo change are themselves involved in reshaping their environment; for their minimal involvement raises the dramatic specter of omniscient, faceless scientists manipulating malleable people against their will. Though this greatly exaggerates behavioral modification, it does call the issue of manipulation to attention and suggests the importance of a contractual relationship in such cases.

The use of fear-arousal techniques consists generally of warning people of their susceptibility to a disease if they do not follow a prescribed behavior.[11] Depending upon the seriousness of the danger and the speed with which it can be reduced, this technique can have immediate effectiveness, but it also has drawbacks that raise ethical questions. Using fear arousal to elicit the greatest possible public response as quickly as possible, for example, may meet the needs of the health professional more than the needs of the public. Especially when coupled with the use of mass communications, it may convey a threat in the strongest terms to all people, including those who are not even vulnerable to the danger.

Moreover, not all people handle threat well. While some are able to respond rationally, others become emotional and may behave in ways injurious to their health. Confusion may result if communications are poor, transmitting the threat but not the prescribed behavior, and the same may occur if there is no access to the treatment resources needed to alleviate the threat. In this case individuals may either respond in reactive or desperate ways that they mistakenly believe to be helpful, or they may mentally block the threat, denying its existence or rationalizing its relevance. Overused, fear techniques only arouse counterproductive distrust and resentment.

For health education, then, there are several ethical dilemmas: (1) the desire to persuade people to behave in ways conducive to good health versus the right of individuals to do as they please with their own health as long as this does not impinge upon the rights of others; (2) the desire to enhance personal freedom and self-determination versus the desire to modify an environment in order to shape more healthful behavior; (3) the use of quick fear-arousal techniques versus the use of slower educational and organizing methods; and (4) the use of win-lose conflict for social change versus the more careful pursuit of win-win strategies.

A professional code

An important measure of any profession is the moral code by which it is guided. For health education, values should be founded above all on respect: respect for human life in all its social manifestations; respect for the dignity and beliefs of the individual; respect for the principles of participatory democracy, including free and open choice, informed consent, and the right to self-determination; respect for the creativity of the learning process; and respect for the highest professional competence at all levels of preparation and practice.

A health educator's code of ethics should emphasize the following:

1. Practicing nondiscrimination against race, religion, age, sex, cultural background, or socioeconomic status both in employment practices and in providing services
2. Respecting obligations to the employing organization, to the clients being served, and to the integrity and rights of coworkers
3. Involving those to be affected by a change effort in its planning and implementation
4. Avoiding manipulative methods to ensure free and open choice among all options.

Like professions themselves, however, values and ethics are not born fully grown but are nurtured by professional preparation, continuing education, and peer review. In their professional preparation, students learn about human needs and individual differences, theories of learning and change, principles of democratic governance, philosophy and logic, and the development of values and ethics in themselves, in health education, and in other professions as well. Continuing education advances knowledge and skills by confronting new issues and permitting a full examination of differing viewpoints with their ethical implications for health education.

Peer review is a quality-control process voluntarily undertaken by the members of a profession—through the American Bar Association for the legal profession and through the American Medical Association for the medical profession. Lawrence W. Green and P. Brooks-Bertram believe that three factors must exist before a satisfactory peer review of health education can be attempted:

1. A national, state, or regional agency or organization having legal au-

thority to grant recognition, authorize governmental payments, or license for business purposes the institutions or programs offering specific professional services within its jurisdiction

2. A professional association or society having a mandate from, or sufficient representation of, members of the profession to provide acceptable peer-review panels

3. Criteria, guidelines, or standards of practice having enough specificity and acceptance by the profession to provide the minimal observable characteristics without which a service or program can be deemed inadequate or inappropriate.[12]

Assuming that these conditions exist, Green and Brooks-Bertram outline seven steps for a peer review.

1. The applicant-organization makes a formal request for review by the legal agency.

2. The agency informs the organization of the procedures for self-evaluation, documentation, and review and asks the appropriate professional association(s) to provide up-to-date guidelines and standards.

3. The association appoints a peer-review panel and provides guidelines and standards to both the applicant-organization and the legal agency.

4. The organization engages in self-evaluation, documenting its strengths and weaknesses in relation to professional standards and its own objectives. This process should include an administration review, budgetary audit, an analysis of consumer participation and of program achievement whenever possible.

5. After reviewing this report, the legal agency asks the professional association to identify problems requiring further study or explanation. The peer-review panel submits specific questions.

6. The legal agency conducts a site visit to the applicant-organization and probes these questions, as well as those raised by consumer groups that have been invited to comment.

7. Finally, the agency takes into account the revised self-evaluation report, the site-visit report, the response of both the organization and the association to this report, and its own judgment of the organization's capacity and commitment to correct its deficiencies.

Looking ahead

Predicting the future is a risky endeavor, not only because the forces that shape the future are never under the control of any one person or institution, but because forces may evolve from future conditions that cannot even be envisaged at present. An unforeseeable breakthrough in medical technology that places the treatment or prevention of a major disease within organizational grasp could greatly alter the future directions of health care, as could the emergence of a devastating new disease or a disruption of ecological balance by some monumental human error.

It can be said, however, that several changes will affect this country's health-care delivery system during the next few years—among them, growing emphasis on the concepts of preventive care, self-care, and wellness, the development of primary health-care services, heightened consumer participation, and national health insurance—all of which will have implications for health education.

One of the key goals of professional leadership during the next few years will be to continue developing national policy and programs for health-education purposes. As the field grows, liaisons with interested organizations will have to be strengthened, for without them much of health education's energy and impact would be fragmented or dissipated. Special attention must also be given to increasing membership in professional associations. Enlisting the energy of as many health-education academicians and practitioners as possible will bring fresh ideas and vitality to these organizations.

Improved funding provisions should result in the creation of new health-education positions. To fill these positions with trained personnel and to meet ongoing replacement needs, training institutions will have to produce many more professionals than they do today and preparation will have to become more differentiated. Individual, organizational, and social change are sufficiently distinct in their theoretical bases and methodological applications to require specialized training, particularly for those who aspire to action research and management.

Standards must be developed for preparation and practice at the bachelor's, master's, and doctoral levels, and professional values and ethics must be continually refined. Continuing education programs will have to be expanded to meet new demands in the behavioral and social sciences and in the areas of organization development, program planning and evaluation, patient education, mass communications, and social change.

Finally, considerable effort should be devoted to promoting job opportunities for health-education specialists in the newer systems and to helping employers understand the contributions that they can make to the field. For health education is a young and highly dynamic profession, and the time for realizing its potential is now.

REFERENCES

1. Society for Public Health Education, "Guidelines for the Preparation and Practice of Professional Health Educators," *Health Education Monographs* 5, no. 1 (Spring 1977): 75–89.

2. Society for Public Health Education, "Guidelines and Standards for Baccalaureate Preparation in Community Health Education," *Health Education Monographs* 5, no. 1 (Spring 1977): 90–98.

3. U.S., Department of Health, Education and Welfare, Public Health Service, Center for Disease Control, *The Priorities of Section 1502: Papers on the National Health Guidelines. Health Education and Public Law 93–641,* prepared for the Bureau of Health Education by H. G. Ogden, HEW Publication no. 77–641, 1977; also listed in idem., *Focal Points,* July 1977.

4. U.S., Department of Health, Education and Welfare, *Model Standards for Community Preventive Health Services,* August 1978: 46–47.

5. P. R. Mico and H. S. Ross, *Health Education and Behavioral Science,* pp. 192–93.

6. Preventive Medicine USA, *Health Promotion and Consumer Health Education,* p. 85. This was a task-force report sponsored by the John E. Fogarty International Center for Advanced Study in the Health Sciences, the National Institutes of Health, and the American College of Preventive Medicine.

7. W. L. French and C. H. Bell, *Organization Development,* p. 144.

8. R. P. Shafer, "Government Control of Individual Behavior: Its Right and Its Proper Role," *American Journal of Public Health* 64, no. 4 (April 1974): 390–93.

9. P. S. German and A. J. Chwalow, "Conflicts in Ethical Problems of Patient Education," *International Journal of Health Education* 19, no. 3 (July-September 1976): 195–201.

10. U.S., Department of Health, Education and Welfare, *Proceedings of the National Heart and Lung Institute Working Conference on Health Behavior,* HEW Publication no. (NIH) 76–868, 12–15 May 1975, p. 37.

11. I. L. Janis and I. Feshback, "Effects of Fear-arousing Communications," *Journal of Abnormal and Social Psychology* 48 (1953): 78–92.

12. L. W. Green and P. Brooks-Bertram, "Peer Review and Quality Control" (Paper presented at Ninth International Conference for Health Education, Ottawa, Ontario, Canada, 30 August 1976).

APPENDIX A

Functions of the health-education specialist

PROGRAM PLANNING

1. Participates in joint program planning for the department, working with administration and other unit directors
2. Identifies and compiles information on existing health problems and related community problems
3. Assists in setting departmental program objectives that are specific enough for progress to be measured
4. Works individually with division chiefs or unit directors to determine their programs' educational needs at the beginning of planning
5. Plans with all division chiefs or unit directors how health-education services can contribute to meeting the educational needs of their programs
6. Works toward clarifying for all staff, especially division chiefs or unit directors, how and where the educational process will contribute to their programs' objectives
7. Works with staff to plan which resources, methods, and materials will be used

SOURCES: Adapted from an undated handout by the California Conference of Local Directors of Health Education.

8. Helps to assure that program plans include keeping records and data and documentation of results for future planning experience

9. Determines priorities for health-education services to different departmental programs, and plans for the scheduling and handling of lower priorities in a manner agreeable to administrative staff

10. Identifies health-education problems requiring additional study or research

PROGRAM EVALUATION

1. Involves appropriate staff in ongoing evaluation and modification of plans as needed

2. Encourages evaluation of joint staff efforts in program planning

3. Involves appropriate staff in measuring progress of departmental work in
   a) Training programs for departmental staff
   b) Case-finding programs
   c) Other ongoing programs
   d) Special projects
   e) Community workshops or conferences

4. Evaluates effectiveness of printed educational materials, audiovisual aids, and other educational tools and materials

5. Evaluates effectiveness of educational methods in selected programs or projects

6. Evaluates progress toward short- and long-range goals for departmental health-education services

COMMUNITY ORGANIZATION SERVICES

1. Has wide knowledge of community health agencies and organizations that are interested in health and have potential influence for health; knows available resources; knows and is in touch with key individuals

2. Compiles selected data that highlight the area's social, economic, and health problems, population characteristics, community ethnic and geographic features, and other needed information; is familiar with and can use methods for community surveys and studies that will yield valid data for planning

3. Has experience working with groups and is able to organize and coordinate community groups for seeking solutions to specific health problems or for support of community effort to solve such problems; involves those affected at an early stage of planning

4. Coordinates work with that of existing community groups and, where indicated, promotes leadership of other groups in achieving important objectives
5. Uses a variety of communication channels to transmit information on health problems and their solution
6. Enlists community volunteers in health department programs as needed
7. Serves on boards, committees, and other groups interested in working on community problems
8. Relates the department's planned educational activities to those of relevant community groups to achieve greater impact on the community and avoid duplication and competition; works toward collaboration and coordination
9. Serves as liaison between school and community health-education programs and alerts health agency personnel to opportunities for using school health services as learning experiences for teachers, students, and parents

TRAINING BY DEPARTMENT STAFF

1. Continually points up needs and opportunities for staff training, especially for professional staff who are carrying on educational activities in all divisions of the department, but excluding none of the department's total staff
2. Helps to plan, supervises, and assists in orientation of new staff, in in-service training, and in the selection of appropriate training methods and materials
3. Provides for training of department staff in skills including
   a) Use of audiovisual equipment
   b) Making posters or other aids
   c) Presentation and use of films in educational programs
   d) Use of materials and educational methods
   e) Use of mass media
   f) Effective speaking
4. Assists directly or indirectly in planning for department's administrative staff meetings
5. Takes leadership, or assists other staff, in preparation for community workshops or conferences
6. Seeks to acquaint all health department staff with opportunities for continuing education outside the department

7. Promotes attendance at conferences and professional meetings that contribute directly or indirectly to staff education
8. Promotes use of available training funds or securing of needed funds from all sources for special staff training

Training by other than department staff

1. Participates in planning and conducting training opportunities for other community groups, agencies, etc., as needs indicate
2. Plans and supervises field training program for health-education students
3. Participates as requested in individual or group teaching

CONSULTATION

1. Advises on needs diagnosis for education, planning of education, selection of methods and materials, use of aids, etc.
2. Periodically reviews with other division chiefs the progress of educational work in their programs; assists in making needed changes
3. Volunteers to assist division chiefs, individual staff members, or departmental committees in order to interpret health education to them
4. Serves on departmental or community committees, especially those working on health problems
5. Cooperates with or assists nursing education director or other staff assigned special educational responsibilities

COMMUNICATION OF HEALTH INFORMATION

1. Prepares and distributes press releases on health department programs
2. Prepares and distributes radio and TV material to promote health department programs; establishes cooperative relationships with TV, radio, and press and supplies appropriate information as needed
3. Collects, maintains supply of, and distributes printed information materials (published by other than the department) on subjects dealing with health department programs and general health education
4. Prepares and supervises pretesting, production, and distribution of printed materials for education as needed by various health department programs
5. Carries out or supervises development, production, and pretesting of audiovisual aids, including posters, slides, charts, exhibits, etc.

6. Circulates pertinent current educational and informational materials to appropriate staff of department

7. Develops and maintains or supervises the maintenance of health-education resource materials

8. Organizes, develops, maintains, and supervises library of public-health books and periodicals

9. Organizes, develops, and maintains a film library; supervises loaning of films and audiovisual equipment; arranges to borrow films from other sources or directs inquiries to other sources

10. Develops or collects, organizes, and distributes materials for health department speakers

11. Assists in selecting educational methods and providing needed materials for orientation sessions, in-service education, conferences, workshops, and community surveys

12. Answers requests for health information from departmental staff and community; prepares reports, memoranda, etc.

13. Prepares or supervises production of regular departmental publications, such as bulletins, newsletters, annual reports, technical articles, etc.

ADMINISTRATION

1. Attends (and promotes the holding of) regular administrative staff meetings

2. Participates in formulating agency goals and policies

3. Performs administrative functions related to the operation of the health-education service; e.g., budgeting, office management, personnel management, evaluation of program progress, etc.

4. Supervises and directs the agency's short- and long-range health-education services

5. Recruits, trains, and supervises health-education staff

6. Obtains and uses funds for training, research, and demonstrations

7. Participates in coordination of special programs and/or directs special projects

APPENDIX B

Health-education resources

The health-education field has diverse organizational resources. Though space limitations do not permit full coverage of these, their breadth can be suggested by a survey of the following areas: governmental agencies, voluntary agencies, international agencies, foundations, educational institutions, and professional organizations. Since hospitals and health centers have been amply discussed throughout the main text, they have been omitted here.

GOVERNMENTAL AGENCIES

U.S. Department of Health, Education and Welfare

At the federal level of government, the Department of Health, Education and Welfare (HEW) has the major responsibility for promoting the health and welfare of the American public.[1] The Office of the Secretary encompasses the Office of the Assistant Secretary, which is in turn responsible for the Public Health Service.

The following discussion will focus on the Office of Health Information and Health Promotion (OHIHP), the Bureau of Health Education, and the Intradepartmental Panel for Health Education of the Public. Health-education activities carried out in other HEW offices (e.g., the Food and Drug Administration, Administration on Aging, Environmental Protection Agency, Social and Rehabilitation Service, etc.) cannot be reviewed here, but they should be documented and evaluated so that successful efforts can be replicated and wasteful ones eliminated.

Office of Health Information and Health Promotion HEW established the OHIHP in the Office of the Assistant Secretary under Section 1706, Title 1, of the National Health Promotion and Disease Prevention Act of 1976 (P.O. 94–317).[2] OHIHP's responsibilities are:

1. To coordinate health information, health promotion, preventive health services and education within the department and the private sector
2. To facilitate coordination and collaboration among Public Health Service components and other federal agencies, professional organizations, and citizens' groups having common interests in health
3. To coordinate the operation of a national clearinghouse on health information, promotion, and prevention activities.

Bureau of Health Education Under authorization by the Secretary of HEW, the Bureau of Health Education was established as part of the Center for Disease Control in 1974. Its charges are:

1. To provide direction and leadership to a comprehensive national health-education program for the prevention of disease, disability, premature death, and unnecessary health problems
2. To provide direction and leadership for a national program to reduce disability and death due to smoking
3. To recommend health-education goals, objectives, and priorities for HEW and to develop collaborative efforts for accomplishing objectives
4. To coordinate HEW's major health-education activities
5. To develop and evaluate standards, criteria, and methodologies for improved health-education programs
6. To participate in, and provide staff support for, the Intradepartmental Panel for Health Education of the Public
7. To maintain liaison with other federal agencies and with public and private organizations engaged in health-education activities
8. To serve as a national clearinghouse on health education
9. To work with and through regional offices, encouraging and assist-

ing in the broader application of effective health-education programs at state and community levels

10. To develop mechanisms for coordinating health-education activities within the private sector.

Under the bureau's Office of the Director are three major divisions: the National Clearinghouse for Smoking and Health, the Community Program Development Division, and the Professional Services and Consultation Division.

The Office of the Director has the following functions:

1. To provide overall administrative services to the bureau
2. To provide leadership in policy formulation and in program planning and development
3. To plan, direct, coordinate, and evaluate bureau activities
4. To participate in, and provide staff support for, the Intradepartmental Panel for Health Education of the Public
5. To maintain liaison with other federal agencies engaged in health-education activities
6. To develop mechanisms for coordinating health-education activities within the private sector
7. To provide consultation and assistance to other organizations in developing and implementing health-education activities.

The National Clearinghouse for Smoking and Health has five broad functions:

1. To administer a national program to reduce smoking-related disability and death
2. To coordinate departmental activities related to smoking and health, maintain liaison with official and voluntary groups concerned with the problem, and conduct surveys assessing the incidence of smoking
3. To develop standards, criteria, and methodologies for improved health-education programs and to evaluate the effectiveness of selected ongoing programs
4. To stimulate and conduct behavioral research
5. To serve as a clearinghouse on health education.

The Community Program Development Division has the following three functions:

1. To develop, conduct, and evaluate health-education demonstration

projects in cooperation with state and local health departments and public and private organizations

2. To develop and apply effective comprehensive programs in selected communities

3. To develop and apply to unmet public health-education needs new combinations of approaches and methods.

Finally, the Professional Services and Consultation Division has three functions:

1. To provide technical advice and consultation to state and local health agencies, and to public and private organizations, in planning and implementing health-education activities

2. To work with and through regional offices, encouraging and assisting in the broader application of effective health-education programs at state and community levels

3. To assist the Office of the Director in coordinating health-education activities within the private sector.

In early 1975 the Bureau of Health Education established seven action priorities for major effort:

1. To assure that health education is included among major developments on the national health scene, such as health-resources planning and development and national health insurance

2. To enhance the effectiveness of antismoking activities

3. To develop and maintain a data-base on health-education efforts in HEW and selected other federal agencies

4. To stimulate cooperation among federal health-education programs that are directed toward common target populations or share common educational goals

5. To encourage the development of effective mechanisms for collaboration among voluntary, professional, industrial, and other private-sector groups with health-education interests

6. To select for direct intervention and support specific projects designed for population groups in special need of health education, e.g., ethnic and linguistic minorities, youth, the aged, the handicapped, and rural and inner-city communities

7. To provide, within financial and staff constraints, technical assistance and consultation to public and private agencies and groups.[3]

Intradepartmental Panel for Health Education of the Public Chaired by HEW's Assistant Secretary for Health, the Intradepartmental Panel for Health Education of the Public was established under the 1974 National Health Education Plan. Its purpose is to establish a central focus for the development and promulgation of department-wide health-education policies and to facilitate the implementation of multiagency health-education activities. Its functions are:

1. To advise and recommend to the Office of the Secretary
2. To develop and recommend throughout the department a set of policies related to health education of the public
3. To recommend consideration of health education in the implementation of major departmental initiatives
4. To recommend attention to health education within each agency's programs
5. To identify educational goals common to two or more agencies and to develop and recommend methods for interagency cooperation in accomplishing them
6. To conduct liaison activities with other federal entities and within the private sector.

State, regional, and local entities

Health departments State, regional, and local health department activities range from intensive media information and community organization programs to innovative demonstration programs. All engage in needs assessment, program planning, implementation, and evaluation, as well as in agency organization, administration, and management. But state and local health departments also perform a number of distinctly different tasks.

State agencies are usually concerned with policy making, planning, legislative activities, local consultation, financial support, and organizational relationships; their services to the public are indirect. In contrast, local health departments conduct immunization programs, operate clinics, inspect and license certain facilities, and monitor air pollution and water and sewage supplies. These services are categorized as follows:

1. Preventive medical and personal health-care services: communicable and chronic disease, maternal and child health, occupational health, dental health
2. Environmental health services: sanitary engineering, food and drug

control programs, pollution control, vector control,* radiologic health, general sanitation

3. Patient-care facilities and services
4. Supportive services: health education, nutrition, social work, laboratory services.

Health-systems agencies Health-systems agencies (HSA) were organized in the United States under the 1974 National Health Planning and Resources Development Act (P.L. 93–641). Thereafter, the Bureau of Health Education funded a project to develop ideas for their use in planning and carrying out effective educational activities. Consumers, health practitioners, civic associations, industrial organizations, and labor groups have all been asked to participate in this project.[4] Some HSAs employ health educators to help develop and coordinate health-education activities within their jurisdictions.

VOLUNTARY AGENCIES

There are approximately 100,000 voluntary organizations in the United States that are concerned either exclusively or partially with matters of health. These are vertically structured—organized on a national basis, with state and local chapters bound together by formal charters—and are not tax-supported; they engage in a variety of fund-raising activities and are financially responsible only to their own membership. Because they are not in the public sector, they are free to influence policy and legislation at all levels of government.

Many voluntary agencies have been active in developing health-education programs—among them, the National Lung Association, American Cancer Society, American Heart Association, American Social Health Association, American Diabetes Association, National Society for the Prevention of Blindness, Planned Parenthood Federation of America, and National Safety Council. Their services include public health education, professional education, a variety of health-care services, and research.

The voluntary health movement has four broad purposes:

1. To heighten public awareness of specific health problems by means of public education campaigns that emphasize prevention, precaution, and the use of medical services

---

*Controlling the growth of insects that convey infection from one body to another.

2. To engender and augment support for community health services by offering practical person-to-person services that build morale and speed recovery among the afflicted

3. To do pioneering research in specific disease categories in order to take swift advantage of medical breakthroughs

4. To encourage volunteers to gain the kind of experience that will enable them to become community leaders.

National Health Council

The National Health Council was founded in 1920 by a group of leaders who foresaw both a vast increase in the then current number of health agencies and the need for a mechanism that would facilitate their working together. The council's principal functions are threefold: (1) to identify and work toward a solution to national health problems, (2) to improve governmental and voluntary health services at state and local levels, and (3) to help member agencies work together more effectively in the public interest. Its activities are guided by a board of directors elected by delegates designated by the member organizations. Dues constitute the major source of income.

The council's membership today numbers more than seventy national organizations. There are three categories of membership, each with its own criteria for eligibility: (1) active members (national voluntary health organizations); (2) associate members (business, labor, civic, consumer, and other organizations or foundations that want to participate in the council's work); and (3) federal agency members (governmental organizations whose advice and assistance are desired).

To assure that member organizations are both efficient and ethically reliable, the council requires of each:

1. Articles of incorporation that specify purposes

2. Programs affecting the broad interests of national health, and activities that are consistent with specified purposes

3. Programs that complement and enhance the work of other organizations in the interests of national health

4. Service to a population large enough, and with problems significant enough, to justify the organization's existence

5. Boards of directors elected by a constituency significantly larger than the number elected, one-half of this number to be from a location outside the organization's geographic headquarters

6. At least one-third of voting members to be in attendance at board

meetings or furnishing written proxies for a valid vote at an annual meeting

7. An annual report, including a list of governing trustees and staff and a complete and accurate financial report

8. Consolidated reporting to the public of financial operations of the national office and all affiliates in conformance with the "Standards of Accounting and Financial Reporting for Voluntary Health and Welfare Organizations"

9. An annual budget examined and approved by the governing board

10. Adherence to ethical fund-raising practices

11. A plan for regularly informing the public how stated purposes are being accomplished.[5]

National Center for Health Education

The National Center for Health Education (NCHE) was created in 1974–75 in response to the principal recommendation of the President's Committee on Health Education and with the assistance of the National Health Council. An independent, nonprofit organization, it relies for its basic financial support on voluntary health agencies, professional societies, industry, labor, and philanthropy.

The NCHE's chief role is to facilitate and energize the efforts of those who are already providing health education to the public. It does this by:

1. Providing a forum for presenting viewpoints about, and objectives for, health education

2. Initiating, conducting, and evaluating research

3. Planning, promoting, evaluating, and improving health-education programs

4. Encouraging the demonstration and application of new approaches

5. Monitoring the impact of public- and private-sector health efforts

6. Serving as a responsible and articulate advocate for the public in matters involving consumer health education

7. Stimulating educational activities that will enable Americans to make their own informed decisions about matters of health.

INTERNATIONAL AGENCIES

All the nations of the world now have health programs that include some amount of health education, the somewhat technically advanced nations sometimes providing assistance to the more disadvantaged ones. Among the principal bodies promoting such programs is the World Health Organization (WHO), whose philosophy is stated in its constitution: "Health is a state of complete physical, mental, and social well-being and not merely the absence of disease or infirmity. . . .Enjoyment of the highest attainable standard of health is one of the fundamental rights of every human being without distinction of race, religion, political belief, economic or social condition. . .Achievement of any state in the promotion and protection of health is of value to all."[6]

WHO serves more than 130 member countries. Its executive board is composed of health experts who are designated by, but do not represent, their governments. Issues and proposals are presented to the annual Health Assembly, which is composed of delegations from all the member countries. WHO has six regional offices:

1. African Region: headquarters in Brazzaville, Republic of Congo; thirty-one member nations and three associate members representing a population of more than 229 million
2. Region of the Americas: headquarters in Washington, D.C.; twenty-six member nations with a population of 488 million
3. Southeast Asia Region: headquarters in New Delhi, India; eight member nations representing a population of 721 million
4. European Region: headquarters in Copenhagen, Denmark; thirty-three member nations representing 753 million people
5. Eastern Mediterranean Region: headquarters in Alexandria, Egypt; twenty-one member nations representing a population of 282 million
6. Western Pacific Region: headquarters in Manila, the Philippines; thirteen member nations representing a population of 278 million.[7]

The World Health Organization's health-education unit has been developing health-education programs throughout the world for many years. Its highest priority at present is to develop programs in relation to primary health-care services in the regions of its various member organizations.

Other international health programs include the United Nations Children's Fund (UNICEF), which provides food and other supplies for child and maternal welfare throughout the world but in developing countries particularly. UNICEF has also been concerned with immunization programs and programs for the control of syphilis, yaws, and malaria.

Finally, the Agency for International Development (AID) of the U.S. Department of State provides military, economic, and technical assistance to other nations but has also provided them with direct services, consultation, and fellowships for training in public health. Some health-education programs carried out under AID's sponsorship have brought health-education professionals from other countries to the United States for further education.[8]

FOUNDATIONS

There are an estimated 5,454 foundations in the United States, and in 1970 alone they gave more than $120 million in grants to the field of health.[9] Recipient projects included family planning, children's health, drug education and therapy, alcoholism, cancer, and health manpower among many others. Prominent foundations interested in health education are the Ford Foundation, Rockefeller Foundation, Kellogg Foundation, Commonwealth Foundation, Millbank Memorial Foundation, Markle Foundation, and Johnson Foundation.[10] The Ford, Rockefeller, and Kellogg foundations have spearheaded health programs in other countries as well. Because they have fewer constraints than other agencies, foundations have been able to introduce innovative, and at times unorthodox, health programs that have kept close pace with the needs of a rapidly changing society.

EDUCATIONAL INSTITUTIONS

Kindergarten through high school

In 1973–74, from kindergarten through the twelfth grade, U.S. school enrollment totaled 45.5 million students in more than 115,000 schools having approximately 2.1 million teachers (not including administrative, supervisory, or service personnel). During these same years, more than 40 percent of U.S. children between the ages of three and five were enrolled in early-childhood education programs. Because no other community setting for health education even approaches the magnitude of this endeavor, school health education should not only continue throughout the life cycle but should be comprehensive, coordinated, and integrated in all community planning for health.[11]

But health education is not concerned with transmitting information alone, for factual data change and, if unrenewed, can be a liability rather than an asset. In its fullest configuration, health education inculcates critical thinking and problem solving, valuing, self-direction, and self-discipline, skills that enhance an individual's lifetime responsibility to participate in community and world concerns. Developing effective health-education programs in schools, then, is the first step in building a life style of beneficial health behavior among America's young people.

For schools, focusing on selected categorical issues can have value if personnel, time, and money are available to sustain the emphasis. It is far better, however, for such efforts to be expanded into an integrated framework that enables learners to gain insights into the personal, social, environmental, political, and cultural implications of issues. Thus, a broad concept of healthful living should form the basis of school health education, and a growing number of states is recognizing this fact. Likewise encouraging is the federal government's interest in a national policy for a comprehensive, sequential program of health education from kindergarten through the twelfth grade.

In sum, effective health education at these grade levels requires:

1. A teaching/learning environment offering opportunities for safe and optimal living and in which a complete and well organized health service is functioning
2. Teachers and supervisors who are professionally qualified in health education
3. Innovative instructional materials and appropriate teaching facilities
4. Time commensurate with that for other subject areas
5. Increased local, state, and national financial support to upgrade the quantity and quality of school health education

Colleges and universities

A 1974 survey revealed that 179 colleges and universities in forty-one states were offering major programs in health education.[12] Baccalaureate-level programs had increased from 87 in 1970 to 165 in 1974, with master's and doctoral programs increasing at a much slower rate. Of eighteen accredited schools of public health today, twelve currently have programs for the preparation of health-education specialists.[13] These schools of public health and programs in community health education, accredited by the Council on Education for Public Health, now account for the bulk of health-education specialists trained at the master's level.

Because health education is among thirty-two major occupational groups within the health field, it is a continuing focus for national data collection on projected manpower needs.[14] At present, a demand for more health-education manpower is anticipated because of the following six developments.[15]

1. *Expansion of hospital-based health education.* Adopted by the American Hospital Association and reflecting recommendations by the President's Committee on Health Education, a 1974 policy statement on personal and community health education provided direction and support to 7,000 member hospitals in developing more comprehen-

sive inpatient, outpatient, staff, and community health-education services. In reality, however, this statement described a process that had already been under way within hospitals and other health-care institutions.

2. *Reimbursement for health education by third-party payers.* The Blue Cross Association and other private insurance companies have released position statements in favor of reimbursement for patient education, and it is anticipated that similar proposals will be developed by other insurance companies and federal health-care programs.

3. *Inclusion of health education in legislation for health maintenance organizations.* Although HMOs have been developing slowly, their mandates require them to provide educational services to their members. Few activities could be more integral to the HMO concept than health education, which is aimed at producing changes in life style and at making effective use of health services.

4. *Increased federal support of health education.* As the 1976–81 Forward Plan for Health has made clear, the federal strategy for improved health requires expanded health-education services. Linked as it is to basic concepts of prevention, health education has become a major tool of health-care planners and providers.

5. *Development of a National Center for Health Education.* The President's Committee on Health Education stated the need for a focal point in the private sector to provide national leadership in health education. The center was formed in 1974–75 and is well on its way to becoming the important national force that was envisaged.

6. *Federal legislation emphasizing health education.* The National Health Planning and Resources Act of 1974, for example, inaugurated a systems approach to regional health-care planning which will not only strengthen existing programs but create new programs and services as well. Likewise, the National Disease Control and Consumer Health Promotion Act of 1975 clearly indicated that the U.S. Senate plans an expansion of health-education services. Although studies suggest that future manpower needs will be great,[16] there is to date insufficient documentation on which to base expanded recruitment and training programs.

PROFESSIONAL ORGANIZATIONS

Professional organizations are formed by people committed to advancing the arts and sciences of their field of practice. Health education has seven such organizations, all committed to the overall field but each concerned with a particular specialty or point of view: the Society of Public Health Education; the Public Health Education and School Health Education sections of the American Public Health Association; the American Association for the Advancement of Health Education; the American School Health Association; the Health Education Section of the American College Health Association; and the American Alliance for Health, Physical Education, and Recreation. Membership in these organizations totals 19,280, though to what extent this figure reflects membership in more than one association is not known.

REFERENCES

1. D. M. Wilner, *Introduction to Public Health*.
2. U.S., Department of Health, Education and Welfare, Bureau of Health Education, *Focal Points*, November 1976.
3. Ibid., August 1975.
4. Ibid., May 1976.
5. National Health Council, "Criteria for Eligibility for Association Membership in National Health Council, Inc.," July 1970.
6. Wilner, *Introduction to Public Health*, p. 65.
7. Ibid., p. 66.
8. Ibid., p. 67.
9. Ibid., pp. 59–60.
10. Ibid., p. 59.
11. American Public Health Association, School Health Section, "Education for Health in the School Community Setting" (Position paper adopted by Governing Council of American Public Health Association, 23 October 1974): D. Oberteuffer, O. A. Harrelson, and M. B. Pollock, *School Health Education*; and C. Mayshark and R. A. Foster, *Health Education in Secondary Schools*.
12. S. K. Simonds, "Health-Education Manpower in the United States," *Health Education Monographs* 4, no. 3 (Fall 1976): 208–25.
13. Ibid., p. 213.
14. Ibid., p. 209.
15. Preventive Medicine USA, *Health Promotion and Consumer Health Education*, pp. 86–103.
16. Ibid., pp. 115–18.

Glossary

Agency   Usually, a tax-supported governmental organization at the federal, state, or local level.

Association   Usually, a group of professionals organized for the purpose of meeting a professional need or goal; also termed *Society*.

Body   Usually, a group of elected or appointed officials who serve as public representatives; e.g., a city council, county board of supervisors, planning commission, etc.

Categorical programs   Programs that receive federal or state funding for a specific purpose, such as heart disease, cancer, alcoholism, drug addiction, etc.

Center   A group of workers organized primarily to deliver health services to a population in a specific area (e.g., a neighborhood health center); also used in reference to a group of professionals, often in an academic setting, who provide specialized services; e.g., Center for Human Services Development, National Center for Health Education, etc.

Community health education   Health-education processes utilizing community organization, intergroup relationships, and communication resources in a specific social system.

Community organization (for health)   Health-education process or method in which the combined efforts of individuals, groups, and organizations are designed to generate, mobilize, coordinate, utilize, and/or redistribute resources to meet unsolved or emergent health needs and problems.

Company Usually, a small, profit-making business owned by a single individual, partners, or a group of share/stockholders.

Consumer participation (in health planning) Involving the consumers of health services in planning the services they are to receive with the intention of making program plans more relevant to their needs.

Control group In research studies, a group that has undergone no change but is used for comparing testing results with an experimental group that has been used in testing an idea. See *Study group*.

Corporation A large, profit-making business or industrial enterprise owned by stockholders and having boards of directors.

Data-base A set of facts determined to be adequate for planning or problem-solving purposes.

Drive Usually, motivational tendencies that provide the energy necessary to initiate behaviors toward a particular objective or end.

Foundation An organization established by philanthropists to distribute financial resources to those who meet its specific eligibility requirements.

Goal A desired end-result target that provides general direction for a long-term program. See *Objective*.

Group process (in health education) The application of educational and communication principles in group situations, designed to facilitate problem solving and decision making through mutual stimulation of creative and critical thinking or to increase the credibility and attractiveness of recommended health practices.

Health education A process with intellectual, psychological, and social dimensions relating to activities that increase the abilities of people to make informed decisions affecting their personal, family, and community well-being. This process, based on scientific principles, facilitates learning and behavioral change in both health personnel and consumers, including children and youth.

Health education of the public A process designed for improvement and maintenance of health, directed to the general population as contrasted with education for the preparation of a health professional.

Health-education program A planned and organized series of health-education activities or procedures implemented with (1) an educational specialist assigned primary responsibility, (2) a budget, (3) an integrated set of objectives sufficiently detailed to allow evaluation, and (4) administrative support.

Health-education resources All the assets, human and material, that may be enlisted in the school organization or community to enrich the health-education experiences of individuals and groups.

Health environment The promotion, maintenance, and utilization of safe and wholesome surroundings, including physical settings, organization of day-by-day experiences, and planned learning procedures to influence favorably emotional, physical, and social health.

Health information Communication of facts about health, designed to develop one's cognitive base for health action.

Health instruction The process of providing a sequence of planned and spontaneously originated learning opportunities comprising the organized aspects of health education in the school or community.

Health science educator Same as *School health educator.* This term is sometimes used in life sciences, medicine, or the allied professions to denote instructors who prepare various health professionals or who teach other than applied science.

Human services Services designed to meet the needs of human beings, such as mental health, social, educational, emergency, and public safety services.

Institution Usually a governmental organization that has a special mandate, certain prescribed procedures for processing people or services, and serves a well-defined population or purpose; e.g., a college, mental hospital, prison, etc.

Macrosystem A large interrelated system, such as a state with its cities or counties or a group of organizations or communities having common alliances or purposes.

Management by Objectives (MBO) A system of management based on the establishment of specific actions to be carried out or end-results to be attained; includes information regarding the resources and time periods necessary to carry out the tasks, as well as the identity of those responsible for implementation.

Mass communications (in health) The transfer of health information to a large and usually heterogeneous population, usually by means of such media as direct mail, newspapers, magazines, radio, television, and motion pictures.

Method A sequence of steps and procedures enabling one to carry out a specific activity toward a specific end with consistency.

Microsystem A small system, such as an organization that exists within a community system.

Model A concept, usually depicted in the form of a chart or drawing, around which a set of principles, relationships, and conclusions can be discussed.

Need Usually used in reference to basic conditions, situations, desires, or inadequacies that relate to human satisfaction or fulfillment.

Norm A pattern of cultural behavior adhered to by members of a group.

Objective A target that provides precise direction for a short-term activity. See *Goal*.

Organization environment The environment within an organization, such as its physical, cultural, and emotional climate.

Patient education Those health experiences designed to influence learning which occur as a person receives preventive, diagnostic, therapeutic, and/or rehabilitative services, including experiences that arise from coping with symptoms, referral to sources of information, prevention, diagnosis and care, and contacts with health institutions, health personnel, family, and other patients.

Primary health care Health-care services provided to people who do not require hospitalization, such as immunizations, dental and diagnostic services, physical examinations, maternal and child health-care services, VD clinics, nutritional counseling, etc.

Private health agency A nongovernmental agency concerned with health, organized as one part of three types: (1) nonprofit incorporated (voluntary), (2) nonprofit unincorporated (voluntary), (3) proprietary (commercial). See also *Voluntary health agency*.

Program Evaluation and Review Technique (PERT) A system of management based on identifying the interrelationships between and among a series of actions necessary to achieve a specific goal; depicted in the form of a flow chart showing the time periods necessary to carry out each step or process in the sequence and distinguishing between those steps that are critical to goal attainment and those that contribute to or make the critical steps possible.

Public health agency An official, governmental, tax-supported organization mandated by law and/or regulation for the protection and improvement of the health of the public.

Public (community) health educator An individual with professional preparation in public health education, including training in the application of selected content from relevant social and behavioral sciences used to influence individual and group learning, mobilization of community health action, and the planning, implementation, and evaluation of health programs.

Role A prescribed set of behaviors performed by a person, carried out consistently, and supported by the shared perceptions of the performer and others whose behaviors are affected by the role.

School health education   That health-education process associated with health-education activities planned and conducted under the supervision of school personnel, with involvement of appropriate community health personnel and utilization of appropriate community resources.

School health-education curriculum   All the health opportunities affecting learning and behavior of children and youth in the total school curriculum. These health experiences are gained in both school and community settings as the individual interacts with his environment, including other students, school personnel, parents, and community members. See also *School health program.*

School health-education curriculum guides   The plans or framework for the curriculum. The plans are developed and implemented cooperatively by health-personnel teachers, administrators, students, parents, and community representatives, preferably under the leadership of a qualified health educator.

School health educator   An individual with professional preparation in health education or health science who is qualified for certification as a health teacher and for participation in the development, improvement, and coordination of school and community health-education programs.

School health program   The composite of procedures and activities designed to protect and promote the well-being of students and school personnel. These procedures and activities include those organized in school health services, providing a healthful environment and health education.

School health services   That part of the school health program provided by physicians, nurses, dentists, health educators, other allied health personnel, social workers, teachers, and others to appraise, protect, and promote the health of students and school personnel. Such procedures are designed to: (1) appraise the health status of pupils and school personnel; (2) counsel pupils, teachers, parents, and others for the purpose of helping pupils obtain health care and for arranging school programs in keeping with their needs; (3) help prevent and control communicable disease; (4) provide emergency care for injury or sudden illness; (5) promote and provide optimum sanitary conditions and safe facilities; (6) protect and promote the health of school personnel; and (7) provide concurrent learning opportunities that are conducive to the maintenance and promotion of individual and community health.

Secondary health care   Services associated with hospitalization, such as surgery, special diagnostic studies, laboratory services, physical therapy, etc.

Society See *Association*.

Standards Translations of functions into specific tasks and measurements which distinguish among various levels of performance.

Store-front clinic Usually, a small health-services program located in a neighborhood for the ready access of residents. See *Center*.

Study group The unit that receives the special treatment or program involved in an experiment being tested. See *Control group*.

Systems analysis A method of evaluating the interrelationships between and among a group of units or organizations in a system.

Tertiary health care Those services involved in posthospitalization care, such as nursing homes, rehabilitation centers, etc.

Voluntary health agency Any nonprofit association organized on a national, state, or local level, composed of lay and professional persons, dedicated to the prevention, alleviation, and cure of a particular disease, disability, or group of diseases and disabilities. It is supported by voluntary contributions, primarily from the general public, and expends its resources for education, research, and service programs relevant to the disease and disabilities concerned.

Bibliography

Alderfer, C. P., and Brown, L. D. *Learning from Changing Organizational Diagnosis and Development.* Beverly Hills, Calif.: Sage Publications, 1975.

Allport, G. W. *Becoming: Basic Considerations for a Psychology of Personality.* New Haven, Conn.: Yale University Press, 1955.

———. *Personality: A Psychological Interpretation.* New York: Holt, Rinehart & Winston, 1937.

American Public Health Association. School Health Section. "Education for Health in the School Community Setting." Position paper adopted by Governing Council at the Annual Meeting of American Public Health Association, New Orleans, 23 October 1974.

Asch, S. E. *Social Psychology.* Englewood Cliffs, N.J.: Prentice-Hall, 1952.

Ashford, N. A. *Summary of Crisis in the Workplace: Occupational Disease and Injury. A Report to the Ford Foundation.* Cambridge, Mass.: MIT Press, 1975.

Bahnson, C. B. "Behavioral Factors Associated with the Etiology of Physical Disease." *American Journal of Public Health* 64, no. 11 (November 1974): 1033–55.

Bandura, A. "Influence of Models' Reinforcement Contingencies on the Acquisition of Initiative Responses." *Journal of Personality and Social Psychology* 1 (1965): 589–95.

Beatty, W. "Emotions: The Missing Link in Education." Paper presented at Conference on Issues in Human Development: Present and Future, at Institute for Child Study, University of Maryland, 20 April 1968.

Becker, M. H., ed. "The Health Belief Model and Personal Health Behavior." *Health Education Monographs* 2, no. 4 (Winter 1974): 409–19.

Beckhard, R. "ABS in Health-Care Systems: Who Needs It?" *Journal of Applied Behavioral Science* 10, no. 1 (1974): 93–106.

Bell, D. *The Cultural Contradictions of Capitalism*. New York: Basic Books, 1976.

Belloc, N. B., and Breslow, L. "Relationship of Physical Health Status and Health Practices." *Preventive Medicine* 1, no. 3 (August 1972): 415–21.

E. Berne. *Games People Play*. New York: Grove Press, 1964.

———. *The Structure and Dynamics of Organizations and Groups*. Philadelphia: J. B. Lippincott Co., 1963.

———. *Transactional Analysis in Psychotherapy*. New York: Grove Press, 1961.

Bernheimer, E., and Clever, L. H. "Experiences Implementing Patient Education in an Outpatient Clinic." Report submitted to California Regional Medical Program, St. Mary's Hospital and Medical Center, San Francisco, 1974–75.

Biddle, B. J., and Thomas, E. J., eds. *Role Theory: Concepts and Research*. New York: John Wiley & Sons, 1966.

Bloom, B. S., ed. *Taxonomy of Educational Objectives. Handbook 1: Cognitive Domain*. New York: David McKay Co., 1956.

Blum, H. L. *Expanding Health-Care Horizons: From a General Systems Concept of Health to a National Health Policy*. Oakland, Calif.: Third Party Associates, 1976.

———. *Planning for Health: Development and Application of Social Change Theory*. New York: Human Sciences Press, 1974.

Bowman, R. A. "Changes in the Activities, Functions, and Roles of Public Health Educators." *Health Education Monographs* 4, no 3 (Fall 1976): 226–45.

Brill, N. I. *Teamwork: Working Together in Human Services*. New York: J. B. Lippincott Co., 1976.

Bryant, N. H. "Practical Considerations in Evaluating Patient/Consumer Health-Education Programs." Paper presented at National Conference on Hospital-based Patient Education, Chicago, 9–10 August 1976.

Buchanan, P. D. *The Leader Looks at Individual Motivation*. Washington, D.C.: Leadership Resources, 1961.

Burke, W. W., and Hornstein, H. A., eds. *The Social Technology of Organization Development*. Washington, D.C.: NTL Learning Resource Corp., 1971.

Campbell, J. P., and Dunnett, M. D. "Effectiveness of T-Group Experience in Managerial Training and Development." *Psychological Bulletin* 70 (1968): 73–104.

Carter, L. F. "On Defining Leadership." In *Group Relations at the Crossroads*, edited by M. Sherif and M. O. Wilson. New York: Harper & Row, 1953.

Cartwright, D., and Zander, A., eds. *Group Dynamics: Research and Theory*. 3d ed. New York: Harper & Row, 1969.

Castile, A. S., and Jerrick, S. J. *School Health in America: A Survey of State School Health Programs*. Kent, Ohio: American School Health Association, 1976.

Cattell, R. B. "Concepts and Methods in the Measurement of Group Syntality." *Psychological Review* 55 (1948): 48–63.

Cline, S. *Alcohol and Drugs and Work*. Washington, D. C.: Drug Abuse Council, 1975.

Coleman, J. C. *Psychology and Effective Behavior*. Palo Alto, Calif.: Scott, Foresman & Co., 1969.

Conant, R. K.; DeLucca, A. J.; and Levin, L. S. "Health Education: A Bridge to the Community." *American Journal of Public Health* 62, no. 9 (September 1972): 1239–44.

Corey, L.; Epstein, M. F.; and Saltman, S. E., eds. *Medicine in a Changing Society*. St. Louis, Mo.: C. V. Mosby Co., 1977.

Corsini, R. J. *Current Personality Theories*. Itasca, Ill.: F. E. Peacock Publishers, 1977.

Craig, R. L.; and Bittel, L. R., eds. *Training and Development Handbook*. New York: McGraw-Hill, 1967.

Crowfoot, J. E., and Chesler, M. A. "Contemporary Perspectives on Planned Social Change: A Comparison." *Journal of Applied Behavioral Science* 10, no. 3 (1974): 278–303.

Danforth, J.; Miller, D. S.; Day, A. L.; and Steiner, G. J. "Group Services for Unmarried Mothers: An Interdisciplinary Approach." *Children* 18, no. 2 (1971): 59–64.

Davis, M. S. "Variations in Patients' Compliance with Doctors' Orders: Analysis of Congruence between Survey Responses and Results of Empirical Investigations." *Journal of Medical Education* 41, no. 11 (1966): 1038–39.

Dayal, I., and Thomas, J. M. "Operation KPE: Developing a New Organization." *Journal of Applied Behavioral Science* 4, no. 4 (1968): 473–506.

Deeds, S. G. "Overview of Evaluation." Paper presented at National Conference on Hospital-based Patient Education, Chicago, 9–10 August 1976.

Delbecq, A. L.; Van de Ven, A. H.; and Gustafson, D. H. *Group Techniques for Program Planning*. Glenview, Ill.: Scott, Foresman & Co., 1975.

Djukanovic, V., and Mach, E. P. *Alternative Approaches to Meeting Basic Health Needs in Developing Countries*. Geneva: World Health Organization, 1975.

D'Onofrio, C. N. *Reaching Our "Hard to Reach": The Unvaccinated*. Berkeley, Calif.: Department of Public Health, 1966.

Doyle, M., and Straus, D. *How to Make Meetings Work: The New Interaction Method*. New York: Wyden Books, 1976.

Doziey, P. W.; Loken, J. O.; and Field, J. A. "T-Group Influence on Feelings of Alienation." *Journal of Applied Behavioral Science* 7, no. 6 (1971): 724–31.

Dubois, R. *Man Adapting*. New Haven, Conn.: Yale University Press, 1965.

Ducanis, S. J., and Gohn, A. K. *The Interdisciplinary Health-Care Team: A Handbook*. Germantown, Md.: Aspen Systems Corp., 1979.

Durbin, R. L., and Springall, W. H. *Organization and Administration of Health Care: Theory, Practice, and Environment*. St. Louis, Mo.: C. V. Mosby Co., 1974.

Egan, G. *Encounter: Group Processes for Interpersonal Growth*. Belmont, Calif.: Brooks/Cole Publishing Co., 1970.

Eisenberg, A., and Eisenberg, H. *Alive and Well: Decisions in Health*. New York: McGraw-Hill, 1979.

Emmerich, W. "Family Role Concepts of Children Ages Six to Ten." *Child Development* 32 (1961): 609–24.

Enelow, A. J., and Henderson, J. B., eds. *Applying Behavioral Science to Cardiovascular Risk: Proceedings of a Conference*. New York: American Heart Association, 1975.

Erikson, E. *Childhood and Society*. 2d ed. New York: W. W. Norton & Co., 1963.

Etzioni, A. *The Active Society.* New York: Free Press, 1968.

Festinger, L. *A Theory of Cognitive Dissonance.* Stanford, Calif.: Stanford University Press, 1957.

Fiori, F. B.; de la Vega, M.; and Vaccaro, M. J. "Health Education in a Hospital Setting: Report of a Public Health Service Project in Newark, New Jersey." *Health Education Monographs* 2, no. 1 (Spring 1974): 11–29.

Frank, F., and Anderson, L. R. "Effects of Task and Group Size upon Group Productivity and Member Satisfaction." *Sociometry* 34 (1971): 135–94.

Franklin, P., and Franklin, R. *Tomorrow's Track Experiments with Learning to Change.* Columbia, Md.: New Community Press, 1976.

French, W. L., and Bell, C. H. *Organization Development: Behavioral Science Interventions for Organization Improvement.* Englewood Cliffs, N.J.: Prentice-Hall, 1973.

Fromm, E. *The Sane Society.* New York: Rinehart & Co., 1955.

Gabriel, R. A. *Program Evaluation: A Social Science Approach.* New York: MSS Information Corp., 1975.

Galiher, C. "Rural Initiatives and Health-Education Needs." *Health Education Monographs* 3, no. 1 (Spring 1975): 109–14.

Galli, N. *Foundations and Principles of Health Education.* New York: John Wiley & Sons, 1978.

Garbus, S. B.; Donohue, T. R.; and Wilson, G. "The Community Workshop as a Stimulus for Hypertension-Control Programs." *American Journal of Public Health* 66, no. 7 (July 1976): 682–83.

Garfield, S. R. "The New Medical Care Delivery System." *Scientific American,* April 1970, pp. 15–23.

Gartner, A., and Riessman, F. "Self-Help Models and Consumer-Intensive Health Practice." *American Journal of Public Health* 66, no. 8 (August 1976): 783–86.

German, P. S., and Chwalow, A. J. "Conflicts in Ethical Problems of Patient Education." *International Journal of Health Education* 19, no. 3 (July-September 1976): 195–201.

Gibbard, G. S.; Hartman, J. J.; Mann, R. D.; eds. *Analysis of Groups.* San Francisco: Jossey-Bass, 1974.

Giglio, R.; Spears, B.; Rumpf, D.; and Eddy, N. "Encouraging Behavior Changes by Client-held Health Records." Paper presented at Annual Meeting of American Public Health Association, Miami, 17–21 October 1976.

Goldstein, K. *The Organism.* New York: American Book Co., 1939.

Golembiewski, R. T. *Approaches to Planned Change: Parts 1 and 2.* New York: Marcel Dekker, 1979.

———. *Sensitivity Training and the Laboratory Approach.* 3d ed. Itasca, Ill.: F. E. Peacock Publishers, 1977.

———. *The Small Group.* Chicago: University of Chicago Press, 1962.

Goodacre, D. M. "The Use of a Sociometric Test as a Predictor of Combat Unit Effectiveness." *Sociometry* 14 (1951): 148–52.

Goodstein, L. D.; Lubin B.; and Lubin, A. W. *Organizational Change Sourcebook II: Cases in Conflict Management.* La Jolla, Calif.: University Associates, 1979.

Gouldner, A. "Some Observations on Systematic Theory, 1945–1955." In *Modern*

Social Theories, edited by C. P. Loomis and B. I. Loomis. New York: D. Van Nostrand Co., 1961.

Grant, R.; Fonaroff, S.; and Levy, L. H., eds. "Issues in Self-Care." *Health Education Monographs* 5, no. 2 (1977): 108–89.

Green, L. W. "Evaluation and Measurement: Some Dilemmas for Health Education." *American Journal of Public Health* 67, no. 2 (February 1977): 155–61.

———. *Status Identity and Prevention Health Behavior.* Berkeley, Calif.: University of California, School of Public Health, 1970; Honolulu: University of Hawaii, School of Public Health, 1970; *Pacific Health Education Reports,* no. 1 (1970), pp. 107–19.

Green, L. W., and Brooks-Bertram, P. "Peer Review and Quality Control." Paper presented at Ninth International Conference for Health Education, Ottawa, Ontario, Canada, 30 August 1976.

Green, L.; Kreuter, M. W.; Deeds, S. G.; and Partridge, K. B. *Health Education Today and the PRECEDE Framework.* Palo Alto, Calif.: Mayfield Publishing Co., 1979.

Griffiths, W. "Health-Education Definitions, Problems, and Philosophies." *Health Education Monograph,* no. 31 (1972), pp. 7–12.

Guilford, J. P. *The Analysis of Intelligence.* New York: McGraw-Hill, 1971.

Harris, T. A. *I'm OK—You're OK.* New York: Harper & Row, 1969.

Harvey, J. B., and Albertson, D. R. "Neurotic Organizations: Symptoms, Causes, and Treatment." In *Contemporary Organization Development: Conceptual Orientations and Interventions,* edited by W. W. Burke. Washington, D.C.: NTL Institute for Applied Behavioral Science, 1972.

Havighurst, R. *Developmental Tasks and Education.* 2d ed. New York: David McKay Co., 1952.

Haythorn, W. W. "The Composition of Groups: A Review of the Literature." *Acta Psychologica* 28 (1968): 97–128.

Heider, F. "Social Perception and Phenomenal Causality." *Psychological Review* 51 (1944): 358–74.

Herzberg, F.; Mausner, B.; and Snyderman, B. *The Motivation to Work.* New York: John Wiley & Sons, 1959.

Holland, G. A. "Transactional Analysis." In *Current Psychotherapies,* edited by R. Corsini. Itasca, Ill.: F. E. Peacock Publishers, 1972.

Homans, G. C. *The Human Group.* New York: Harcourt, Brace & World, 1950.

Horn, D. "A Model for the Study of Personal-Choice Health Behavior." *International Journal of Health Education* 19, no. 2 (1976): 89–98.

Hornstein: H. S.; Bunker, B. B.; Burke, W. W.; Gindes, M.; and Lewicki, R. J. *Social Intervention: A Behavioral Science Approach.* New York: Free Press, 1971.

House, R. J. "T-Group Education and Leadership Effectiveness: A Review of the Empirical Literature and a Critical Evaluation." *Personnel Psychology* 20 (1967): 1–32.

Hovland, C. I., and Weiss, W. "The Influence of Source Credibility on Communication Effectiveness." *Public Opinion Quarterly* 15 (1951): 635–50.

Insel, P. M., and Roth, W. T. *Health in a Changing Society.* Palo Alto, Calif.: Mayfield Publishing Co., 1976.

Janis, I. L., and Feshback, I. "Effects of Fear-arousing Communications." *Journal of Abnormal and Social Psychology* 48 (1953): 78–92.

Johnson, R. L. "Health Education: Ramifications and Consequences." *Health Education Monographs*, no. 31 (1972), pp. 19–21.

Kanaaneh, H. A. K.; Rabi, S. A.; and Badarneh, S. M. "The Eradication of a Large Scabies Outbreak Using Community-wide Health Education." *American Journal of Public Health* 66, no. 6 (June 1976): 564–67.

Katz, D., and Kahn, R. L. *The Social Psychology of Organizations*. New York: John Wiley & Sons, 1966.

Katz, E., and Lazarsfeld, P. F. *Personal Influence: The Part Played by People in the Flow of Mass Communication*. Glencoe, Ill.: Free Press, 1955.

Keeton, M. T., and Associates. *Experiential Learning: Rationale, Characteristics, and Assessment*. San Francisco: Jossey-Bass, 1977.

Knutson, A. L. *The Individual, Society, and Health Behavior*. New York: Russell Sage Foundation, 1965.

Kolb, D. A., and Fry, R. "Toward an Applied Theory of Experiential Learning." In *Theories of Group Processes*, edited by C. L. Cooper. New York: John Wiley & Sons, 1975.

Kouzes, J. M., and Mico, P. R., "Domain Theory: An Introduction to Organizational Behavior in Human Service Organizations." *Journal of Applied Behavioral Science* 15, no. 4 (1979): 449–69.

Krathwahl, D. K.; Bloom, B. S.; and Masia, B. B. *Taxonomy of Educational Objecives. Handbook 2: Affective Domain*. New York: David McKay Co., 1964.

Krech, D.; Crutchfield, R. S.; and Levson, N. *Elements of Psychology*. New York: Alfred A. Knopf, 1970.

Kuhn, A. *The Logic of Social Systems*. San Francisco: Jossey-Bass, 1974.

Laughlin, P. R.; Branch, L. G.; and Johnson, H. H. "Individual versus Triadic Performance on a Unidimensional Complementary Task as a Function of Initial Ability Level." *Journal of Personality and Social Psychology* 12 (1969): 144–50.

Lazes, P. M., ed. *The Handbook of Health Education*. Germantown, Md.: Aspen Systems Corp., 1979.

Levin, L. S.; Katz, A. H.; and Holst, E. *Self-Care: Lay Initiatives in Health*. New York: Prodist, 1976.

Levy, L. H. "Forces and Issues in the Revival of Interest in Self-Care: Impetus for Redirection in Self-Care." *Health Education Monographs* 5, no. 2 (1977): 115–20.

———. "Self-Help Groups: Types and Psychological Processes." *Journal of Applied Behavioral Science* 12, no. 3 (1976): 310–22.

Lewin, K. "Group Decision and Social Change." In *Readings in Social Psychology*, edited by G. Swansom, T. M. Newcomb, and Z. L. Harlety. New York: Henry Holt, 1952.

———. "Quasi-Stationary Social Equilibria and the Problem of Permanent Change." In *The Planning of Change*, edited by W. G. Bennis, K. D. Benne, and R. Chin. New York: Holt, Rinehart & Winston, 1961.

———. *Resolving Social Conflicts*. New York: Harper & Brothers, 1948.

Lewin, K.; Lippitt, R.; and White, R. K. "Patterns of Aggressive Behavior in Experientially Created Social Climates." *Journal of Social Psychology* 10 (1939): 271–99.

Likert, R. *The Human Organization: Its Management and Value.* New York: McGraw-Hill, 1967.

———. *New Patterns of Management.* New York: McGraw-Hill, 1961.

Lindzey, G.; Hall, C. S.; and Thompson, R. F. *Psychology.* New York: Worth Publishers, 1975.

Lippitt, R., and White, R. K. "The 'Social Climate' of Children's Groups." In *Child Behavior and Development,* edited by R. G. Barker, J. Kownin, and H. Wright. New York: McGraw-Hill, 1943.

Lubin, B.; Goodstein, L. D.; and Lubin, S. W. *Organization Change Sourcebook I: Cases in Organization Development.* La Jolla, Calif.: University Associates, 1979.

Luft, J. *Group Processes: An Introduction to Group Dynamics.* 2d ed. Palo Alto, Calif.: National Press Books, 1970.

MacKinnon, D. W. "Assessing Creative Persons." *Journal of Creative Behavior* 1, no. 3 (1967): 291–304.

McAlister, A. L.; Farquhar, J. W.; Thoresen, C. E.; and Maccoby, N. "Behavioral Science Applied to Cardiovascular Health: Progress and Research Needs in the Modification of Risk-taking Habits in Adult Populations." *Health Education Monographs* 4, no. 1 (Spring 1976): 45–74.

McGregor, D. *The Human Side of Enterprise.* New York: McGraw-Hill, 1960.

McGuire, W. J. "The Nature of Attitudes and Attitude Change." In *The Handbook of Social Psychology.* Vol. 3, *The Individual in theSocial Context,* edited by G. Lindzey and E. Aronson. Reading, Mass.: Addison-Wesley Publishing Co., 1969.

Marieskind, H. I., and Ehrenreich, B. "Toward Socialist Medicine: The Women's Health Movement." *Social Policy* 6, no. 2 (September–October 1975): 34–42.

Marklund, R. E., and Durand, D. E. "An Investigation of Sociopsychological Factors Affecting Infant Immunization." *American Journal of Public Health* 66, no. 2 (February 1976): 168–72.

Maslow, A. H. *Toward a Psychology of Being.* 2d ed. New York: D. Van Nostrand Co., 1968.

Mayer, J. *Health.* New York: D. Van Nostrand Co., 1974.

Mayshark, C., and Foster, R. A. *Health Education in Secondary Schools.* 3d ed. St. Louis, Mo.: C. V. Mosby Co., 1972.

Mechanic, D. "Social-Psychological Factors Affecting the Presentation of Bodily Complaints." *New England Journal of Medicine* 21 (1972): 1132–39.

Merwin, D. J. "The National Center for Health Education." Speech presented at National Conference on Hospital-based Patient Education, Chicago, 9–10 August 1976.

Michael, D. N. *On Learning to Plan and Planning to Learn.* San Francisco: Jossey-Bass, 1973.

Mico, P. R. *First Tango in Boston.* Washington, D. C.: National Training and Development Service, 1973.

———. *Problem-Oriented Applied Behavioral Science: Toward Newer Technologies for Improving the Processes of Social Problem Solving.* Washington, D.C.: NTL Institute for Applied Behavioral Science, 1972.

———. *Program Budgeting for California Cities.* Sacramento, Calif.: League of California Cities, 1976.

Mico, P. R., and Ross, H. S. *Health Education and Behavioral Science*. Oakland, Calif.: Third Party Associates, 1975.

Milio, N. *The Care of Health in Communities: Access for Outcasts*. New York: Macmillan Co., 1975.

Minkler, M. "The Uses of Incentives in Family Planning Programmes: A Study of Competing Theories Regarding Their Influence on Attitude Change." *International Journal of Health Education* 19 (supp.), no. 3 (July-September 1976): 1–11.

Nisbet, R. "Public Opinion versus Popular Opinion." In *The American Commonwealth, 1976*, edited by N. Glazer and I. Kristol. New York: Basic Books, 1976.

Oberteuffer, D.; Harrelson, O. A.; and Pollock, M. B. *School Health Education*. 5th ed. New York: Harper & Row, 1972.

Ogden, H. G. "The Bureau of Health Education." Speech presented at National Conference on Hospital-based Patient Education, Chicago, 9–10 August 1976.

Olmsted, M. S., and Hare, P. A. *The Small Group*. 2d ed. New York: Random House, 1978.

Palmiere, D. "Types of Planning in the Health-Care System." *American Journal of Public Health* 62, no. 8 (August 1972): 1112–15.

Pearson, C. "Education for Health in the Workplace." Paper presented at Tenth International Conference on Health Education, London, England, 2–7 September 1979.

Pine, G., and Horne, P. "Principles and Conditions for Learning in Adult Education." *Adult Leadership* 18, no. 4 (October 1969): 108–34.

Pratt, L. "Changes in Health-Care Ideology in Relation to Self-Care by Families." *Health Education Monographs* 5, no. 2 (Summer 1977): 121–35.

President's Committee on Health Education. *The Report of the President's Committee on Health Education*. New York: 801 Second Ave., 1973.

Preventive Medicine USA. *Health Promotion and Consumer Health Education*. New York: Prodist, 1976.

Radelfinger, S. "Some Effects of Fear-arousing Communications on Preventive Health Behavior." *Health Education Monographs*, no. 19 (1965), pp. 2–15.

Reiff, R. "The Control of Knowledge: The Power of the Helping Professions." *Journal of Applied Behavioral Science* 10, no. 3 (1974): 451–61.

Roberts, B. J. "A Framework for Consideration of Forces in Achieving Earliness of Treatment." *Health Education Monographs*, no. 19 (1965), pp. 16–32.

Rogers, C. R. *On Becoming a Person: A Therapist's View of Psychotherapy*. Boston: Houghton Mifflin Co., 1961.

Rokeach, M. "Attitude Change and Behavior Change." *Public Opinion Quarterly* 30 (1966–67): 529–50.

Rosenstock, I. M. "Historical Origins of the Health Belief Model." *Health Education Monographs* 2, no. 4 (Winter 1974): 328–35.

Ross, H. S. "Changes Effected in Cross-Cultural T-Groups." Doctoral dissertation, University of California at Berkeley, 1971.

Ross, H. S.; Collen, F. B.; and Soghikian, K. "Health-Education Discussion Groups for 'Worried Well' Patients in an Ambulatory Setting." *Health Education Monographs* 5, no. 1 (Spring 1977): 51–61.

Rubin, I. M.; Plovnick, M. S.; and Fry, R. E. *Improving the Coordination of Care: A*

Program for Health Team Development. Cambridge, Mass.: Ballinger Publishing Co., 1975.

———. "Initiating Planned Change in Health-Care Systems." *Journal of Applied Behavioral Science* 10, no. 1 (1974): 107–24.

Rueveni, U. "Using Sensitivity Training with Junior High School Students." *Children* 18, no. 2 (1971): 69–72.

Schein, E. H. *Organizational Psychology*. 2d ed. Englewood Cliffs, N.J.: Prentice-Hall, 1970.

———. *Process Consultation: Its Role in Organization Development*. Reading, Mass.: Addison-Wesley Publishing Co., 1969.

Schein, E. H., and Bennis, W. G. *Personal and Organizational Change through Group Methods: The Laboratory Approach*. New York: John Wiley & Sons, 1965.

Schell, R. E., and Hall, E. *Developmental Psychology Today*. 3d ed. New York: Random House, 1979.

Schutz, W. C. *FIRO: A Three-dimensional Theory of Interpersonal Behavior*. New York: Rinehart & Co., 1958.

———. *FIRO-B Questionnaire*. Palo Alto, Calif.: Consulting Psychologists Press, 1959.

———. *Joy: Expanding Human Awareness*. New York: Grove Press, 1967.

Shafer, R. P. "Government Control of Individual Behavior: Its Right and Proper Role." *American Journal of Public Health* 64, no. 4 (April 1974): 390–93.

Shafritz, J. M., and Whitbeck, P. H. *Classics of Organization Theory*. Oak Park, Ill.: Moore Publishing Co., 1978.

Shapiro, I. S. "HMOs and Health Education." *American Journal of Public Health* 65, no. 5 (May 1975): 469–73.

Shaw, M. E. *Group Dynamics: The Psychology of Small Group Behavior*. 2d ed. New York: McGraw-Hill, 1976.

Simmons, J., ed. "Making Health Education Work." *American Journal of Public Health* 65 (supp.) (October 1975): 1–49.

Simmons, J., and Skiff, A. F. *Report of the Committee on Manpower Education Proceedings: Federal Focus on Health Education*. Atlanta, Ga.: Center for Disease Control, Bureau of Health Education, 1974.

Simonds, S. K. "Emerging Challenges in Health Education." *International Journal of Health Education* 19 (supp.), no. 4 (October–December 1976): 1–19.

———. "Health Education as Social Policy." *Health Education Monographs* 2, no. 1 (1974): 1–10.

———. "Health-Education Manpower in the United States." *Health Education Monographs* 4, no. 3 (Fall 1976): 208–25.

Skinner, B. F. *Science and Human Behavior*. New York: Macmillan Co., 1953.

Sleet, D. A. "The Use of Games and Simulations in Health Instruction." *California School Health* 9 (January 1975): 11–14.

Smelzer, N. J. *Essays in Sociological Explanation*. Englewood Cliffs, N.J.: Prentice-Hall, 1968.

Smolensky, J., and Haar, F. B. *Principles of Community Health*. 3d ed. Philadelphia: W. B. Saunders Co., 1972.

Society for Public Health Education. "Guidelines and Standards for Baccalaureate

Preparation in Community Health Education." *Health Education Monographs* 5, no. 1 (Spring 1977): 90–98.

———. "Guidelines for the Preparation and Practice of Professional Health Educators." *Health Education Monographs* 5, no. 1 (Spring 1977): 75–89.

———. "SOPHE Position Statement on Patient and Family Education." *SOPHE News & Views* 5, no. 2 (April 1976): 2–3.

Sommer, R. *Personal Space: The Behavioral Basis of Design.* Englewood Cliffs, N.J.: Prentice-Hall, 1969.

Steiner, I. D. *Group Process and Productivity.* New York: Academic Press, 1972.

Stock, D. "A Survey of Research on T-Groups." In *T-Group Theory and Laboratory Method,* edited by L. P. Bradford, J. R. Gibb, and K. K. Benne. New York: John Wiley & Sons, 1964.

Storms, M. D., and Nisbett, R. E. "Insomnia and the Attribution Process." *Journal of Personality and Social Psychology* 16 (1970): 319–28.

Strodtbeck, F. L., and Hook, L. H. "The Social Dimensions of a Twelve-Man Jury Table." *Sociometry* 24 (1961): 397–415.

Sullivan, D. "Model for Comprehensive, Systematic Program Development in Health Education." *Health Education Report* 1, no. 1 (November-December 1973): 4–5.

Tannenbaum, R., and Schmidt, W. H. "How to Choose a Leadership Pattern." *Harvard Business Review* (reprint no. 73311), May-June 1973, pp. 1–10.

Tannenbaum, T. H. "Initial Attitude toward Source and Concepts as Factors in Attitude-Change through Communication." *Public Opinion Quarterly* 20 (1956): 413–25.

Thibaut, J. W., and Kelley, H. H. *The Social Psychology of Groups.* New York: John Wiley & Sons, 1959.

Thompson, J. D. *Organizations in America.* New York: McGraw-Hill, 1967.

Ulrich, M. "How Hospitals Evaluate Patient-Education Programs." Paper presented at National Conference on Hospital-based Patient Education, Chicago, 9–10 August 1976.

U.S. Congress. House. Committee on Interstate and Foreign Commerce. *Report No. 94–1007: National Health Promotion and Disease Prevention Act of 1976.* 94th Cong., 2d sess., 1976.

U.S. Department of Health, Education and Welfare. *Forward Plan for Health FY 1977–81.* HEW Publication No. (OS) 76–50024, June 1975.

———. *Forward Plan for Health FY 1978–82.* HEW Publication No. (OS) 76–50046, August 1976.

———. *Patient Education Workshop.* Atlanta, Ga.: Center for Disease Control, 1976.

———. *Proceedings of the National Heart and Lung Institute Working Conference on Health Behavior.* HEW Publication No. (NIH) 76–868, 12–15 May 1975.

———. Public Health Service, Center for Disease Control. *The Community and Its Involvement in the Study-Planning Action Process.* Prepared for the Bureau of Health Education and Bureau of State Services, Atlanta, Ga. HEW Publication No. (CDC) 78–8355, 1977.

———. *HEIRS: Thesaurus of Health-Education Terminology.* Prepared for the Bureau of Health Education by the editorial staff of *Health Education Monographs*, Johns Hopkins University School of Hygiene and Public Health, Baltimore, Md., 1965.

————. *The Priorities of Section 1502: Papers on the National Health Guidelines. Health Education and Public Law 93–641*. Prepared for the Bureau of Health Education by H. G. Ogden. HEW Publication No. 77–641, 1977.

————. *Using a Nutrition Clinic's Waiting Room for Patient Education*. Prepared for the Health Resources Administration by J. M. Scanlan, 1976.

United Way of America. *UWASIS II: A Taxonomy of Social Goals and Human Service Programs*. 2d ed. Alexandria, Va.: 1976.

Warren, R. *Perspectives on the American Community*. Chicago: Rand McNally & Co., 1961.

Wechsler, H.; Gurin, J. A.; and Cahill, G. F. *The Horizons of Health*. Cambridge, Mass.: Harvard University Press, 1977.

Weisbord, M. R. "Why Organization Development Hasn't Worked (So Far) in Medical Centers." *Health Care Management Review*, Spring 1976, pp. 17–28.

Williams, S. J. *Issues in Health Services*. New York: John Wiley & Sons, 1980.

Williams, S. J., and Torrens, P. R. *Introduction to Health Services*. New York: John Wiley & Sons, 1980.

Wilner, D. M. *Introduction to Public Health*. 6th ed. New York: Macmillan Co., 1960.

Witte, J. J. "Recent Advances in Public Health." *American Journal of Public Health* 64, no. 10 (October 1974): 939–44.

World Health Organization. *Health Education: A Programme Review*. Offset Publication No. 7. Geneva: 1974.

Zaltman, G., and Duncan, R. *Strategies for Planned Change*. New York: John Wiley & Sons, 1977.

Zaltman, G.; Kotler, P.; and Kaufman, I., eds. *Creating Social Change*. New York: Holt, Rinehart & Winston, 1972.

Index